An Aid to the
MRCP Short Cases

'MRCP; Member of the Royal College of Physicians . . .
They only give that to crowned heads of Europe'.

From *The Citadel* by A. J. Cronin

An Aid to the MRCP Short Cases

R. E. J. RYDER

M. A. MIR

E. A. FREEMAN

Department of Medicine
University Hospital of Wales and
University of Wales College of Medicine, Cardiff
and
Department of Geriatric Medicine
University Hospital of Wales, Cardiff and
St Woolos Hospital, Newport

Blackwell Scientific Publications

OXFORD LONDON EDINBURGH

BOSTON MELBOURNE

One-third of the royalties from this book will be donated to the
Missionaries of Charity of Mother Teresa of Calcutta

© 1986 by
Blackwell Scientific Publications
Editorial offices:
Osney Mead, Oxford, OX2 0EL
8 John Street, London, WC1N 2ES
23 Ainslie Place, Edinburgh, EH3 6AJ
3 Cambridge Center, Suite 208, Cambridge,
    Massachusetts 02142, USA
107 Barry Street, Carlton, Victoria 3053, Australia

First published 1986
Reprinted 1988, 1989

Typeset by CCC, printed and bound in Great Britain
by William Clowes Limited, Beccles and London

DISTRIBUTORS

Marston Book Services Ltd
PO Box 87
Oxford OX2 0DT
(*Orders:* Tel: 0865 791155
            Fax: 0865 791927
            Telex: 837515)
USA
  Year Book Medical Publishers
  200 North LaSalle Street,
  Chicago, Illinois 60601

Canada
  The C.V. Mosby Company
  5240 Finch Avenue East, Scarborough, Ontario

Australia
  Blackwell Scientific Publications (Australia) Pty Ltd
  107 Barry Street, Carlton, Victoria 3053

British Library
Cataloguing in Publication Data

Ryder, R. E. J.
An aid to the MRCP short cases.
1. Medicine—Problems, exercises, etc.
I. Title   II. Mir, M.A.   III. Freeman, E.A.
610′.76   R834.5

ISBN 0-632-01451-2

Contents

Preface, vii

Acknowledgements, viii

Introduction, xi

Section 1: Preparation, 1

Section 2: Examination *routines*, 9

Section 3: 150 Short case *records*, 59

Section 4: Experiences, anecdotes, tips, facts and figures, quotations, 325

Appendices

Preface

The short cases part of the examination for the membership of the Royal College of Physicians (MRCP) is, by tradition, considered to be the most critical test of bedside behaviour and diagnostic competence. It forms an important milestone in the development of practising physicians. There is, however, no formal syllabus or tutoring and, despite the high failure rate, there is a notable lack of books specifically written to help candidates with this test.

The spectrum of clinical conditions used in the short cases examination is determined by a variety of interchanging factors such as the availability of patients with demonstrable physical signs, the prejudice of the doctors choosing the cases, that of the examiners taking part in the examination and, occasionally, the speciality bias of the examination centre. The cases chosen by the examiners from those assembled on the day in turn determine the problems presented to the candidates and the clinical skills required of them. For this reason we decided to build this book around an extensive survey conducted amongst successful candidates. Our questionnaires yielded information about the cases presented, the questions asked, answers given and the reactions of the examiners. We have thus been able to identify the chief difficulties of candidates in dealing with this practical examination and have attempted to help with these. The advice in Section 1 on how to prepare for the short cases is based on, and illustrated by, the comments received from the candidates. Section 2 is written around the clinical instructions given by the examiners to the candidates, the likely diagnoses under each instruction as revealed in the survey, and details of the examination steps suitable for each command. Section 3 forms the bulk of the book and presents the clinical features of 150 short cases in order of the frequency of their occurrence in the examination as derived from our survey. Thus, priorities are sorted out for the candidates preparing for the examination. In the final section we pass on the experiences and advice of some of the candidates in our survey which we felt would be of interest.

In fulfilling our main task of helping candidates to improve their performance in clinical examinations we have used three learning techniques which are rather novel to this field. Firstly, the iterative approach which exploits the retentive potential of reinforcement by repeating the main clinical features of a number of conditions whenever any reference to these is made. It is hoped that this method will not only reinforce, but will also alert the candidates to other diagnostic possibilities when looking at a related condition. Secondly, in the examination methods suggested by us we have individualized the inspection to the examination of each subsystem, and have provided a *visual survey* to note the features most likely to be present. This enriches the usual advice to look for everything which often accomplishes nothing unless a specific sign is being looked for. Thirdly, we have reduced our suggested clinical methods to simple steps (*checklists*) which, if practised, may become spontaneous clinical habits, easy to recall and execute.

In the age of superspecialization, the task of summarizing and streamlining a subject as vast and diverse as general medicine to the needs of the short cases examinee has been formidable. We are in no doubt that our attempt will have its inadequacies and would be pleased if you would write to us (c/o Blackwell Scientific Publications) about any errors of fact, or with any suggestions which might be helpful for a future edition, or indeed with any other comments. We would also be interested to hear of any short cases which have occurred in the examination and which are not included on our lists (please give us an idea of your confidence that the case was indeed the condition concerned and why—clinical details, invigilator's confirmation, etc.) or of any membership experiences which might be of interest.

Medical student note

Although this book has concentrated exclusively on the needs of MRCP candidates, it is noteworthy that the cases included in undergraduate medical short cases examinations are drawn from the same pool as those used in the MRCP examination. Furthermore, physicians are all MRCP trained and tend to use the MRCP style in these examinations. Though clearly the required standard of performance is lower, we feel that medical students preparing for their short cases examinations would also benefit from using this book. It would be a supplement to information gained from more comprehensive textbooks (we assume much basic knowledge) and an aid to practice on the wards.

Acknowledgements

We are indebted to Dr Ralph Marshall and his team (especially Paul Crompton, Keith Bellamy, Steve Young and Adrian Shaw) in the Department of Medical Illustration at the University Hospital of Wales, and Nigel Pearce and Steve Cashmore at the Department of Medical Illustration at the Royal Gwent Hospital. A large proportion of the photographs in the book are from the archives of these departments.

We are grateful to all the patients who gave their consent to the publication of the photographs depicting their medical conditions. Our thanks are due to many colleagues who have allowed us to use photographs from their own collections and photographs of their patients including: T. M. Hayes, C. E. C. Wells, M. S. J. Pathy, R. Marks, R. Hall, J. G. Graham, B. H. Davies, P. J. A. Holt, J. Jessop, M. H. Pritchard, N. W. D. Walshaw, I. S. Petheram, J. M. Swithenbank, M. D. Mishra, B. D. Williams, I. N. F. McQueen, P. E. Hutchinson, J. Rhodes, C. A. R. Pippen, A. J. Birtwell, P. M. Smith, A. G. Knight, S. Richards, A. G. Karseras, J. P. Thomas, C. N. A. Matthews, P. J. Sykes, M. L. Insley, P. I. Williams, B. S. D. Sastry, J. H. Jones, M. Y. Khan, J. D. Spillane, K. Tayton, G. M. Tinker, A. Compston, B. A. Thomas, H. J. Lloyd, G. B. Leitch, B. Calcraft, O. M. Gibby, G. O. Thomas, E. Graham Jones, Byron Evans, D. J. Fisher, G. S. Kilpatrick, L. E. Hughes, P. Harper, G. Griffiths, A. D. Holt-Wilson, D. B. Foster, D. L. T. Webster, J. H. Lazarus, D. Beckingham, J. E. Cawdery, R. Prosser, M. F. Scanlon, I. A. Hughes, O. P. Gray, E. Waddington and L. Beck. Fig. 3.42b has already been published in 'An Atlas of Clinical Neurology' by Spillane and Spillane (Oxford University Press) and Figs. 3.97b and 3.114 from the UHW Medical Illustration archives are also published in 'A Picture Quiz in Medicine' by Ebden, Peiras and Dew (Lloyd-Luke (Medical Books) Ltd.). Figs. 3.115a (i) and (ii) are published with the permission of the Department of Medical Photography, Leicester Royal Infirmary and Fig. 3.110 with the permission of the University of Newcastle upon Tyne, holders of the copyright.

Our thanks go to colleagues who advised us on points of uncertainty in their fields of interest; especially A.C., B.H.D., M.J.D., L.G.D., R.H., T.M.H., M.H., T.P.K., I.N.F.M., M.D.M., M.F.S., H.S., P.M.S., S.S. and B.D.W.

We are obliged to: Andrea Hill for typing and retyping the manuscript; Janet Roberts for secretarial help with the survey; Jill Manfield for telephoning, chasing and writing again in pursuit of patient consents and for numerous minor secretarial chores; Alan Peiras for some nifty detective work in Edinburgh during the survey; Steve Young for the cover photograph for the book; and to certain pharmaceutical companies for financial assistance (including Astra Pharmaceuticals Ltd., CIBA Laboratories, May and Baker Ltd., Roche Products Ltd., Merck Sharp and Dohme Ltd. and Thomas Morson Pharmaceuticals). Our particular thanks to Bayer UK Ltd. for sponsoring the colour photographs are recorded on p. 370.

Most of all we thank our long-suffering families without whose forebearance and help the book would never have been finished.

Introduction

*'The result comes as a particular shock when
you have been sitting exams for many years
without failing them.'*

The candidate who reaches the MRCP 'clinical' examination has already demonstrated considerable knowledge of medicine by passing the MRCP Part I and MRCP Part II written examinations. The clinical is divided into viva, long case and short cases. The failure rate in the viva and long case is of the order of 30% (and the vast majority of these candidates also fail the short cases). You can compensate for a borderline failure in one of these by a good performance in the other parts of the examination. The failure rate for the short cases examination is about 70% (figure from a Membership examiner) and there is no compensation. Thus all are agreed that the short cases examination is the major hurdle in MRCP Part II. The fact is that the majority of Part II candidates pass the written, viva and long case but the majority fail the short cases. For many it would be the first examination they have ever failed and it may also be the only examination they have taken that does not have some form of syllabus.

The short cases examination is a practical test which assesses various facets of clinical competence in many subtle ways. Although it is generally accepted that clinical competence cannot be acquired from textbooks, a book such as this can provide indirect help towards that objective. We hope that the examination *routines* (Section 2) together with the *checklists* (Appendix 1) may assist candidates in developing a keen sense of clinical search and detection. The short case *records* (Section 3) should provide the framework, i.e. the main clinical features, the discipline of how to look for them, how to differentiate the diagnostic from the incidental or associated findings, and how and when to be alert to other possibilities. By basing our book on the results of a survey of successful MRCP candidates (see below) we have *created a form of syllabus* which we hope will be of value to future candidates. Not only do the results of the survey advise as to what you are required to know and do, but they also grade these requirements in order of importance.

The short cases examination

'I am sure they assess you very quickly—whether they would like you to be in charge of their patients.'†

Two examiners will take you for approximately fifteen minutes each. The College asks them each to record a separate, as well as a combined, mark. Nowadays examiners are encouraged to introduce each case, e.g.: 'This is Mr Smith. His doctor found a heart murmur on routine examination. Please would you examine his heart'. Nonetheless, the old system often prevails: 'Examine this patient's heart'. A striking feature of the examination is the absence of a discussion. The cases are examined, the findings given, and perhaps one or two causes

*p. 349.   †p. 353.

sought whilst moving on to the next case. Only in a minority of the cases is a little time given for the occasional question or brief discussion of causes or complications. The examiners are constantly testing your ability to *elicit and interpret physical signs*. Many examiners say that, in the final analysis, whether a candidate will pass or fail depends very much on the general air of competence or incompetence which prevails during his clinical performance.

The survey of MRCP short cases

*'Certain "favourite" topics seem to recur. Make sure you know these.'**

The survey has been introduced in the preface. In the first part of this survey, questionnaires were obtained from a number of doctors who had gained the MRCP during the last ten years. In the second part all the successful candidates at a recent sitting were circulated. The questionnaires obtained in the two parts of the survey included both the pass and the previous fail attempts of these candidates. Altogether we collected accounts of 248 attempts at the MRCP short cases, covering over 1300 'main focus' short cases as well as over 500 'additional' short cases (see Section 3 for an explanation of these terms). The diagnoses given by these candidates were graded according to the confidence each candidate had in his retrospective assessment. Pass attempt diagnoses were given more weight than fail attempt ones. As a result we hope that the rather complex analysis performed has produced a picture which is as near to the truth as possible. Analysis of the first part of the survey covering candidates' attempts over several years was essentially the same as analysis of the second part. This suggests that the cases used and the skills tested tend to remain constant. This comparison also gives some support to the accuracy of our method of analysis. The main figures from the survey are given in Sections 2 and 3. Some additional figures of interest are collected together under 'Facts and Figures' in Section 4. Apart from figures, the organization of our suggested examination *routines* (Section 2) and the contents of our short case *records* (Section 3) have been closely guided by the survey. For light entertainment, but with ingrained lessons, a number of experiences, anecdotes and quotations from the survey are given in Section 4.

*p. 348.

Section 1
Preparation

'Expressionless and without comment they led me away.'*

The clinical skills required for the MRCP examination, particularly in relation to the short cases, can only be acquired by thoughtful preparation, experience and purposeful practice. Tutors and examiners alike agree that it is more important to spend time examining patients than reading textbooks. The examiners are not looking for encyclopaedic knowledge, they are just anxious to ascertain that you can be trusted to carry out an adequate clinical examination and make a competent clinical assessment. This book aims to help you organize your overall preparation to meet that objective. We have provided preparatory aids including examination *routines* and short case *records* (see below). We also aim to give you some insight into what most candidates experience in the examination and we hope to help you prepare psychologically. We would like to stress that though the written examination may appear a formidable hurdle, you are very much more likely to pass it than the short cases. You would be wise to err on the side of safety and prepare for the short cases before, during and after your preparations for the written. Thus, we begin with some basic principles of practice and preparations at work.

Clinical experience in everyday work

'Imagine you are seeing the cases in a clinic and carrying out a routine examination.'*

The intention of the College in the examination is to gain a reflection of your usual working day clinical competence for the examiners to judge. In arriving at their final verdict the examiners may take particular note of factors such as your approach to the patient, your examination technique, spontaneity of shifting from system to system in pursuit of relevant clinical signs, fluidity in giving a coherent account of all the findings and conclusions, and your composure throughout. Though you can acquire all this for the day only, as some successful candidates do who are experts at passing examinations, it would be preferable if you could adopt many of these good habits into your everyday clinical approach. In either event, a long, diligent and disciplined practice is required if your aim is to be able to perform a smooth and polished clinical examination, to display the subtle confidence of a skilled performer, and to suppress all signs of anxiety.

One simple approach to the task is that, whatever your job, you should consider all the patients you see as short or long cases (or even viva questions!). Such a practice should not only improve your readiness for the examination but also improve your standard of patient care—the primary objective of every clinician. Look out for all the 'good signs' passing through your hospital and use as many of these as possible as practice short cases. Ask your colleagues to let you know of every heart murmur, every abnormal fundus, every case with abnormal neurology, etc. If you are in, or can get to, a teaching hospital, make regular trips not only to clinical meetings and demonstrations but also, more importantly, to *visit the specialist wards*—neurology, cardiology, chest, rheumatology, dermatology, etc. It is useful to study the signs and conditions even when you know the diagnosis in order to further

*p. 353

familiarize yourself with them. It is also a good practice to see cases 'blind' to the diagnosis and to try to simulate the examination situation. Imagine that two examiners are standing over you and there is a need to complete an efficient, once-only examination followed by an immediate response to the anticipated question: 'What are your findings?' or 'What is the diagnosis?'

Simulated examination practice

'I had a lot of practice presenting short cases to a "hawk" of an S.R. This experience was invaluable.'*

If a constant effort is made to improve your clinical skills by seeing as many cases as possible, there is no reason why the spontaneity and competence so acquired should not show up on the day. As with all examinations, however, much can be learned about the deficiencies requiring special attention when you put your composite clinical ability to the test in 'mock' examinations. In most district general, and all teaching, hospitals the local postgraduate clinical tutors organize membership teaching and 'mock' examination sessions, and you should find out about, and join in, as many of these as you can manage. Unfortunately, a lot of these, though useful, tend to teach in groups and discuss management or look at X-rays, rather than provide the intensive 'on the spot' practice on patients that is the ideal preparation for the MRCP short cases. It is, therefore, advisable to supplement these sessions with simulated examination practice arranged by yourself. This requires the cooperation of a 'mock' examiner (consultant, senior registrar or experienced registrar and, on occasion, a fellow examinee) on a *one-to-one basis*. If you can arrange such practice with a variety of 'mock' examiners, you will not only broaden the assessment of your imperfections but also learn to respond to the varied approaches of different examiners.

Examination *routines*

'The most important point is to look professional—as if you have done it a hundred times before.'†

The short cases part of the test is very important for the membership examination because it is designed to test critically two major areas of clinical competence. The first and more important of these is your ability to detect abnormal physical signs, interpret them correctly and put them together into a reasonable diagnosis or differential diagnosis. The second is your competence to conduct a professional and efficient clinical examination (see experience 34, p. 334). As said above, these are generally considered to arise from day-to-day work and your conduct in the examination will reflect your experience in performing clinical tasks, presenting your assessments of patients to your seniors and getting their constant constructive criticism. If you are lucky enough to have worked with a good teacher you may have acquired a firm foundation upon which you could build a structured clinical examination for all systems. As most candidates are engaged in busy clinical jobs and their seniors are often over-burdened by administrative chores, etc., useful clinical dialogue between them may be limited. As a result there may be little improvement in the weaknesses acquired during the

*p. 348   †p. 348

undergraduate years. The enormous task of preparing for the membership examination provides an ideal opportunity to remedy any deficiencies in one's clinical methods. We would suggest that you work out the exact number and sequence of clinical steps for the examination of each subsystem, particularly those you would need to take in response to a particular command from the examiner; then practise going through these steps. Practise them over and over again on your spouse, or any other willing person, until all the steps become as automatic as driving a car. Practise them on patients until you are confident of being able to pick up or demonstrate any abnormal physical signs. You should be able to maintain the same sequence and run through it rapidly and comprehensively in a way that is second nature to you. The sequence of clinical steps required for the examination of each system or subsystem is collectively referred to as the examination *routine* in this book. In Section 2 we suggest various examination *routines* (which you may wish to adopt or adapt) for you to practise in response to particular commands. In Appendix 1 we provide *checklists* which summarize the major points in each examination *routine*. The *checklists* are designed to help in practising the *routines*.

Short case *records*

> *'The more practice at presenting short cases the better.'**

A knowledge of the possible short cases that may be used in the examination is important so that you can become familiar with the physical signs associated with each and know what you are looking for as you work through the examination *routine*. Having a good grasp of the clinical features of the case may enable you to score extra marks by looking for additional signs which may be present. Such extra marks identify the above-average candidate from the average ones. Furthermore, by becoming acquainted with descriptions of typical cases you will find it easier to present the case to the examiner using acceptable descriptive terms. In this book, under each short case, we have presented the typical clinical features for you to remember, and to 'regurgitate' what you see (hence the descriptive term *record*), omit what you do not find, and add what you find new. Thus, when confronted with the face of a man with Parkinson's disease which you diagnose at once on seeing his tremor, instead of stuttering and stumbling as you try to think of the right words to describe his face, the terms depressed, expressionless, unblinking, drooling and titubation will immediately surface for you to use. In Section 3 we have covered the overwhelming majority of cases which could occur and we have put them in order of priority according to the likelihood of occurrence as assessed from our survey.

Getting 'psyched up'

> *'Do not be distracted by mistakes made (or imagined) in preceding cases or the examiners' mannerisms or approach (I was and suffered for it). Being very nervous does not necessarily fail you and one bad case should not put you off.'†*

It is common to hear candidates agonizing over their feeling that they failed to give a performance commensurate with their actual capabilities, simply because they were

*p. 348   †Quotations 37, 61, 38, pp. 350, 352

discouraged by the 'examination ordeal'. Though it is true that knowledge and competence tend to generate confidence and capability, it is also true that extreme anxiety can seriously impair the performance of even the most knowledgeable and competent candidate.

The downward spiral syndrome

> *'After the first case there was a long pause as if they were waiting for me to say more—I went to pieces after this.'**

The candidate, an otherwise able and experienced doctor, enters the short cases room extremely anxious and lacking in confidence. He is just hovering on the edge of despair and the slightest upset is going to push him over. On one or more of the cases he convinces himself that he is doing badly (whether or not he actually is) and over the edge he goes. The first stage of a rapid 'downward spiral' sets in; the dispirited candidate get worse and worse and actually gives up before the end in the certainty that he has failed. Months of intensive bookwork and bedside practice, not to mention the examination fee, go to waste because of *inadequate psychological preparation*. To avoid this there are four basic rules which are well worth noting.

1. You never know you have failed until the list is published

> *'Don't be put off if you get a few things wrong. I made a lot of mistakes that I know of and still passed.'†*

In the same way as it is said of the greatest saints that they considered themselves to be the greatest sinners, many successful candidates leave the examination centre feeling certain that they have failed. Good candidates may have a heightened awareness of the imperfections of their performance and thereby may exaggerate the impact of their mistakes on the examiner. Furthermore, the 'hawk' examiner may make you feel that you are doing badly, or you may deduce it from his mannerism, regardless of your performance. By the same token the newcomer may slide through the short cases unaware of any errors and with the examiner's acting benignly, and then express great surprise as the inevitable 'thin' envelope arrives. It is not really important whether or not you think you have failed during the days between the examination and the arrival of the result. However, if you become convinced that you are failing while you are still sitting the examination, the thought can be disastrous and impair your performance to the extent that your conviction becomes a reality (see experiences 1, 2, pp. 327, 328, anecdote 12, p. 342 and quotation 39, p. 350)

2. Do not be put off by the examiners or their reactions

> *'The most off-putting aspect of each case is the lack of feedback from the examiners as to whether you are right or wrong. This is much more disconcerting than outright criticism.'‡*

Many first-timers, despite excellent clinical experience, are stunned by the sombre and restrained atmosphere of the examination which is unlike anything in their past experience

---

*p. 350
†p. 350
‡p. 90. This quotation refers to the 'poker-face' examiner. The candidates in our survey give similar warnings regarding the

'hawk' ('The examiners may appear irritable and unsympathetic—don't worry'—p. 350) and the 'dove' ('Don't be fooled by the apparent relaxed nature of the examiners'—p. 348)

(except perhaps the driving test!). It is as well, therefore, to be aware that the examiners tend to wear a 'poker-face' and usually give no feedback or encouragement. The 'hostile hawk' may appear dissatisfied by everything you do and say, but this is not necessarily a guide as to whether you are doing badly or not. A positive atmosphere is no guide either: the smiling ('smiling death'!) and pleasant ('deadly dove'!) examiner (and the apparently uninterested one), can be as deadly as a black widow spider if you get yourself into a diagnostic maze! Bear in mind that 'hawks' and 'doves' tend to have similar rates of passing and failing candidates. Disregard the atmosphere and concentrate on what the examiner asks you to do rather than on what he looks like, and recall your *routines* and *records*.

3. The cases are easy and you have seen it all before

> '*My cases were more straightforward than I had been led to believe. Nothing was particularly rare.*'*

The psychological scenario of the examination is such that many candidates enter it with the distorted view that behind every case and every question there will be some catch, some clever trap, something never seen before, or a diagnosis never heard of. In fact these suspicions are rarely justified. The *vast majority* of cases and questions are straightforward and a realization of this is likely to produce a confident, straightforward answer from the start instead of the hesitancy born of a mind filled with suspicion and struggling to solve the hidden catch. A study of membership short cases† reveals that there are two broad groups. The first group includes common conditions which you are well used to seeing in everyday clinical practice such as rheumatic heart disease, cirrhosis of the liver, rheumatoid hands and so on. These should surely present little difficulty (especially if you have tailor-made *routines* and *records*). In the second broad group are the rarities with good physical signs such as Osler–Weber–Rendu syndrome, pseudoxanthoma elasticum, Peutz–Jeghers syndrome, etc. You should be well used to these from the study of colour atlases, etc. that you will have done for the MRCP 'slides'. These too, therefore, should be easy (once you recognize the condition all you have to do is 'play the record'!).

4. You have already passed and you have just got to keep it that way

> '*It's like skating on thin ice—if you keep going and don't fall through, you make it.*'‡

Confidence in one's ability is a very important ingredient in any form of competition. As you go into the examination imagine that you have a clean sheet with 100% mark and that you just have to keep it that way as the examiner shows you a few simple cases such as psoriatic arthropathy, mitral stenosis, cerebellar signs, clubbing, splenomegaly and diabetic retinopathy (a typical combination). Such an attitude should replace the more usual: 'Everybody fails this examination; it's too difficult; how can I possibly pass'. The short cases examination has been well described (Royal Northern course) as 'like walking up a path full of puddles without stepping in the puddles; and you make the puddles yourself'. Remember the way to success is '*Readiness, Routines, Records* and *Right frame of mind*'.

---

*p. 352
† The 150 covered in this book form a list far more comprehensive than you probably need in order to pass. If you have studied all 150 it would be excessively rare for you to be surprised by a condition not met before.
‡p. 351

Section 2
Examination *Routines*

*'Work out the best method for examination and
practise it until it is second nature to you.'**

*p. 348

In this chapter *routines* are suggested for the clinical assessment of various subsystems. These are readily adaptable to your individual methods. The subsystems are arranged according to the examiners' standard instructions (e.g. examine the heart, abdomen, hands, etc.). The choice and order of subsystems have been governed by our survey. We have worked out the frequencies of the various instructions and have presented these in their order of priority. Some of the variations of the instruction are also given. Under each subsystem a list of the possible short cases is presented in order of their occurrence in the survey. The percentages given represent our estimate of your chances of each diagnosis being present when you hear the particular instruction.* These lists of diagnoses have guided our suggested *routines*. The latter are broken down into numbered constituents to aid memory and *checklists* are given in Appendix 1 which match up to the numbered points in the examination *routine*. The *checklists* are to help your practice with each subsystem. The idea is to develop a controlled, spontaneous and flawless technique of examination for each subsystem, so that you do not have to keep pausing and thinking what to do next and so that you do not miss out important steps (see experience 36, p. 335). Often you will not need the complete sequence in the examination (for example, it will be rare for you to carry out all the steps in the 'Examine this patient's arms' *routine*) but it will certainly increase your confidence if you enter the examination armed with the complete *routines* so that you can adapt them as necessary. The examination methods are supplemented with appropriate hints to avoid common pitfalls and to simplify the diagnostic maze.

Before dealing with the individual subsystems we would make some general points. You should avoid repeating the examiner's command or echoing the last part of it. Refrain from asking questions like: 'Would you like me to give you a running commentary or give the findings at the end?' Such a response wastes invaluable seconds which could be used running through the *checklist* and completing your *visual survey*. It is like a batsman asking a bowler in a cricket match whether he would like his ball hit for a six or played defensively! You must do what you are best at and hope that the examiner does not ask you to do otherwise. As suggested below, a well rehearsed procedure suited to each subsystem should make it possible for you to start purposefully without delay. Your approach to the patient is of great importance; you should introduce yourself to him and ask his permission to examine him. Permission should also be sought for various manoeuvres, such as adjusting the backrest when examining the heart, or before removing any clothing. These polite exchanges will not only please most examiners and patients, but will also provide you with an opportunity to calm your nerves, collect your thoughts and recall the appropriate *checklist*. Although we have continually emphasized the value of looking for signs peripheral to the examiner's instruction (e.g. examine this patient's heart, abdomen, chest), we would like to emphasize

*As with all our survey analyses, we graded the confidence of each candidate in his retrospective diagnosis of each short case seen. The percentages are not meant to add up to 100% because: (i) there are always missing percentages representing those short cases we could not be certain about; (ii) sometimes more than one diagnosis was considered worth counting for one instruction (for example, in order to give you the percentage of 'heart' cases with clubbing, when clubbing was present it was counted as well as the underlying cardiac condition). The figures are best used to give an index of the *relative importance* of the different conditions in terms of frequency of occurrence when you hear a given instruction.

too that *dithering* may be counterproductive. In the *visual survey* you should be scanning the patient rapidly and purposefully with a trained eye, not gazing helplessly at him for a long period while you try to decide what to do next. While you are feeling the pulse (heart) or settling the patient lying flat (abdomen), a quick look at the hands should establish whether there are any abnormalities or not. Pondering over normal hands from all angles at great length looks as unprofessional as, indeed, it is. It is of paramount importance to be gentle with the patient. Rough handling (e.g. roughly and abruptly digging deep into the patient's abdomen so that he winces with pain) can bring you instantly to the pass/fail borderline or below it (see also experience 73, p. 340). Make sure that you cover the patient up when you have finished examining him, and thank him.

1 / 'Examine this patient's heart'

Frequency of instruction:

97% of candidates in our survey were asked to do this

Variations of instruction:

Listen to this patient's heart
Examine this praecordium
Feel the pulse, then listen to the apex and the base
Examine the heart/cardiovascular system. Don't worry about peripheral pulses—concentrate
    on the heart
Auscultate the chest
Listen to the apex beat
This patient is short of breath due to cardiovascular disease—examine her
Feel the pulse—listen to the heart sounds
Examine the heart—just listen
This patient has a problem with heart valves—please examine
Listen to the heart. No, don't do that, just listen to the heart
Palpate the apex beat and listen to the heart only
Examine the JVP, apex beat and listen to the apex
Assess the cardiovascular system
Examine the cardiovascular system
This patient has TIAs. Examine the cardiovascular system to elicit a cause
This patient recently had an infarct. Examine the cardiovascular system
This patient has something wrong with his cardiovascular system. Find out in the most
    expeditious way
Examine the cardiovascular system bit by bit
Examine the cardiovascular system and talk me through it

Diagnoses from survey in order of frequency:

1. Mitral stenosis (lone) 16%
2. Mixed mitral valve disease 13%
3. Combinations of mitral and aortic valve disease 9%
4. Mixed aortic valve disease 8%
5. Aortic incompetence (lone) 7%
6. Mitral incompetence (lone) 5%
7. Aortic stenosis (lone) 5%
8. Ventricular septal defect 3%
9. Prosthetic valves 2%
10. Tricuspid incompetence 2%
11. Mitral valve prolapse 2%
12. Clubbing 2%
13. Patent ductus arteriosus 1%
14. Eisenmenger's syndrome 1%

Other diagnoses were: atrial septal defect ($<1\%$), coarctation of the aorta ($<1\%$), chronic liver disease due to tricuspid incompetence ($<1\%$), Fallot's tetralogy with a Blalock shunt ($<1\%$), pulmonary stenosis ($<1\%$), cor pulmonale ($<1\%$), complete heart block ($<1\%$), transposition of the great vessels ($<1\%$), repaired thoracic aortic aneurysm ($<1\%$), dextrocardia ($<1\%$), left ventricular aneurysm ($<1\%$).

Examination *routine*

When asked to 'examine this patient's heart' candidates are often uncertain as to whether they should start with the pulse or go straight to look at the heart. On the one hand it would be absurd to feel all the pulses in the body and leave the object of the examiner's interest to the last minute, whilst on the other hand it would be impetuous to palpate the praecordium straight away. Repeating the examiner's question in the hope that he might clarify it, or asking for a clarification, does nothing but communicate your dilemma to the examiner. You should not waste any time. Bear in mind that our survey has confirmed that the diagnosis is usually mitral and/or aortic valve disease. Approach the right-hand side of the patient and adjust the backrest so that he reclines at 45° to the mattress. If the patient is wearing a shirt you should ask him to remove it so that the chest and neck are exposed. *Meanwhile*, you should complete a *quick*

1 *visual survey.* Observe whether the patient is
(a) breathless,
(b) *cyanosed*,
(c) pale, or
(d) whether he has a *malar flush* (mitral stenosis).
Look at the *neck* for *pulsations*—
(e) forceful carotid pulsations (Corrigan's sign in aortic incompetence; vigorous pulsation in coarctation of the aorta), or
(f) tall, sinuous venous pulsations (congestive cardiac failure, tricuspid incompetence, pulmonary hypertension, etc.).

Run your eyes down onto the chest looking for

(g) a *left thoracotomy scar* (mitral stenosis*) or a midline sternal scar (valve replacement†), and then down to the feet looking for

(h) ankle oedema. As you take the arm to feel the pulse complete your *visual survey* by looking at the hands (a quick look; don't be ponderous) for

(i) clubbing of the fingers (cyanotic congenital heart disease, SBE) and splinter haemorrhages (infective endocarditis).

If the examiner does not want you to feel the pulse he may intervene at this stage—otherwise you should proceed to

2   note the *rate* and *rhythm* of the **pulse**.

3   Quickly ascertain whether the pulse is **collapsing** or not (make sure you are seen lifting the arm up—see experience 36, p. 335).

Next may be an opportune time to look for

4   **radio-femoral delay** (coarctation of the aorta), though this can be left until after auscultation if you prefer and are sure you will not forget it (see experience 1, p. 327).

5   Feel the brachial pulse followed by the carotid pulses to see if the pulse is a **slow rising** one.

If the pulsations in the neck present any interesting features you may have already noted these during your initial *visual survey*. You should now proceed to confirm some of these impressions. The Corrigan's sign in the neck (forceful rise and quick fall of the carotid pulsation) may already have been reinforced by the discovery of a collapsing radial pulse. The individual waves of a large venous pulse can now be timed by palpating the opposite carotid. A large *v* wave, which sometimes oscillates the earlobe, suggests tricuspid incompetence and you should later on demonstrate the peripheral oedema and the pulsatile liver using the bimanual technique. If the venous wave comes before the carotid pulsation it is an *a* wave suggestive of pulmonary hypertension (mitral valve disease, cor pulmonale) or pulmonary stenosis (rare). After

6   assessing the height of the **venous pressure** in centimetres vertically above the sternal angle you should move to the praecordium‡ and

7   localize the **apex beat** with respect to the midclavicular line and ribspaces, first by inspection for visible pulsation and secondly by *palpation*. If the apex beat is vigorous you should stand the index finger on it, to localize the point of maximum impulse (PMI) and *assess* the extent of its thrust. The impulse can be graded as just palpable, lifting (diastolic overload, i.e. mitral or aortic incompetence), thrusting (stronger than lifting), or heaving (outflow obstruction).

8   Palpation with your hand placed from the lower left sternal edge to the apex will detect a **tapping** impulse (mitral stenosis) or *thrills* over the mitral area (mitral valve disease), if present.

9   Continue palpation by feeling the **right ventricular lift** (left parasternal heave). To do this place the flat of your right palm parasternally over the right ventricular area and apply *sustained* and gentle pressure. If right ventricular hypertrophy is present you will feel the heel of your hand lifted by its force (pulmonary hypertension).

---

*NB experiences 4, 7, pp. 329, 330.
†Other scars may also be noted during your *visual survey*—those of previous cardiac catheterizations may be visible over the brachial arteries.
‡The *visual survey* and the examination steps 2-6 should be completed *quickly* and efficiently particularly if you have been asked to examine the *heart*. The objective should be not only to avoid irritating an impatient examiner but also to accommodate as many short cases as possible in the allotted time.

10   Next, you should **palpate** the pulmonary area for a *palpable second sound* (pulmonary hypertension), and the aortic area for a palpable *thrill* (aortic stenosis).

If you feel a strong right ventricular lift quickly recall, and sometimes recheck, whether there is a giant *a* wave (pulmonary hypertension, pulmonary stenosis) or *v* wave (tricuspid incompetence, congestive cardiac failure) in the neck. A palpable thrill over the mitral area (mitral valve disease), or palpable pulmonary second sound over the pulmonary area (pulmonary hypertension) should make you think of, and check for, the other complementary signs. You should by now have a fair idea of what you will hear on auscultation of the heart but you should keep an open mind for any unexpected discovery.

11   The next step will be **auscultation** and you should only stray away from the heart (examiner's command) if you have a strong expectation of being able to demonstrate an interesting and relevant sign (such as a pulsatile liver to underpin the diagnosis of tricuspid incompetence). *Time* the first heart sound with either the apex beat, if this is palpable, or by feeling the carotid pulse (see experience 69, p. 339). It is important to listen to the expected murmurs in the most favourable positions. For example, mitral diastolic murmurs are best heard by turning the patient *onto the left side*, and the early diastolic murmur of aortic incompetence is made more prominent by asking the patient to *lean forwards* with his breath held in expiration.* For low-pitched sounds (mid-diastolic murmur of mitral stenosis, heart sounds) use the bell of your chest-piece but do not press hard, or else you will be listening through a diaphragm formed by the stretched skin! The high-pitched early diastolic murmur of aortic incompetence is very easily missed (see anecdote 20, p. 343). Make sure you specifically listen for it.

If the venous pressure is raised you should check for

12   **sacral oedema** and, if covered, expose the feet to demonstrate any *ankle oedema*. Auscultation over

13   the **lung bases** for inspiratory crepitations (left ventricular failure), though an essential part of the routine assessment of the cardiovascular system, is seldom required in the examination. You may make a special effort to do this in certain relevant situations such as a breathless patient, aortic stenosis with displaced PMI or if there are any signs of left heart failure (orthopnoea, pulsus alternans, gallop rhythm, etc.). Similarly, after examination of the heart itself it may (on rare occasions only) be necessary to

14   palpate the **liver** especially if you have seen a large *v* wave and heard a pansystolic murmur over the tricuspid area. In such cases you may be able to demonstrate a *pulsatile* liver by placing your left palm posteriorly and the right palm anteriorly over the enlarged liver. Finally, you should offer to

15   measure the **blood pressure**. This is particularly relevant in patients with aortic stenosis (low systolic and narrow pulse pressure), and aortic incompetence (wide pulse pressure).

For *checklist* see p. 357.

---

*With the diaphragm of your chest-piece *ready* in position: 'Take a deep breath in; now out; hold it'. Listen intently for the absence of silence in early diastole. Ask the patient to repeat the exercise if necessary.

2 / 'Examine this patient's abdomen'

Frequency of instruction:

79% of candidates in our survey were asked to do this

Variations of instruction:

What abnormal structure can you feel in this abdomen?
Palpate this abdomen
Examine this patient's abdomen—look for signs of hepatic failure
Briefly examine the upper abdomen of this man
Examine the abdomen and anything else relevant
Examine this abdomen by palpation only

Diagnoses from survey in order of frequency:

1   Hepatosplenomegaly (not chronic liver disease) 19%
2   Splenomegaly 13%
3   Polycystic kidneys 12%
4   Chronic liver disease 11%
5   Hepatomegaly (without chronic liver disease or splenomegaly) 9%
6   Ascites 6%
7   Single palpable kidney 5%
8   Miscellaneous abdominal masses 4%
9   Hepatosplenomegaly and generalized lymphadenopathy 3%
10 Hepatomegaly and generalized lymphadenopathy 2%
11 Primary biliary cirrhosis 2%

Other diagnoses were: Crohn's disease (1%), aortic aneurysm (1%), haemochromatosis (<1%), polycystic kidneys and a transplanted kidney (<1%), splenomegaly and generalized lymphadenopathy (<1%), abdominal lymphadenopathy (<1%), post-splenectomy (<1%) and normal abdomen (<1%).

Examination *routine*

Analysis of the above list reveals that in nearly 80% of cases the findings in the abdomen relate to a palpable spleen, liver or kidneys. Bearing this in mind you should approach the right-hand side of the patient and position him so that he is lying supine on one pillow (if comfortable), with the whole abdomen and chest in full view. Ideally the genitalia should also be exposed but to avoid embarrassment to patients, who are volunteers and whose genitals are usually normal, we suggest that you ask the patient to lower his garments and ensure that these are pulled down to a level about halfway between the iliac crest and the symphysis pubis. While these prepararations are being made you should be performing
1   a *visual survey* of the patient. Amongst the many relevant physical signs that you may observe in these few seconds are pallor, pigmentation, jaundice, spider naevi, xanthelasma,

parotid swelling, gynaecomastia, scratch marks, abdominal distension, distended abdominal veins, an abdominal swelling, herniae and decreased body hair. If you use the following *routine* most of these will also be noted during your subsequent examination but at this stage you should particularly note any

2 **pigmentation.** As the patient is being correctly positioned,

3 *quickly* **examine the hands*** for

(a) Dupuytren's contracture,

(b) clubbing,

(c) leuconychia,

(d) palmar erythema,

(e) a flapping tremor (if relevant).

After asking you to examine the abdomen many examiners would like, and *expect*, you to concentrate on the abdomen itself without delay, and yet they will not forgive you for missing an abnormal physical sign elsewhere. This emphasizes the importance of a good *visual survey*; a trained eye will miss nothing important on the face or in the hands while the patient is being properly positioned with the hands by his side. Thus, steps 1–3 need not occupy you for more than a few seconds; you may wish to omit steps 5 and 6 if there is no visible abnormality, and steps 7–11 can be completed as part of the *visual survey*.

4 Pull down the **lower eyelid** to look for *anaemia*. At the same time check the sclerae for *icterus* and look for *xanthelasma*. The guttering between the eyeball and the lower lid is the best place to look for pallor or for any discolouration (e.g. cyanosis, jaundice, etc.).

5 Look at the lips for cyanosis (cirrhosis of the liver) and shine your pen torch into the **mouth†** looking for swollen lips (Crohn's), telangiectasis (Osler–Weber–Rendu), patches of pigmentation (Peutz–Jeghers) and mouth ulcers (Crohn's).

6 **Palpate the neck** and supraclavicular fossae for *cervical lymph nodes*. If you do find lymph nodes you should then proceed to examine the axillae and groins for evidence of generalized lymphadenopathy (lymphoma, chronic lymphatic leukaemia). As you move from the neck to the chest, check for

7 **gynaecomastia** (palpate for glandular breast tissue in obese subjects),

8 **spider naevi** (may have been noted already on hands, arms and face and may also be present on the back) and

9 **scratch marks** (may have been noted on the arms, and may also be found on the back and elsewhere). Next,

10 look at the chest (in the male) and in the axillae for **paucity of hair** (if diminished note facial hair in the male; pubic hair if not visible, may be noted later).

11 **Observe the abdomen** in *three segments* (epigastric, umbilical and suprapubic) for any visible signs such as *pulsations*, generalized *distension* (ascites) or a *swelling* in one particular area. Look for distended *abdominal veins* (the flow is away from the umbilicus in portal hypertension but upwards from the groin in inferior vena cava obstruction).

With practice the examination to this point can be completed very rapidly and will provide valuable information which may be overlooked if proceeding carelessly straight to palpation of the abdomen (see experience 2, p. 328). If the examiner insists that you start with

---

*For a full list of the signs that may be visible in the hands in chronic liver disease see p. 78.

†Though a brief examination of the mouth is usefully included as part of the full 'examine the abdomen' *routine*, it is worth noting that in our survey when there were the findings mentioned, the candidates were given a more specific instruction such as 'Look at this patient's mouth'.

abdominal palpation* it suggests that there is little to be found elsewhere, but you should nevertheless be prepared to use your 'wide-angled lenses' in order not to miss any of the above features.

12 **Palpation** of the abdomen should be performed in an orthodox manner; any temptation to go straight for a visible swelling should be resisted. Put your palm gently over the abdomen and ask the patient if he has any tenderness and to let you know if you hurt him. First systematically examine the whole of the abdomen with *light palpation*. Palpation should be done with the *pulps* of the fingers rather than the tips, the best movement being a gentle flexion at the metacarpophalangeal joints with the hand flat on the abdominal wall. Next, examine specifically for the *internal organs*. For both liver and spleen start in the right iliac fossa (you cannot be frowned upon for following this orthodox procedure), working upwards to the right hypochondrium in the case of the *liver* and diagonally across the abdomen to the left hypochondrium in the case of the *spleen*. The organs are felt against the radial border of the index finger and the pulps of the index and middle fingers as they descend on inspiration, at which time you can gently press and move your hand upwards to meet them. The *kidneys* are then sought by bimanual palpation of each lateral region. Palpation of the internal organs may be difficult if there is ascites. In this case the technique is to press quickly, flexing at the wrist joint, to displace the fluid and palpate the enlarged organ ('dipping'). In a patient well chosen for the examination, a mass in the left hypochondrium may present a problem of identification (see experiences 23, 30, 53, pp. 332, 333, 337 and anecdotes 12, 15, p. 342); the examiner (testing your confidence) may ask you if you are sure that it is a spleen and not a kidney or vice versa. Do not forget to establish whether you can *get above* the mass and *separate* it from the costal edge, whether you can *bimanually* palpate it and whether the percussion note over it is *resonant* (all features of an enlarged kidney, see also p. 74). Palpate *deeply* with the pulps to look for the *ascending* and *descending colons* in the flanks, and use *gentle* palpation to feel for an *aortic aneurysm* in the midline. Complete palpation by feeling for *inguinal lymph nodes*, noting obvious herniae and, at the same time, adding information about the distribution and thickness of pubic hair to that already gained about the rest of the body hair.

13 Heavy **percussion** must be used from the nipple downwards on both sides to locate the upper edge of the liver on the right and the spleen on the left (NB the left lower lateral chest wall may become dull to percussion before an enlarged spleen is palpable). The lower palpable edges of the spleen and liver should be defined by percussion in an orthodox manner, proceeding from the resonant to dull areas. If you suspect free fluid in the peritoneum you must establish its presence by demonstrating

14 **shifting dullness.** Initially check for *stony dullness* in the flanks. There is no need to continue with the procedure of demonstrating shifting dullness if this is not present. By asking the patient with ascites to turn on his side you can shift the dullness from the upper to the lower flank. Before you conclude the palpation and percussion of the abdomen, ask yourself whether you have found anything abnormal. If there are no abnormal physical signs make sure that you have not missed a polycystic kidney or a palpable splenic edge (or occasionally a mass in the epigastrium or iliac fossae); during your auscultation listen carefully for a bruit over the aorta and renal vessels. Generally speaking

---

*Some examiners admit to being irritated at seeing candidates examine normal hands for a long time after being asked to examine the abdomen. They argue that the information obtainable from the face, mouth and hands can be gathered without delay during the inspection part of the examination (see anecdote 13, p. 342).

15 **auscultation** has very little to contribute in the examinaion setting, but as part of the full *routine* you should listen to the bowel sounds, check for renal artery bruits and for any other sounds such as a rub over the spleen or kidney or a venous hum (both excessively rare). Examination of the

16 **external genitalia** is not usually required in the examination for the reasons given above, and we have never heard of a case where

17 **a rectal examination** was required. You should, however, comment that you would like to complete your examination of the abdomen by examining the external genitalia (especially in the male with chronic liver disease—small testes; or cervical lymphadenopathy—drainage of testes to para-aortic and cervical lymph nodes) and rectum. You may of course never get this far since the examiner may interrupt you at an appropriate stage to ask for your findings. If you are allowed to conclude the examination and you have found nothing abnormal despite your careful search, on rare occasions the diagnosis of a normal abdomen will be accepted (see p. 322).

For *checklist* see p. 357.

3 / 'Examine this patient's fundi'

Frequency of instruction:

67% of candidates in our survey were asked to do this

Variations of instruction:

Examine the left eye with the ophthalmoscope provided
Look at the normal fundus on the left, then look at the abnormal fundus on the right
Examine the ocular movements and fundi

Diagnoses from survey in order of frequency:

1 Diabetic retinopathy 36%
2 Optic atrophy 14%
3 Hypertensive retinopathy 9%
4 Retinitis pigmentosa 5%
5 Papilloedema 5%
6 Cataracts 4%
7 Choroidoretinitis 4%
8 Retinal vein thrombosis 3%
9 Myelinated nerve fibres 2%
10 Retinal artery occlusion 1%

Other diagnoses were: normal fundi in a patient with multiple sclerosis (<1%), large optic cup due to glaucoma (<1%), retinal detachment (<1%), iridodonesis (fluttering of the iris) due to a removed lens (<1%), lupus retinopathy (<1%), calcified embolus (<1%).

Special note

Two-thirds of the candidates in our survey received this instruction. Though there are only a limited number of possibilities, it is clear from the survey that a lot of candidates experience more difficulty with a fundus than with any other short case. On our questionnaire a considerable number of candidates reported 'I said optic atrophy . . .', or 'I said diabetic retinopathy . . . but I hadn't got a clue what it was' (see experiences 50, 51, pp. 336, 337). Clearly there is not a lot that a book like this can do to help other than to warn you in advance of the problem, to provide you with a list of the likely conditions and to describe them (see individual short cases). Other than this the art of fundoscopy and fundal diagnosis can only be acquired with practice. With a moderate degree of clinical expertise and common sense most candidates ought to be able to overcome this hurdle.

Examination *routine*

Almost invariably if you are asked to look at the fundus the diagnosis must be in the fundus. However, it is a good practice to precede fundoscopy with

1   a **quick general look** at the patient (this will rarely help but the occasional diabetic in the examination may also have *foot ulcers* or *necrobiosis lipoidica* or may be wearing a *medic-alert* bracelet or neck chain), at his eyes (*arcus lipidus* at an inappropriately young age may suggest diabetes), and at his pupils (usually, but not always, dilated for the examination).

   Turning to ophthalmoscopy, it may be your practice to focus immediately on the fundus and, in the vast majority of cases, this will provide the diagnosis. However, it would be preferable to cultivate the habit (if you can gain sufficient expertise to do it quickly and efficiently) of looking first at

2   the structures in front of the fundus, particularly the **lens** (diabetics will often reward you with early *cataract* formation; your examiner will sometimes not have noticed it, but as long as you are right when he checks you may score points). Adjust the lenses of the ophthalmoscope so that you move down through

3   the **vitreous** noting any *opacities* or *haemorrhages* or *new vessel formation* (diabetes) until you get to

4   the **fundus.** Localize the disc and examine it and its margins for *optic atrophy**, *papillitis* (p. 76) or *papilloedema* (p. 152) and for *myelinated nerve fibres* (p. 229). Trace the

5   **arterioles** and **venules** out from the disc noting particularly their calibre, light reflex (*silver wiring*) and a-v crossing points (*a-v nipping*—see p. 128).

6   Examine **each quadrant** of the fundus and especially the **macular area** and its temporal aspect. You are looking particularly for *haemorrhages* (dot, blot, flame-shaped), *microaneurysms, exudates* both hard (well-defined edges; increased light reflex) and soft (fluffy with ill-defined edges; cotton wool spots). If hard exudates are present see if these form a ring (*circinates* in diabetes).

   If you see haemorrhages you must look specifically for

(a) dot haemorrhages/microaneurysms;

---

*There are normal variations in disc colour; in both infancy and old age it is naturally pale, as is the enlarged disc of a myopic eye. The advice of a well known neurologist and experienced MRCP teacher to his MRCP candidates was: 'Don't diagnose optic atrophy unless it is a "barn door" optic atrophy'. It is well worth bearing this advice in mind (see experience 51, p. 337). Temporal pallor of the disc due to a lesion in the papillomacular bundle is often seen in multiple sclerosis. However, temporal pallor is not always pathological.

(b) new vessel formation;

(c) photocoagulation scars.

If you diagnose diabetic retinopathy your examiner will expect you to be able to comment on the presence or absence of all of these (see experiences 52, 71, pp. 337, 340). If you cannot find these diagnostic clues you may have noted the features that suggest hypertensive rather than diabetic retinopathy (silver wiring, a-v nipping, more soft exudates than hard, haemorrhages which are mainly flame-shaped, early disc swelling with loss of venous pulsation* or frank papilloedema).

It would be useful if you knew that the patient was a diabetic (see experience 75, p. 340 and quotation 33, p. 350) but if you remain in doubt remember that diabetes and hypertension often coexist in a patient, and that it is more important that you have checked comprehensively for the above features, and report your findings honestly (mentioning the features in favour of one diagnosis or the other), than to guess or make up findings.

We leave you to master the findings of the other fundal short cases and to ensure that you would recognize each (see individual short cases). The final point in this important *routine* is to

7 **stay examining until** you have finished and are **ready** to present your findings. Do not be put off by the impatient words or mumblings of your examiner; these will be forgotten when you present accurate findings and get the diagnosis right. On the other hand it is too late to go back and check if the examiner asks whether you saw a . . . and you are not sure (experiences 52, 71, pp. 337, 340). You need to be able to give a clear and unequivocal 'yes' or 'no'. Thus, the best tip we can offer as you look around the fundus is to stop at the disc, the macula, and in each quadrant of each eye and ask yourself the question: 'Are there any abnormalities? What are they?' before moving on to the next area.

For *checklist* see p. 357.

4 / 'Examine this patient's hands'

Frequency of instruction:

58% of candidates in our survey were asked to do this

Variations of instruction:

Look at this man's hands

Look at this patient's hands and then, after you have made a diagnosis, look at the face

Examine this man's hands, commenting on positive or negative features as you go

Examine the wrists and hands

What do you think of these hands? Describe them to me

---

*Observation of venous pulsation is an expertise which comes with much practice of looking at normal as well as abnormal fundi. Though it could be useful if you have acquired this expertise before the examination, do not get bogged down studying the venous pulsation for too long if you are not used to it. See also p. 152.

Diagnoses from survey in order of frequency:

1   Rheumatoid hands 22%
2   Systemic sclerosis (CRST) 13%
3   Wasting of the small muscles of the hand 12%
4   Psoriatic arthropathy/psoriasis 11%
5   Ulnar nerve palsy 9%
6   Clubbing 7%
7   Raynaud's 3%
8   Vasculitis 3%
9   Steroid changes (especially purpura) 3%
10 Acromegaly 2%
11 Motor neurone disease 2%
12 Xanthomata 2%
13 Cyanosis 2%
14 Chronic liver disease 2%
15 Thyroid acropachy 2%
16 Carpal tunnel syndrome 2%
17 Osteoarthrosis 2%
18 Osler–Weber–Rendu syndrome 1%
19 Tophaceous gout 1%

Other diagnoses were: neurofibromatosis (<1%), systemic lupus erythematosus (<1%), cervical myelopathy (<1%), dermatomyositis ('examine hands and face'—<1%), nail-patella syndrome ('examine hands and knees'—<1%), Charcot–Marie–Tooth disease (<1%), superior vena cava obstruction (<1%), facio-scapulo-humeral muscular dystrophy (<1%), Addison's disease (<1%), Marfan's syndrome (<1%).

Examination *routine*

Analysis of the list given above suggests that when you hear this instruction, rheumatoid arthritis is likely to be present in about a quarter of the cases, and either scleroderma, wasting of the small muscles of the hand, psoriasis, ulnar nerve palsy or clubbing in about a further half. As you approach the patient you should bear this in mind and look specifically at
1   the **face** for the typical expressionless facies, with adherent shiny skin, sometimes with telangiectasis (*systemic sclerosis*). It is clear from the survey list that a variety of other conditions may show signs in either the face or in the general appearance, particularly *Cushingoid* facies (steroid changes in a patient with rheumatoid arthritis), *acromegalic* facies, *arcus senilis* or *xanthelasma* (xanthomata), *icterus* and *spider naevi* (chronic liver disease), or *exophthalmos* (thyroid acropachy). We leave you to consider the changes you may note as you approach the patient with the other conditions on the list (see individual short cases). Even if the diagnosis is not immediately clear on looking at the face it is likely that in many cases it will become rapidly apparent as you
2   **inspect the hands.** Run quickly through the six main conditions that make up 75% of cases:
(a) *rheumatoid arthritis* (proximal joint swelling, spindling of the fingers, ulnar deviation, nodules);

(b) *systemic sclerosis* (sclerodactyly with tapering of the fingers, sometimes with gangrene of the fingertips, tight, shiny, adherent skin, calcified nodules, etc.);

(c) generalized *wasting* of the small muscles of the hand, perhaps with dorsal guttering;

(d) *psoriasis* (pitting of the nails, terminal interphalangeal arthropathy, scaly rash);

(e) *ulnar nerve palsy* (may be a typical claw hand or may be muscle wasting which spares the thenar eminence; often this diagnosis will only become apparent when you have made a sensory examination);

(f) *clubbing*.

The changes that you may see in the other conditions in the list are dealt with under the individual short cases, but if in these first few seconds you have not made a rapid spot diagnosis, study first the dorsal and then the palmar aspects of the hands, looking specifically at

3   the **joints** for swelling, deformity or Heberden's nodes;

4   the **nails** for pitting, onycholysis, clubbing, nail fold infarcts (vasculitis—usually rheumatoid) or splinter haemorrhages (unlikely);

5   the **skin** for *colour* (pigmentation, icterus, palmar erythema), for *consistency* (tight and shiny in scleroderma; papery thin, perhaps with purpuric patches in steroid therapy; thick in acromegaly), and for *lesions* (psoriasis, vasculitis, purpura, xanthomata, spider naevi, telangiectasis in Osler–Weber–Rendu and systemic sclerosis, tophi, neurofibromata, other rashes);

6   the **muscles** for isolated *wasting* of the thenar eminence (median nerve lesion), for generalized wasting especially of the first dorsal interosseous but sparing the thenar eminence (ulnar nerve lesion), for generalized wasting from a T_1 lesion or other cause (p. 148) or for *fasciculation* which usually indicates motor neurone disease, though occasionally it can occur in other conditions such as syringomyelia, old polio or Charcot–Marie–Tooth disease.

Before leaving the inspection it is worth looking specifically for *skin crease pigmentation* (see experience 65, p. 339) before moving to

7   **palpation** of the hands for Dupuytren's contracture, nodules (may be palpable in the palms in rheumatoid arthritis), calcinosis (scleroderma/CRST), xanthomata, Heberden's nodes or tophi. In the vast majority of cases you will have, by now, some findings demanding either specific further action (see below) or a report with a diagnosis. Nonetheless, you should be prepared to continue with a full neurological examination of the hands to confirm a suspected neurological lesion, or if you have still made no diagnosis. If the hands appear normal it may be that there is a sensory defect. In these cases, it is more efficient, therefore, to commence the examination by testing

8   **sensation.** If you feel the examiners will not object, ask the patient if there has been any numbness or tingling in his hands and if so, when (?worse at night—carpal tunnel syndrome) and where. Bearing in mind the classical patterns of sensory defect in ulnar and median nerve lesions (Fig. 2.1) and the dermatomes (see Fig. 2.3, p. 41) seek and define an area of deficit to *pinprick* and *light touch* (dab cotton wool lightly), and check the *vibration* and *joint position* sense. With incomplete sensory loss due to either an ulnar or a median nerve defect, if you stroke the medial border of the little finger and the lateral border of the index finger with your fingers simultaneously, the patient may sense that the one side feels different from the other.

9   Check the **tone** of the muscles in the hand by flexing and extending all the joints including the wrist in a 'rolling wave' fashion.

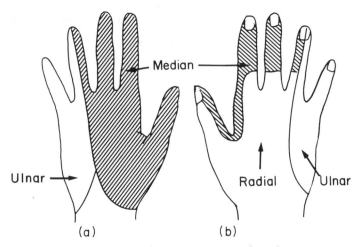

Fig. 2.1. Dermatomes in the hand.

10   The **motor** system of the hands can be tested with the instructions:

(i) 'Open your hands; now close them; now open and close them quickly' (dystrophia myotonica).

(ii) 'Squeeze my fingers'—offer two fingers (C8, T1).

(iii) 'Hold your fingers out straight' (demonstrate); 'stop me bending them' (C7).

(iv) 'Spread your fingers apart' (demonstrate); 'stop me pushing them together' (dorsal* interossei—ulnar nerve).

(v) 'Hold this piece of paper between your fingers; stop me pulling it out' (palmar* interossei—ulnar nerve).

(vi) 'Point your thumb at the ceiling; stop me pushing it down' (abductor pollicis brevis—median nerve).

(vii) 'Put your thumb and little finger together; stop me pulling them apart' (opponens pollicis—median nerve).

Finally, for the sake of completeness, check the

11   **radial pulses**.

The action you take after finding an abnormality at any stage during the above *routine* will depend on what you find. Most commonly an abnormality found during the inspection will lead to most of the above being skipped in favour of a search for other evidence of the condition you suspect. It is worth emphasizing that there may be clues at

12   the **elbows** in several of the common conditions: rheumatoid arthritis (nodules), psoriatic arthropathy (psoriatic plaques), ulnar nerve palsy (scar, filling of the ulnar groove, restriction of range of movement at the elbow or evidence of fracture) and xanthomata. On the evidence of our survey you will need to examine the elbows in over 40% of cases (do not be put off by rolled-down sleeves). It is worth considering where else you would look, what for and what other tests you would do with the other conditions on the list (see individual short cases), but in particular remember to look for *tophi* on the ears if you suspect gout, and if you have diagnosed acromegaly seek an associated *carpal tunnel syndrome* (see experience 9, p. 330). If on inspection you suspect a neurological deficit in the hand, you may wish to confirm it by performing only that part of the above *routine* relevant to that lesion, e.g. testing abduction

*Remember DAB and PAD: DAB=dorsal abduct, PAD=palmar adduct.

and opposition of the thumb and seeking the classical sensory pattern if you see lone wasting of the thenar eminence and suspect carpal tunnel syndrome.

For *checklist* see p. 357.

For *checklist* see p. 357.

5 / 'Examine this patient's legs'

Frequency of instruction:

54% of candidates in our survey were asked to do this

Variations of instruction:

Examine this patient's lower limbs
Examine this patient's legs neurologically
Look at these legs
Look at these legs and make a few general observations
Examine this patient's legs. What else would you like to examine?
Show me how you would examine the reflexes in the legs
Examine the motor system of this man's legs
Examine this man's legs from the end of the bed

Diagnoses from survey in order of frequency:

Group 1 (Spot)
Paget's disease 13%
Erythema nodosum 4%
Pretibial myxoedema 4%
Diabetic foot 3%
Necrobiosis lipoidica diabeticorum 3%
Erythema ab igne 2%
Vasculitis 2%
Swollen knee 1%
Pemphigoid/pemphigus <1%
DVT/ruptured Baker's cyst <1%
Ankle swelling (nephrotic syndrome) <1%
Multiple thigh abscesses <1%
Vasculitic leg ulcers <1%
Pyoderma gangrenosum <1%
Stigmata of sickle-cell disease <1%
Mycosis fungoides <1%
Diabetic ischaemia <1%
Ehlers–Danlos syndrome <1%
Bilateral below knee amputation <1%

Group 2 (Neurological)
Spastic paraparesis 13%
Peripheral neuropathy 12%
Hemiplegia 5%
Cerebellar syndrome 4%
Cervical myelopathy 4%
Diabetic foot 3%
Motor neurone disease 3%
Old polio 3%
Absent leg reflexes and extensor plantars 3%
Friedreich's ataxia 2%
Subacute combined degeneration of the cord 2%
Charcot–Marie–Tooth disease 1%
Polymyositis <1%
Lateral popliteal nerve palsy <1%
Tabes <1%
Diabetic amyotrophy <1%

Examination *routine*

An analysis of the conditions in our survey shows that they roughly fall into the two broad groups shown above:
Group 1: a spot diagnosis
Group 2: a neurological diagnosis.
Either way initial clues may be gained by first performing a brief

1 *visual survey* of the patient as a whole. Look at the head and face for signs such as *enlargement* (Paget's disease), *asymmetry* (hemiparesis), *exophthalmos* with or without *myxoedematous facies* (pretibial myxoedema), or obvious *nystagmus* (cerebellar syndrome). Run your eyes over the patient for other significant signs such as thyroid *acropachy* (pretibial myxoedema), *rheumatoid hands* (swollen knee), nicotine-stained fingers (leg amputations), *wasted hands* (motor neurone disease, Charcot–Marie–Tooth disease, syringomyelia), and for muscle *fasciculation* (usually motor neurone disease).

Turning to the legs, look at the skin, joints and general shape and for any

2 **obvious lesion,** especially from the list of disorders in Group 1. If such a lesion is visible a further full examination of the legs will not be required in most cases. You will be able to begin your description and/or diagnosis immediately (see individual short cases). If there is no obvious lesion look again specifically for

3 **bowing** of the tibia (see experience 61, p. 338), with or without enlargement of the skull. Though the changes of vascular insufficiency (absence of hair, shiny skin, cold pulseless feet, peripheral cyanosis, digital gangrene, painful ulcers) barely occurred in our survey, these should be *briefly* looked for (because they will direct you to examine the pulses, etc. rather than the neurological system).

Observing the legs from the neurological point of view note whether there is

4 **pes cavus** (Friedreich's ataxia, Charcot–Marie–Tooth disease) or

5 **one leg smaller** than the other (old polio, infantile hemiplegia). Next note

6 **muscle bulk.** Bear in mind that some generalized disuse atrophy may occur even in a limb with upper motor neurone weakness (e.g. severe spastic paraparesis—see experience 2, p. 328). There may be unilateral loss of muscle bulk (old polio), muscle wasting that stops part of the way up the leg (Charcot–Marie–Tooth disease), isolated anterior thigh wasting (e.g. diabetic amyotrophy) or generalized proximal muscle wasting (polymyositis) or muscle wasting confined to one peroneal region (lateral popliteal nerve palsy). Look specifically for

7 **fasciculation** (nearly always motor neurone disease).

8 Examine the **muscle tone** in each leg by passively moving it at the hip and knee joints (with the patient relaxed roll the leg sideways, backwards and forwards on the bed; lift the knee and let it drop, or bend the knee and partially straighten in an irregular and unexpected rhythm).

9 Test **power**:
(i) 'Lift your leg up; stop me pushing it down' (L1,2).
(ii) 'Bend your knee; don't let me straighten it' (L5,S1,2).
(iii) (Knee still bent) 'Push out straight against my hand' (L3,4).
(iv) 'Bend your foot down; push my hand away' (S1).
(v) 'Cock up your foot; point your toes at the ceiling. Stop me pushing your foot down' (L4,5).
Moving smoothly into testing

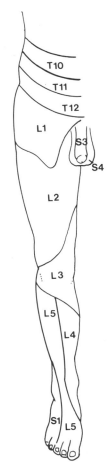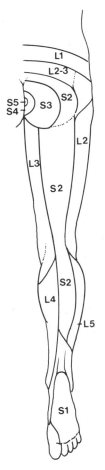

Fig. 2.2. Dermatomes in the lower limb (after Foerster [1933], Oxford University Press, *Brain*, **56**, 1). There is considerable variation and overlap between the cutaneous areas supplied by each spinal root so that an isolated root lesion results in a much smaller area of sensory impairment than the diagram indicates.

10 **coordination**, take your hand off the foot and run your finger down the patient's shin below the knee saying

(vi) 'Put your heel just below your knee then run it smoothly down your shin; now up your shin, now down . . .' etc.*

11 Check the knee (L3,4) and ankle (S1,2) **jerks** and if there is any possibility of pyramidal disease try to demonstrate *ankle clonus* (and patellar clonus).

12 Test the **plantar response** remembering that in slight pyramidal lesions an extensor plantar is more easily elicited on the outer part of the sole than the inner.†

13 Turning to **sensation**, dermatomes L2 to S1 on the leg (Fig. 2.2) are tested if you examine *light touch* (dab cotton wool lightly), and *pinprick* once each on the outer thigh (L2), inner thigh (L3), inner calf (L4), outer calf (L5), medial foot (L5) and lateral foot (S1). The most

*If there is possible or definite cerebellar disease, you may wish to demonstrate dysdiadochokinesis in the foot by asking the patient to tap his foot quickly on your hand.
†In slight pyramidal disease the extensor plantar is first elicited on the dorsilateral part of the foot (*Chaddock's manoeuvre*). As the degree of pyramidal involvement increases the area in which a *Babinski's sign* may be elicited increases first to cover the whole sole and then spreads beyond the foot until *Oppenheim's sign* (extensor response when the inner border of the tibia is pressed heavily—Fig. 3.68b, p. 199) or *Gordon's reflex* (extensor response on pinching the Achilles tendon) can be elicited. In such cases the big toe may be seen to go up as the patient takes his socks off.

common sensory defect is a peripheral neuropathy with stocking distribution loss. Demonstrate this with light touch (usually the most sensitive indicator) and pin prick:
Test above the sensory level:
    'Does the pin feel sharp and prickly'—'Yes'.
Test on the feet:
    'Does the pin feel sharp and prickly'—'No'.
    'Tell me when it changes'.
Work up the leg to the sensory level and confirm afterwards by demonstrating the same level medially and laterally.* The level of the peripheral neuropathy may be different on the two legs. *Vibration* should be tested on the medial malleoli (and knee, iliac crest, etc. if it is impaired), and *joint position* sense in the great toes (remember to explain to the patient what you mean by 'up' and 'down' in his toes before you get him to close his eyes; whilst testing the position sense hold the toe by the lateral aspects).

    Sometimes the examiner will stop you before you get this far. If the lesion is predominantly motor he may break in before you have tested sensation, and if predominantly sensory he may lead you to test sensation earlier or stop you at this point. You should however be sufficiently deft to perform the full examination described above quickly and efficiently, and be prepared to complete it by examining the patient's

14 **gait** (check the patient can walk by asking for either his or the examiner's permission to examine the gait). First, watch his *ordinary walk* to a defined point and back (see p. 170) and then watch him walk *heel-to-toe* (ataxia), on his *toes* and on his *heels* (foot-drop). Finally perform

15 **Romberg's** test with the feet together and the arms outstretched. You must be ready to catch the patient if there is any possibility of ataxia. Romberg's test is only positive (sensory ataxia, e.g. subacute combined degeneration, tabes dorsalis) if the patient is more unsteady with the eyes closed than open.

For *checklist* see p. 358.

6 / 'Examine this patient's chest'

Frequency of instruction:

49% of candidates in our survey were asked to do this

Variations of instruction:

Listen to this man's chest
Examine the respiratory system of this man's chest. Is there anything else you would look for
Examine the right side of this man's chest
Listen to the back of this patient's chest
Examine this lady's chest but could you confine yourself to her back

---

*The same method can be used for rapid demonstration of a higher sensory level: normal sensation is demonstrated above the lesion, e.g. on the shoulder or chest. The pin is then rapidly moved up the whole body from the foot until the patient announces that the sensation is changing to normal. That area is then worked over rapidly to detect the actual sensory level.

Listen to and percuss the posterior aspect of this gentleman's chest
Examine this man's chest from the front
This lady is short of breath. Examine the respiratory system from behind
Listen to the back of the chest. What two other signs would you seek?

Diagnoses from survey in order of frequency:

1   Dullness at the lung base 27%
2   Fibrosing alveolitis 15%
3   Old tuberculosis 12%
4   Carcinoma of the bronchus 10%
5   Bronchiectasis 8%
6   Chronic bronchitis and emphysema 8%
7   Radiation burn on the chest 4%
8   Pneumonia or chest infection 4%
9   Heart murmurs* 2%
10 Ankylosing spondylitis 2%
11 Cor pulmonale 1%
12 Superior vena cava obstruction <1%
13 Pancoast's syndrome <1%
14 Pneumothorax <1%
15 Systemic sclerosis <1%
16 (Kypho)scoliosis <1%

Examination *routine*

While approaching the patient, asking for his permission to examine him and settling him reclining at 45° to the bed with his chest bare, you should observe

1   his **general appearance**. Note any evidence of *weight loss*. The features of conditions such as superior vena cava obstruction (p. 224), systemic sclerosis (p. 90) and lupus pernio (p. 210) may be readily apparent as should be severe kyphoscoliosis. However, *ankylosing spondylitis* is easily missed with the patient lying down (see experiences 3, 31, pp. 329, 334). Observe specifically whether the patient

2   is **breathless** at rest or from the effort of removing his clothes,

3   **purses** his lips (chronic small airways obstruction), or

4   has central **cyanosis**† (cor pulmonale, fibrosing alveolitis, bronchiectasis). Central cyanosis may be difficult to recognize; it is always preferable to look at the oral mucous membranes (see below). Observe

5   if the **accessory muscles** are being used during breathing (chronic small airways obstruction, pleural effusion, pneumothorax, etc.),

*Though a small number of candidates in our survey reported that they were asked to 'examine the chest' in patients with heart murmurs, we suspect that the examiners gave some further suggestive clue that they meant the heart to be examined.
†Occurs with mean capillary concentration of ≥ 4 g dl^{-1} of deoxygenated haemoglobin (or 0.5 g dl^{-1} methaemoglobin). Alternatively, the presence of cyanosis may be confirmed by demonstrating a low arterial oxygen saturation (<85%) noninvasively with a Hewlett–Packard ear oximeter applied to the antihelix of the ear. Central cyanosis is more readily detected in patients with polycythaemia than in those with anaemia—because of the low haemoglobin, patients with anaemia require a much lower oxygen saturation to have 4 g dl^{-1} of unsaturated haemoglobin in capillary blood.

6   if there is generalized **indrawing** of the intercostal muscles or supraclavicular fossae (hyperinflation) or if there is indrawing of the lower ribs on inspiration (due to low, flat diaphragms in emphysema). Localized indrawing of the intercostal muscles suggests bronchial obstruction.

   Listen to the breathing with unaided ears whilst you observe the chest wall and hands (but do not dither). This will allow a dual input whereby a collaboration of what you hear and what you see may help you form a diagnostic impression. You should listen to whether *expiration* is more *prolonged* than inspiration (normally the reverse), and difficult (chronic small airways obstruction), whether it is *noisy* (breathlessness) and if there are any additional noises such as *wheezes* or *clicks*. Difficult and noisy inspiration is usually caused by obstruction in the major bronchi (mediastinal masses, retrosternal thyroid, bronchial carcinoma, etc.) while the more prolonged, noisy and often wheezy expiration is caused by chronic small airways obstruction (asthma, chronic bronchitis). While you are listening observe

7   the *movement* of the **chest wall**. It may be mainly *upwards* (emphysema), or *asymmetrical* (fibrosis, collapse, pleural effusion, pneumothorax). In the context of the examination it is particularly important to look for localized *apical flattening* suggestive of underlying fibrosis due to old tuberculosis. You may also note a thoracotomy or thoracoplasty *scar* (pp. 102 and 132) or the presence of *radiotherapy field markings* (Indian ink marks) or radiation *burns* on the chest (intrathoracic malignancy—p. 272).

   Check the hands for

8   **clubbing** (p. 188), *tobacco staining*, coal dust tattoos, or other conditions which affect the hands and may be associated with lung disease such as rheumatoid arthritis (nodules, p. 68) or systemic sclerosis (p. 90).

9   Feel the **pulse** and if it is bounding, or if the patient is cyanosed, check for a *flapping tremor* of the hands (CO_2 retention). If there is doubt about the presence of cyanosis you could at this point check the tongue and the buccal mucous membranes over the premolar teeth before moving to the neck to look for

10   **raised venous pressure** (cor pulmonale) or fixed distension of the neck veins (superior vena cava obstruction). Next examine

11   the **trachea**. Place the index and ring fingers on the manubrium sternae over the prominent points on either side. Use the middle finger as the exploring finger to feel the tracheal rings to detect either *deviation* or a *tracheal tug* (i.e. the middle finger being pushed upwards against the trachea by the upward movement of the chest wall). Check the *notch–cricoid* distance.*

12   Feel for **lymphadenopathy** (carcinoma, tuberculosis, lymphoma, sarcoidosis) in the cervical region and axillae. As the right hand returns from the left axilla look for

13   the **apex beat** (difficult to localize if the chest is hyperinflated) which in conjunction with tracheal deviation may give you evidence of mediastinal displacement (collapse, fibrosis, effusion, scoliosis).

14   To look for **asymmetry** rest one hand lightly on either side of the front of the chest to see if there is any diminution of movement (effusion, fibrosis, collapse, pneumothorax). Next grip the chest symmetrically with the fingertips in the rib spaces on either side and approximate the thumbs to meet in the middle in a straight horizontal line in order

15   to assess **expansion** first in the inframammary and then in the supramammary regions.

---

*The length of trachea from the suprasternal notch to the cricoid cartilage is normally three or more finger breadths. Shortening of this distance is a sign of hyperinflation.

Note the distance between each thumb and the midline (may give further information about asymmetry of movement) and between both thumbs and try to express the expansion in centimetres (it is better to produce a tape measure for a more accurate assessment of the expansion in centimetres). Comparing both sides at each level

16 **percuss** the chest from above downwards starting with the clavicles and do not forget to percuss over the axillae. Few clinicians now regularly map out the area of cardiac dullness. In healthy people there is dullness behind the lower left quarter of the sternum which is lost together with normal liver dullness in hyperinflation. Complete palpation by checking for

17 **tactile vocal fremitus** with the ulnar aspect of the hand applied to the chest.

18 Auscultation of the **breath sounds** should start *high* at the apices and you should remember to listen in the *axillae*. You are advised to cover both lung fields first with the bell before using the diaphragm (if for no other reason than that this allows you a chance to check the findings without appearing to backtrack!). In the nervousness of the examination harsh breathing heard with the diaphragm near a major bronchus (over the second intercostal space anteriorly or below the scapula near the midline posteriorly) may give an impression of bronchial breathing, particularly in thin people. Compare corresponding points on opposite sides of the chest. Ensure that the patient breathes with the mouth open, regularly and deeply, but not noisily (see experience 55, p. 337). Auscultation is completed by checking

19 **vocal resonance** in all areas; if you have found an area of bronchial breathing (the sounds may resound close to your ears—aegophony) check also for whispering pectoriloquy. The classical timings of crackles/crepitations of various origins are

Early inspiratory: chronic bronchitis, emphysema, asthma
Early and mid inspiratory and recurring in expiration:
    bronchiectasis (altered by coughing)
Late inspiratory: restrictive lung disease (e.g. fibrosing
    alveolitis*) and pulmonary oedema.

20 To **examine** the **back** of the chest sit the patient forward (it may help to cross the arms in front of the patient to pull the scapulae further apart) and repeat steps 14–19. You may wish to start the examination of the back by palpating for cervical nodes from behind (particularly the scalene nodes between the two heads of sternomastoid).

Though with sufficient practice this whole procedure can be performed rapidly without loss of efficiency, often in the examination you will only be asked to perform some of it— usually 'examine the back of the chest'. As always when forced to perform only part of the complete *routine*, be sure that the partial examination is no less thorough and professional. Be prepared to put on your 'wide-angled lenses' so as not to miss other related signs (see experience 1, p. 327 and anecdote 2, p. 340)

Though by now you will usually have sufficient information to present your findings, occasionally you will wish to check other features on the basis of the findings so far. Further purposeful examination gives an impression of confidence but it should not be overdone. For example, looking for evidence of Horner's syndrome, or wasting of the muscles of one hand† in a patient with apical dullness and a deviated trachea, will suggest professional keenness; whereas routinely looking at the eyes and hands after completion of the examination may

---

*In fibrosing alveolitis late inspiratory crackles may become reduced if the patient is made to lean forward; thereby the compressed dependent alveoli (which crackle-open in late inspiration) are relieved of the pressure of the lungs.

†A good *visual survey* may reveal such signs at the beginning.

only suggest to the examiner that you do not have the diagnosis and are hoping for inspiration! If you suspect airways obstruction the examiner may be impressed if you perform a bedside respiratory function test—the *forced expiratory time (FET)**

For *checklist* see p. 358.

For *checklist* see p. 358.

7 / 'What is the diagnosis?'

Frequency of instruction:

41% of candidates in our survey were asked to do this

Variations of instruction:

First, look generally at this man. What do you notice?
What is wrong with this patient?
Ask the patient to look at the ceiling—what is the diagnosis?
Look at this patient
Look at this man and at his hands
I would like you to look at him and tell me what's the matter
What do you notice from here? (end of the bed)
Look at this patient. What other specific things would you like to examine?
Observe this patient
What is that?
Comment on this patient's appearance
Diagnosis please
Give me as many diagnoses as you can and listen to the heart
What do you think this man is suffering from and why?
What do you think?
Do you notice anything about this patient's appearance?
Come and have a look at this man
What do you notice? Now examine the abdomen
On general appearance what's wrong with this man?
This man is breathless. Observe him
What observations do you make?
What do you notice looking at this patient that is in the MRCP curriculum?
Look at this man from the end of the bed. What would you like to do now?
Look at this patient and then examine the relevant parts

---

*Ask the patient to take a deep breath in and then, on your command (timed with the second hand of your watch), to breathe out as hard and as fast as he can until his lungs are completely empty. A normal person will empty his lungs in less than six seconds (one second for every decade of age—e.g. a normal thirty-year-old will do it in three seconds). An FET of > six seconds is evidence of airways obstruction. You need to practise this test with patients if it is to be slick. As with PFR and FEV_1 etc. it is important to make sure that certain patients, particularly females, *are* blowing as hard and as fast as they can ('don't worry about what you look like—give it everything you've got—like this'—give a demonstration) and empty their lungs completely ('keep going, keep going . . . keep going, well done!')

Diagnoses from survey in order of frequency:

1 Acromegaly 11%
2 Parkinson's disease 5%
3 Hemiplegia 5%
4 Goitre 5%
5 Jaundice 5%
6 Dystrophia myotonica 4%
7 Pigmentation 4%
8 Graves' disease 4%
9 Exophthalmos 4%
10 Paget's disease 3%
11 Ptosis 3%
12 Choreoathetosis 3%
13 Drug-induced Parkinsonism 3%
14 Breathlessness 2%
15 Purpura 2%
16 Hypopituitarism 2%
17 Addison's/Nelson's 2%
18 Cushing's syndrome 2%
19 Psoriasis 2%
20 Hypothyroidism 2%
21 Systemic sclerosis/CRST 2%
22 Sturge–Weber syndrome 2%
23 Spider naevi and ascites 1%
24 Marfan's syndrome 1%
25 Neurofibromatosis 1%
26 Cyanotic congenital heart disease 1%
27 Pretibial myxoedema 1%
28 Uraemia and dialysis scars 1%
29 Horner's syndrome 1%
30 Cachexia 1%
31 Osler–Weber–Rendu syndrome 1%
32 Ankylosing spondylitis 1%
33 Ulnar nerve palsy 1%
34 Turner's syndrome 1%
35 Down's syndrome 1%
36 Bilateral parotid enlargement/Mikulicz's syndrome 1%
37 Old rickets 1%
38 Torticollis 1%
39 Congenital syphilis 1%
40 Syringomyelia <1%
41 Herpes zoster <1%
42 Pemphigoid/pemphigus <1%
43 Bell's palsy <1%

44 Necrobiosis lipoidica diabeticorum <1%
45 Primary biliary cirrhosis <1%

Examination *routine*

Advice commonly given by the candidates in our survey as a result of their Membership experiences was to 'keep calm'. When you stand before a patient with a condition from the above list and hear the instruction under consideration you are being asked to do what you do every day of your medical life. There are two differences, however, between everyday medical life and the examination: (i) The patients in the examination usually have classical, often florid, signs and should be easier to diagnose than most patients seen in the clinic. (ii) In the examination, you may be overwhelmed by nerves and as a result make the most fundamental errors. You must indeed try to keep calm and remind yourself that this is likely to be an easy case, and that you will not only make a diagnosis (as you would with ease in the clinic), but will also find a way of scoring some extra marks. Unlike some of the instructions requiring long examination *routines*, the 'spot diagnosis' may be solved in seconds leaving time for something extra which you may be able to dictate, rather than leaving it to the examiner to lead. You should start with

1   a *visual survey* of the patient, running your eyes from the head via the neck, trunk, arms and legs to the feet, seeking the areas of abnormality, and thereby the diagnosis. We would suggest that you rehearse presenting the *records* for the various possibilities on the list (see individual short cases). If you are well prepared with the features of these short cases, then in the majority of instances you should be able to make a diagnosis, or likely diagnosis, which you can confirm or highlight by demonstrating additional features (see below). If you have scanned the patient briefly and not found any obvious abnormality, then

2   **retrace** the same ground scrutinizing each part more thoroughly and asking yourself at each stage, 'Is the head normal?', 'Is the face normal?' etc. If it is not normal describe the abnormality to yourself in the mind trying to match it up with one of the short case *records*. In this way cover the

(i) head (think especially of *Paget's* and *dystrophia myotonica* with frontal balding);
(ii) face (think especially of *acromegaly, Parkinson's,* the facial asymmetry of *hemiplegia*, the long lean look of dystrophia myotonica, tardive dyskinesia, hypopituitarism, Cushing's, hypothyroidism, systemic sclerosis);
(iii) eyes (*jaundice, exophthalmos*, ptosis, Horner's, xanthelasma);
(iv) neck (*goitre*, Turner's, ankylosing spondylitis, torticollis);
(v) trunk (pigmentation, ascites, purpuric spots, spider naevi, wasting, pemphigus, etc.);
(vi) arms (choreoathetosis, psoriasis, Addison's, spider naevi, syringomyelia);
(vii) hands (acromegaly, *tremor*, clubbing, sclerodactyly, arachnodactyly, claw hand, etc.);
(viii) legs (bowing, purpura, pretibial myxoedema, necrobiosis);
(ix) feet (pes cavus).

If you still do not have the diagnosis

3   specifically consider **abnormal colouring** such as *pigmentation, icterus* or pallor, and then cover the same ground again but in even more detail

4   **breaking down each part into its constituents,** scrutinizing them, and continually asking yourself the question: 'Is it normal?' This procedure is most profitable on the face (see p. 38).

Once you have the diagnosis, the natural impulse for most people is to give it in one word, and then stand back and wait for the applause. However, it is worth remembering that the majority of the candidates, who have all worked hard and prepared for the examination, are likely to 'spot' the diagnosis and yet only a few end up with the diploma. Do not let this opportunity pass you by; try to make more of the case yourself by proceeding to

5   look for **additional** and **associated features**, and then by making your presentation more elaborate. Describe the findings in detail (see individual short cases) and highlight the key features to support your diagnosis (lenticular abnormalities in dystrophia myotonica and Marfan's; thyroid bruit in Graves' disease; webbed neck in Turner's syndrome, and so on). It is worth going through the diagnoses on the list yourself, and considering what additional features you would look for, and how you could really go to town on an easy case. For example, if you diagnose acromegaly you could demonstrate the massive sweaty palms, commenting on the increased skin thickening and on the presence or absence of thenar wasting (carpal tunnel syndrome—see experience 9, p. 330), and then proceed to test the visual fields. If you suspect Parkinson's disease, take the hands and test for cog-wheel rigidity at the wrist, demonstrate the glabellar tap sign (despite its unreliability) and then ask the patient to walk. If you diagnose hemiplegia, confirm that the VIIth nerve lesion is upper motor neurone (see p. 100), and then check for atrial fibrillation. If you see a goitre, examine it and then assess the thyroid status.

For *checklist* see p. 358.

8 / 'Examine this patient's eyes'

Frequency of instruction:

32% of candidates in our survey were asked to do this

Variations of instruction:

Tell me about this patient's eyes
Look at these eyes
Examine the eye movements

Diagnoses from survey in order of frequency:

1   Exophthalmos 27%
2   Ocular palsy 23%
3   Nystagmus 11%
4   Diabetic retinopathy 8%
5   Optic atrophy 7%
6   Myasthenia gravis 4%
7   Visual field defects 3%
8   Ptosis 3%
9   Retinitis pigmentosa 2%
10   Horner's syndrome 2%
11   Holmes–Adie pupil 1%
12   Argyll Robertson pupils 1%

13   Cataracts 1%
14   Papilloedema 1%

Other diagnoses were: buphthalmos in a patient with Sturge–Weber syndrome (1%), normal eyes in a patient who was supposed to have internuclear ophthalmoplegia (1%), retinal detachment (< 1%).

Examination *routine*

A study of the above list maps out your examination steps when you hear this instruction. It is basically going to be a part of your cranial nerves *routine* but carried out in slightly more detail. It should be your habit to commence all examination *routines* by *scanning* the whole patient. The patient with nystagmus due to cerebellar disease (p. 130) may have an *intention tremor* which will occasionally be noticeable even with minor movements. The patient with exophthalmos may have *pretibial myxoedema* or *thyroid acropachy*. A number of other conditions with stigmata elsewhere on the body may cause eye signs. Though these conditions were not prominent in our survey, they should be borne in mind as you complete this *visual survey*: face and hands of acromegaly, foot ulcers in diabetes, pes cavus in Friedreich's ataxia, the long, lean look of dystrophia myotonica, etc. As you finish your *visual survey* briefly look again at
1   the **face** (e.g. myasthenic facies, tabetic facies, facial asymmetry in hemiparesis), and then concentrate on
2   the **eyes**. Ask yourself if there is
(a) exophthalmos,
(b) strabismus,
(c) ptosis
or other abnormalities such as xanthelasma or arcus senilis. Look at
3   the **pupils** for inequality of size and shape; whether one or both are small (Argyll Robertson, Horner's) or large (Holmes–Adie, IIIrd nerve palsy). Next, it is traditional to check
4   the **visual acuity** by asking the patient to read a newspaper or other print which you hold up, and by asking him to look at the clock on the wall (see p. 55); alternatively it would be preferable to pull out a pocket-sized Snellen's chart.* In the traditional *routine* you should next test
5   **visual fields** (see p. 48). However in the majority of cases the important findings are on testing
6   **eye movements** (see p. 55). We leave you to decide if you wish to follow the traditional *routine* or check eye movements before acuity and visual fields (see experience 37, p. 335 and quotation 42, p. 350). You are looking for
(a) ocular palsy (p. 110),
(b) diplopia,
(c) nystagmus,
(d) lid lag.
In order to test

*We advise you to take a pocket-sized Snellen's chart (like the one provided in Appendix 5). It will enable you to put an approximate value on the patient's visual acuity while taking no extra time.

7 the **pupillary light reflex**, take out your pen torch and shine the light twice (*direct* and *consensual*) in each eye. Then test

8 the **accommodation-convergence reflex**—hold your finger close to the patient's nose:

'Look into the distance';

then suddenly

'Now look at my finger'.

Finally, examine

9 the **fundi**.

As usual, when you have the diagnosis, think what else you could look for (e.g. cerebellar signs in a patient with nystagmus; sympathectomy scar over the clavicle in a patient with Horner's syndrome; absent limb reflexes in Holmes–Adie pupil) before shouting out the diagnosis even if it is obvious (e.g. exophthalmos).

For *checklist* see p. 358.

9 / 'Examine this patient's face'

Frequency of instruction:

20% of candidates in our survey were asked to do this

Variations of instruction:

Look at this patient's face

What is wrong with this patient's face?

Comment on the facial appearance

You are good at looking at the face and making a diagnosis; can you do that in this patient?

Diagnoses from survey in order of frequency:

1   Lower motor neurone VIIth nerve lesion 12%
2   Lupus pernio 8%
3   Ptosis 7%
4   Sturge–Weber syndrome 7%
5   Hypothyroidism 7%
6   Osler–Weber–Rendu syndrome 7%
7   Dystrophia myotonica 4%
8   Jaundice 4%
9   Horner's syndrome 4%
10 Systemic sclerosis/CRST 3%
11 Peutz–Jeghers syndrome 3%
12 Upper motor neurone VIIth nerve lesion 3%
13 Systemic lupus erythematosus 3%
14 Parkinson's disease 3%
15 Cushing's syndrome 2%

16 Neurofibromatosis 2%
17 Superior vena cava obstruction 2%
18 Plethora (polycythaemia rubra vera) 2%
19 Hypopituitarism 2%
20 Vitiligo and a goitre 2%
21 Cyanosis 2%
22 Paget's disease 1%
23 Bilateral parotid enlargement 1%
24 Exophthalmos 1%
25 Acromegaly 1%
26 Dermatomyositis (hands and face) 1%
27 Xanthelasma and arcus senilis 1%
28 Acne rosacea 1%
29 Dermatitis herpetiformis 1%
30 Malar flush 1%

Examination *routine*

This instruction is really just a variation on the 'spot diagnosis' theme, only easier because you are told where the abnormalities lie. In a way similar to that described in the 'What is the diagnosis?' *routine*,

1 *survey* the patient from head to foot and then

2 **scan the face** and skull. The abnormality will usually be obvious (see above list) but if you find none then proceed to

3 **break down the parts** of the face into their constituents and scrutinize each, asking the question to yourself: 'Is it normal?'. Thus if you have scanned the eyes and have not been struck by any obvious abnormality (e.g. ptosis or an abnormal pupil), you should look at all the structures such as the eyelids (mild degree of ptosis, heliotrope rash on the upper lid in dermatomyositis), eyelashes (sparse in alopecia*), cornea (arcus senilis, ground glass appearance in congenital syphilis), sclerae (icteric, congested in SVC obstruction and polycythaemia), pupils (small, large, irregular, dislocated lens in Marfan's, cataract in dystrophia myotonica) and iris ('muddy iris' in iritis)† on both sides. Look at the face for any erythema or infiltrates (lupus pernio, SLE, dermatomyositis, malar flush), around the mouth for tight, shiny, adherent skin (systemic sclerosis) or pigmented macules (Peutz–Jeghers) and, if indicated, in the mouth for telangiectases (Osler–Weber–Rendu), cyanosis or pigmentation (Addison's). The whole face can be rapidly covered in this manner. Having spotted the abnormality and, you hope, made the diagnosis you should, if appropriate, try to score extra points by demonstrating

4 **additional features** in the same way as described under 'What is the diagnosis?' Go through each diagnosis on the list and work out what additional features you would see elsewhere. Thus, if you find a lower motor neurone VIIth nerve lesion, demonstrate the weakness in the upper as well as the lower part of the face (see p. 184), then be seen to examine the ears for evidence of herpes zoster (Ramsay Hunt syndrome).

---

*May be associated with the organ-specific autoimmune diseases—see p. 254.
†Another uncommon but important sign which may occur in the iris is neovascularization in diabetes (rubeosis iridis). However, it is unlikely that this would occur in the context of 'examine this patient's face' at the examination.

If despite carrying out the above routine there is still no apparent abnormality then examine the facial musculature (see 'Examine this patient's cranial nerves') for evidence of a VIIth nerve lesion which is not obvious.

For *checklist* see p. 359.

For *checklist* see p. 359.

10 / 'Examine this patient's arms'

Frequency of instruction:

15% of candidates in our survey were asked to do this

Variations of instruction:

This lady has noticed weak arms. Examine her
Look at this patient's forearms
Examine this patient's forearms

Diagnoses from survey in order of frequency:

1   Wasting of the small muscles of the hand 26%
2   Motor neurone disease 19%
3   Hemiplegia 7%
4   Cerebellar syndrome 6%
5   Cervical myelopathy 6%
6   Neurofibromatosis 4%
7   Muscular dystrophy 4%
8   Psoriasis 4%
9   Purpura due to steroids 4%
10   Parkinson's disease 3%
11   Syringomyelia 3%
12   Hemiballismus 3%
13   Lichen planus 3%
14   Pseudoxanthoma elasticum 3%
15   Old polio 3%
16   Rheumatoid arthritis 3%
17   Axillary vein thrombosis 3%
18   Contracture of the elbow in a case of haemophilia 3%
19   Ulnar nerve palsy 1%
20   Pancoast's syndrome 1%
21   Herpes zoster 1%
22   Mycosis fungoides 1%
23   Polymyositis 1%

Examination *routine*

Consideration of the above list from the survey reveals that the vast majority (over 80%) of conditions behind this instruction are neurological with a handful of spot diagnoses which will usually be obvious. If the diagnosis is not an obvious 'spot' (and you should make sure that you would recognize each on the list—see individual short cases) your *routine* should commence in the usual way by scanning the whole patient but in particular looking at

1   the **face** for obvious abnormalities such as *asymmetry* (hemiplegia), *nystagmus* (cerebellar syndrome), *wasting* (muscular dystrophy), sad, immobile, unblinking facies (*Parkinson's disease*), or *Horner's* syndrome (syringomyelia, Pancoast's syndrome). You may return to seek a less obvious Horner's or nystagmus later, if necessary. In search of obvious abnormalities run your eyes down to

2   the **neck** (pseudoxanthoma elasticum, lymph nodes), and then scan down the arms looking in particular at

3   the **elbows** which should be particularly inspected for *psoriasis, rheumatoid nodules* and *scars* or *deformity* underlying an ulnar nerve palsy. Before picking up the hands look for

4   a **tremor** (Parkinson's disease), then briefly inspect

5   the **hands** in the same way as you have practised under 'Examine this patient's hands', looking at
(a) the joints (swelling, deformity);
(b) nail changes (pitting, onycholysis, clubbing, nail fold infarcts);
(c) skin changes (colour, consistency, lesions).
      If you have not already been led towards a diagnosis requiring specific action, start a full neurological examination by studying first

6   the **muscle bulk** in the upper arms, lower arms and hands, bearing in mind that in about one-quarter of cases there will be wasting of the small muscles of the hands (see p. 148), and in one-fifth of cases there will be motor neurone disease which means wasting and

7   **fasciculation**.

8   Test the **tone** in the arms by passively bending the arm (with the patient relaxed) to and fro in an irregular and unexpected fashion, and in the hands by flexing and extending all the joints, including the wrist in the classic 'rolling wave' fashion used to detect cog-wheel rigidity (Parkinson's disease).

9   Ask the patient:
'Hold your **arms out in front** of you' (look for *winging* of the scapulae); 'Now close your eyes' (look for *sensory wandering*).
Next test

10   **power**:
(i) 'Put your arms out to the side' (demonstrate this to the patient yourself—arms at 90° to your body with elbows flexed); 'Stop me pushing them down' (deltoid—C5).
(ii) 'Bend your elbow; stop me straightening it' (biceps—C5,6).
(iii) 'Push your arm out straight'—resist elbow extension (triceps—C7).
(iv) 'Squeeze my fingers'—offer two fingers (C8,T1)
(v) 'Hold your fingers out straight' (demonstrate);
'Stop me bending them' (if the patient can do this there is nothing wrong with motor C7 or the radial nerve).

(vi) 'Spread your fingers apart' (demonstrate); 'stop me pushing them together' (dorsal interossei—ulnar nerve).

(vii) 'Hold this piece of paper between your fingers; stop me pulling it out' (palmar interossei—ulnar nerve).

(viii) 'Point your thumb at the ceiling; stop me pushing it down' (abductor pollicus brevis—median nerve).

(ix) 'Put your thumb and little finger together; stop me pulling them apart' (opponens pollicis—median nerve).

11   Test **coordination**

(i) 'Can you do this?'—demonstrate by flexing your elbows at right angles and then pronating and supinating your forearms as rapidly as possible.

(ii) 'Tap quickly on the back of your hand' (demonstrate).

(iii) 'Touch my finger; touch your nose; backwards and forwards quickly and neatly' (demonstrate if necessary—vary the target).

This test may be compared with the eyes open and closed if you suspect sensory ataxia.

12   Check the biceps (C5,6), triceps (C7) and supinator (C5,6) **reflexes**.

13   Finally perform a **sensory screen** with *light touch* and *pinprick* bearing in mind the dermatomes shown in Fig. 2.3 and the areas of sensation covered by the ulnar, median and radial nerves in the hand (see Fig. 2.1, p. 24). Finally, check *vibration* and *joint position* sense.

We leave you to consider where else you could look with each of the conditions given on the list in order to find additional information (see individual short cases). For example, you could look for nystagmus should you find cerebellar signs, or for a Horner's syndrome should you suspect syringomyelia or Pancoast's syndrome.

For *checklist* see p. 359.

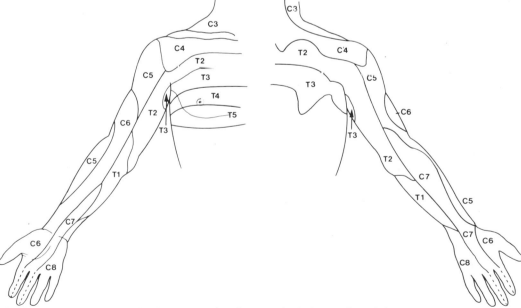

Fig. 2.3. Dermatomes in the upper limb (after Foerster [1933], Oxford University Press, *Brain*, **56**, 1). There is considerable variation and overlap between the cutaneous areas supplied by each spinal root so that an isolated root lesion results in a much smaller area of sensory impairment than the diagram indicates.

11 / 'Examine this patient's neck'

Frequency of instruction:

12% of candidates in our survey were asked to do this

Variations of instruction:

Examine this patient's neck. Do you think she is euthyroid?
Feel the mass in this patient's neck

Diagnoses from survey in order of frequency:

1 Goitre 46%
2 Generalized lymphadenopathy 17%
3 Graves' disease 12%
4 JVP abnormality 6%
5 Bilateral parotid enlargement/Mikulicz's syndrome 4%
6 Supraclavicular mass with a Horner's syndrome 4%
7 Facio-scapulo-humeral muscular dystrophy 4%
8 Ankylosing spondylitis 2%
9 Hypothyroidism 2%

Examination *routine*

As usual the first step is to
1 *survey* the patient quickly from head to foot (exophthalmos, myxoedematous facies, ankle oedema, etc.) and then to
2 **look at the neck**. According to the survey the reason for the instruction in half of the cases will be a *goitre*. If another abnormality is visible your further action will be dictated by what you see and we suggest you go through the list and establish a sequence of actions for each abnormality (e.g. if you see giant *v* waves you would wish to examine the heart and liver—see p. 201). If you do see a goitre, offer a drink to the patient:
    'Take a sip of water and hold it in your mouth';
look at the neck:
    'Now swallow'.
Watch the movement of the goitre, or the *appearance* of a *nodule* not visible before swallowing (behind sternomastoid—see Fig. 3.29c, p. 119). Next ask the patient's permission to feel the neck, and then approach him from behind. If there has been no evidence of a goitre so far you may wish to palpate the neck for lymph nodes *before* feeling for a goitre. Otherwise
3 **palpate** the thyroid. With the right index and middle finger feel below the thyroid cartilage where the isthmus of the thyroid gland lies over the trachea. Then palpate the two lobes of the thyroid gland which extend laterally behind the sternomastoid muscle. Ask the patient to swallow again while you continue to palpate the thyroid, ensuring that the neck is slightly flexed to ease palpation. Remember that if there is a goitre, when you give your presentation you are going to want to comment on its *size*, whether it is *soft*, or *firm*, whether

it is *nodular* or *diffusely enlarged*, whether it *moves* readily on swallowing, whether there are *lymph nodes* (see below) and whether there is a vascular *murmur* (see below). Extend palpation upwards along the medial edge of the sternomastoid muscle on either side to look for a *pyramidal lobe* which may be present. Apologize for any discomfort you may cause because the deep palpation necessary to feel the thyroid gland causes pain, particularly in patients with Graves' disease. Next palpate laterally to examine

4   for **lymph nodes**. If you find lymph node enlargement check not only in the *supraclavicular fossae* and right up the neck but also in the *submandibular, postauricular* and *suboccipital* areas, ensuring that the head is slightly flexed on the side under palpation to allow access and scrutiny of slightly enlarged lymph nodes. Ascertain whether the lymph nodes are *separate* (reactive hyperplasia, infectious mononucleosis, lymphoma, etc.) or *matted* together (neoplastic, tuberculous), *mobile* or *fixed* to the skin or deep tissues (neoplastic), or whether they are *soft, fleshy, rubbery* (Hodgkin's disease) or *hard* (neoplastic). Particularly if you find lymph nodes without a goitre, examine for lymph nodes in the axillae and groins (lymphoma, chronic lymphatic leukaemia, etc.) and, if allowed, feel for the spleen.

5   **Auscultate** over the thyroid for evidence of increased vascularity. You may need to occlude venous return to rule out a venous hum, and listen over the aortic area to ensure that the thyroid bruit you hear is not, in fact, an outflow obstruction murmur conducted to the root of the neck.

6   If there is any evidence of thyroid disease begin an assessment of **thyroid status** (see 'Examine this patient's thyroid status') by feeling and counting the pulse (NB do not miss *atrial fibrillation* whether slow or fast). The examiner will soon stop you if he wishes to hear your description of a multinodular goitre in a euthyroid patient.

For *checklist* see p. 359.

12 / 'Ask this patient some questions'

Frequency of instruction:

8% of candidates in our survey were asked to do this

Variations of instruction:

Talk to this patient
Examine this patient's speech
Converse with this patient

Diagnoses from survey in order of frequency:

1   Dysphasia 24%
2   Cerebellar dysarthria 16%
3   Raynaud's 11%
4   Systemic sclerosis/CRST 8%
5   Pseudobulbar palsy 8%

6   Myxoedema 5%
7   Graves' disease 5%
8   Crohn's disease 5%
9   Ankle oedema due to nephrotic syndrome 5%
10 Senile dementia 5%
11 Parkinson's disease 3%

Examination *routine*

Inspection of the list of cases in our survey which provoked this instruction reveals that they fall into four groups, each with a very different reason for the instruction:

Group 1: To spot the diagnosis and then confirm it by eliciting *revealing answers* 39%
Group 2: To demonstrate and diagnose the type of a dysarthria 32%
Group 3: To diagnose a dysphasia 24%
Group 4: To assess higher mental function 5%

With the Group 1 patients you may have been given a lead such as 'look at the hands' (Raynaud's) or 'look at the face' (systemic sclerosis, myxoedema, etc.) before the instruction 'ask this patient some questions'. At any rate you should start your examination as usual with

1   a ***visual survey*** of the patient from head to foot, particularly looking for evidence of: (i) the spot diagnosis in Group 1 patients (Raynaud's, systemic sclerosis/CRST, hypo- or hyperthyroidism, Crohn's, nephrotic syndrome), (ii) a *hemiplegia* which may be associated with dysphasia, or (iii) any of the conditions associated with dysarthria (see p. 238) especially *nystagmus* or *intention tremor* (which may be revealed by even minor movements) in cerebellar diseases, *pes cavus* in Friedreich's ataxia and the *facies/tremor* of Parkinson's disease.

In the Group 1 patients once you are on to the diagnosis the sort of
2   **specific questions** the examiners are looking for (see also the individual short cases) are:
Raynaud's (see also anecdote 8, p. 341):

'Do your fingers change colour in the cold?'
'What colour do they go?' ('Is there a particular sequence of colours?')
'How long have you had the trouble?'
'What is your job?' (vibrating tools, etc.)

and if there is any possibility of connective tissue disease

'Do you have any difficulty with swallowing?' etc.

Systemic sclerosis:

'Do you have any difficulty with swallowing?'
'Do your fingers change colour in the cold?'
'Do you get short of breath?' (on hills? on flat? etc.)

We leave you to work out the straightforward questions you would ask the slow croaking patient with *myxoedematous facies*, the patient with *exophthalmos*, or the one who has *lid retraction* and is *fidgety*, or the patient who has *multiple scars* and *sinuses* on his abdomen. In the young patient who may have nephrotic syndrome you would be looking for the history of a sore throat.

If there are no features suggesting a Group 1 patient, it is likely that the problem is either a dysarthria or dysphasia, and, as already mentioned, there may be clues pointing to one of these. You need to ask the patient

3 some **general questions** to get him *talking*:
   'My name is . . . Please could you tell me your name?'
   'What is your address?'

If you still need to hear a patient speak further ask

4 **more questions** which require *long answers* such as
   'Please could you tell me all the things you ate for breakfast/lunch.'

To test

5 **articulation** ask the patient to repeat the traditional words and phrases such as 'British Constitution', 'West Register Street', 'Biblical criticism' and 'artillery'. As well as testing articulation such

6 **repetition** is useful for assessing speech when the patient only gives one-word answers to questions. If necessary ask the patient to repeat long sentences after you. Information gained from repetition may also be useful in your assessment of dysphasia (see below).

If the problem is *dysarthria*, it is really a spot diagnosis to test your ability to recognize and demonstrate the features of the different types (see p. 238). It is recommended that you find as many patients as possible with the conditions causing the various types of dysarthria and listen to them speak so that, as with murmurs, the diagnosis is a question of instant recognition. This is particularly true of the ataxic dysarthria of cerebellar disease. When you have heard enough to make the diagnosis, you should either describe the speech (p. 238) and, with supporting signs seen on inspection, give the diagnosis, or proceed to look for

7 **additional signs** (in the same way as you might do after the 'What is the diagnosis' instruction).

If the patient has a *dysphasia* (see p. 239) you may wish to demonstrate that

8 **comprehension** is good (expressive dysphasia) or impaired (receptive dysphasia):
   'Put your tongue out'.
   'Shut your eyes'.
   'Touch your nose'.
   'Smile', etc.

By asking the patient to repeat a sentence you may wish to demonstrate that repetition is better than spontaneous speech in expressive dysphasia, whereas receptive dysphasia results in paraphasic distortions and irrelevant insertions (see p. 239). Test for

9 **nominal dysphasia.** Hold up your keys:
   'What is this?'—Patient does not answer
   'Is this a spoon?'—'No'.
   'Is it a pen?'—'No'.
   'Is it a key?'—'Yes'.

Our survey showed that it is extremely rare for candidates to be asked to assess

10 **higher mental functions.*** This is, however, an assessment which every Membership candidate should be equipped to make. The following is the 'Abbreviated Mental Test' (AMT)—more than four of the questions wrong suggests a well-established dementia:

*Rare at the time of writing (see anecdote 21, p. 343): it is conceivable that any examiners who see this book will be given ideas as to the areas they are neglecting!

1 Age.
2 Time (to nearest hour).
3 Address for recall at end of test—this should be repeated by the patient to ensure it has been heard correctly: 42 West Street.
4 Year.
5 Name of this place.
6 Recognition of two persons (doctor, nurse, etc.).
7 Date of birth (day and month sufficient).
8 Year of First World War.
9 Name of present Monarch.
10 Count backwards from 20 to 1.

Agnosia, apraxia, dyslexia, dysgraphia and dyscalculia are considered on p. 100.

For *checklist* see p. 359.

13 / 'Examine this patient's pulse'

Frequency of instruction:

7% of candidates in our survey were asked to do this

Variations of instruction:

Feel this pulse
Examine this patient's pulse—look for the cause
Examine this patient's pulses

Diagnoses from survey in order of frequency:

1 Irregular pulse 44%
2 Slow pulse 12%
3 Graves' disease 12%
4 Aortic stenosis 9%
5 Complete heart block 9%
6 Brachial artery aneurysm 9%
7 Impalpable radial pulses due to low output cardiac failure 9%
8 Tachycardia 6%
9 Takayasu's disease 3%
10 Hypothyroidism 3%
11 Fallot's tetralogy with a Blalock shunt 3%

Examination *routine*

As you approach the patient from the right and ask for his permission to examine him you should
1 look at his **face** for a *malar flush* (mitral stenosis, myxoedema) or for any signs of *hyper-*

or *hypothyroidism*. As you take the arm to examine the right radial pulse, continue the *survey* of the patient by looking at

2   the **neck** (Corrigan's pulse, raised JVP, thyroidectomy scar, goitre) and then the *chest* (thoracotomy scar). Quickly run your eyes down the body to complete the *survey* (ascites, clubbing, pretibial myxoedema, ankle oedema, etc.) and then concentrate on

3   the **pulse** and note

4   its **rate** (count for at least 15 seconds) and

5   its **rhythm**. A common diagnostic problem is presented by *slow atrial fibrillation* which may be mistaken for a regular pulse. To avoid this concentrate on the *length of the pause* from one beat to another and see if each pause is equal to the succeeding one (see also p. 174). This method will reveal that the pauses are variable from beat to beat in controlled slow atrial fibrillation.

6   Assess whether the **character** (wave-form) of the pulse (information to be gained from radial, brachial and carotid) is normal, *collapsing, slow rising*, or jerky. To determine whether there is a collapsing quality put the palmar aspect of the four fingers of your left hand on the patient's wrist just below where you can easily feel the radial pulse. Press gently with your palm, lift the patient's hand above his head and then place your right palm over the patient's axillary artery. If the pulse has a *waterhammer* character you will experience a flick (a sharp and tall up-stroke and an abrupt down-stroke) which will *run* across all four fingers and at the same time you may also feel a flick of the axillary artery against your right palm. The pulse does not merely become palpable when the hand is lifted but its character changes and it imparts a sharp knock. This is classical of the pulse that is present in haemodynamically significant aortic incompetence and in patent ductus arteriosus. If the pulse has a collapsing character but is not of a frank waterhammer type then the flick runs across only two or three fingers (moderate degree of aortic incompetence or patent ductus arteriosus, thyrotoxicosis, fever, pregnancy, moderately severe mitral incompetence, anaemia, atherosclerosis). A *slow rising* pulse can best be assessed by palpating the brachial pulse with your left thumb and, as you press *gently*, you may feel the anacrotic notch (you will need practice to appreciate this) on the up-stroke against the pulp of your thumb. In mixed aortic valve disease the combination of plateau and collapsing effects can produce a bisferiens pulse. Whilst feeling the brachial pulse look for any catheterization *scars* (indicating valvular or ischaemic heart disease).

7   Proceed to feel the **carotid** where either a slow rising or a collapsing pulse can be confirmed.

8   Feel the **opposite radial pulse** and determine if both radials are the same (e.g. Fallot's with a Blalock shunt—p. 258), and then feel

9   the **right femoral pulse** checking for any *radio-femoral delay* (coarctation of the aorta). If you are asked to examine the pulses (as opposed to the pulse) you should continue to examine

10   all the other **peripheral pulses**. It is unlikely that the examiner will allow you to continue beyond what he thinks is a reasonable time to spot the diagnosis that he has in mind. However, should he not interrupt continue to look for

11   **additional diagnostic clues.** Thus, in a patient with atrial fibrillation and features suggestive of thyrotoxicosis you should examine the thyroid and/or eyes. In a patient with atrial fibrillation and hemiplegia or atrial fibrillation and a mitral valvotomy scar, proceed to examine the heart.

For *checklist* see p. 359.

14 / 'Examine this patient's visual fields'

Frequency of instruction:

6% of candidates in our survey were asked to do this

Variation of instruction:

See p. 366.

Diagnoses from survey in order of frequency:

1   Homonymous hemianopia 25%
2   Optic atrophy 21%
3   Bitemporal hemianopia 21%
4   Unilateral hemianopia 7%
5   Partial field defect in one eye due to retinal artery branch occlusion 7%
6   Bilateral homonymous quadrantic field defect 4%
7   Acromegaly 4%

Examination *routine*

Ask the patient to sit upright on the side of the bed while you position yourself in visual confrontation about a metre away. This apposition will help you to test the visual fields of his left and right eyes against those of your right and left respectively. As he is doing this perform

1   a *visual survey* (acromegaly, hemiparesis, cerebellar signs in multiple sclerosis) of the patient. Ask him to cover his right eye with his right index finger, and close your left eye:
    'Keep looking at my eye'.
2   Examine his **peripheral visual fields.** Test his left temporal vision against your right temporal by moving your wagging finger from the periphery towards the centre:
    'Tell me when you see my finger move'*.
Indicate to the examiner whether or not the patient's field matches your own each time the patient reports. The temporal field should be tested in the horizontal plane and by moving your finger through the upper and lower temporal quadrants. Change hands and repeat on the nasal side. By comparing his visual field with your own, any areas of field defect are thus mapped out. The visual fields of his right eye are similarly tested.
3   A **central scotoma** is tested for with a red-headed hat pin. If you have already found a field defect which does not require further examination, or if the examiner does not wish you to continue, he will soon stop you. Otherwise comparing your right eye with his left, as before, move the red-headed pin from the temporal periphery through the central field to the nasal periphery, asking the patient:
    'Can you see the head of the pin? What colour is it? Tell me if it disappears or changes colour.'

---

*This will pick up most gross visual field defects rapidly. Moving objects are more easily detected and therefore your moving finger will be immediately noticed by the patient as it moves out of the blind area into his field of vision. Remember that his area of blindness to a stationary object may be greater than that to a moving object.

If there is no scotoma find his blind spot and compare it with your own.

Having found the field defect, look for

4 **additional features** (e.g. acromegaly, hemiparesis, nystagmus and cerebellar signs) if appropriate. Recall the possible causes for each type of field defect as this question, at the end of the case, is almost inevitable (see p. 124).

For *checklist* see p. 360.

15 / 'Examine this patient's skin'

Frequency of instruction:

5% of candidates in our survey were asked to do this

Variations of instruction:

Look at this skin
Examine the skin
Look at this skin lesion

Diagnoses from survey in order of frequency:

1   Psoriasis 15%
2   Vitiligo 10%
3   Systemic sclerosis/CRST 10%
4   Radiation burn on the chest 10%
5   Epidermolysis bullosa dystrophica 10%
6   Purpura 5%
7   Pseudoxanthoma elasticum 5%
8   Localized scleroderma 5%

Examination *routine*

This instruction is a rather more specific variation of the 'spot diagnosis' *routine*. You should
1   perform a *visual survey* of the patient, from scalp to sole, with a particular regard to the fact that most dermatological lesions have a predilection for certain areas. It is as well to remember some of the regional associations as you *survey* the patient:

Scalp   Psoriasis (look especially at the hairline for redness, scaling, etc.), alopecia,*
            ringworm (very uncommon).

---

*Some causes of alopecia:
(a) Diffuse—male pattern baldness, cytotoxic drugs, hypothyroidism, hyperthyroidism, iron deficiency.

(b) Patchy—alopecia areata, ringworm; with scarring—discoid lupus erythematosus, lichen planus.

Face	Systemic sclerosis (tight shiny skin, pseudorhagades, beaked nose, telangiectasis), discoid lupus erythematosus (raised, red, scaly lesions with telangiectasis and altered pigmentation), xanthelasma, dermatomyositis (heliotrope colour to eyelids), Sturge–Weber, rodent ulcer (usually below the eye or on the side of the nose, raised lesion with central ulcer, the edges being rolled and having telangiectatic blood vessels).
Mouth	Osler–Weber–Rendu, Peutz–Jeghers, lichen planus (white lace-like network on mucosal surface), pemphigus, candidiasis (white exudate inside the mouth usually associated with a disease requiring multiple antimicrobial therapy, or an immunosuppressive disorder, e.g. leukaemia etc.), herpes simplex, Behçet's.
Neck	Pseudoxanthoma elasticum, tuberculous adenitis with sinus formation (?ethnic origin).
Trunk	Radiotherapy stigmata, morphoea, neurofibromatosis, dermatitis herpetiformis (itching blisters over scapulae, buttocks, elbows, knees), herpes zoster along the intercostal nerves, pityriasis rosea, Addison's (areolar and scar pigmentation), pemphigus (trunk and limbs).
Axillae	Vitiligo, acanthosis nigricans (pigmentation and rugosity of axillary skin, perianal, areolar and lateral abdominal skin, 'tripe palms', mucous membranes involved, maybe underlying malignancy).
Elbows	Psoriasis (extensor), pseudoxanthoma elasticum (flexor), xanthomata (extensor), rheumatoid nodules (extensor), atopic dermatitis (flexor), olecranon bursitis, gouty tophi.
Hands	Systemic sclerosis (sclerodactyly, infarcts of finger pulps, prominent capillaries at nail folds), lichen planus (wrists), dermatomyositis (linear psoriasiform lesions on the dorsum of the fingers/hands, nail fold capillary dilatation and infarction), Addison's (skin crease pigmentation), granuloma annulare, erythema multiforme (polymorphic eruption, mucous membrane involvement, macules, vesicles, bullae, etc.), scabies (not in MRCP clinical!).
Nails	Psoriasis (pitting, onycholysis), iron deficiency (koilonychia), fungal dystrophy, tuberous sclerosis.
Genitalia	Behçet's (iridocyclitis, uveitis, pyodermes, ulcers, etc.), lichen sclerosis, candidiasis.
Legs	Leg ulcer (diabetic, venous, ischaemic, pyoderma gangrenosum), necrobiosis lipoidica diabeticorum, pretibial myxoedema, erythema nodosum, Henoch–Schönlein purpura, tendon xanthomata in Achilles, erythema ab igne, pemphigoid (legs and arms), lipoatrophy.
Feet	Pustular psoriasis, eczema, verrucae, keratoderma blenorrhagica (?eyes, joints, etc.).

During this *survey* you should consider

2   the **distribution** of the lesions (psoriasis on extensor areas, lichen planus in flexural areas, candidiasis in mucous membranes, tuberous sclerosis on nails and face, necrobiosis lipoidica diabeticorum usually bilateral, gouty tophi in the joints of hands, elbows and on the ears, etc.). Then after the *survey* (which should take a few seconds)

3   examine the **lesions** (see 'Examine this patient's rash') looking in particular for the *characteristic* features, e.g. scaling in psoriasis, shiny purple polygonal papules with

Wickham's striae in lichen planus, etc. If you have made a diagnosis consider whether you need to look for any

4 **associated lesions** (arthropathy and nail changes with psoriasis, evidence of associated autoimmune disease with vitiligo, etc.). Go through the skin conditions which our survey has suggested occur in the exam (see also Appendix 6) and make sure that you would recognize each, would know what else to look for, and what to say in your presentation.

For *checklist* see p. 360.

16 / 'Examine this patient's gait'

Frequency of instruction:

4% of candidates in our survey were asked to do this

Variations of instruction:

Look at this patient's gait
Watch this patient walk
Watch this patient walk. What do you think the diagnosis is?

Diagnoses from survey in order of frequency:

1 Ataxia 45%
2 Spastic paraparesis 20%
3 Parkinson's disease 10%
4 Charcot–Marie–Tooth disease 5%
5 Ankylosing spondylitis 5%

Examination *routine*

As you approach the patient perform

1 a *quick* **visual survey** noting any *cerebellar signs* (nystagmus, intention tremor) or obvious signs of conditions such as *Parkinson's* disease (facies, tremor), *Charcot–Marie–Tooth* disease (peroneal wasting, pes cavus, etc.) or *ankylosing spondylitis*. Introduce yourself to the patient and ask him

2 **whether he can walk** without help (*cerebellar dysarthria* heard during his reply may be a useful clue). If he reports difficulty reassure him that you will stay with him in case of any problems.

3 **Ask him to walk** to a defined point and back whilst you look for any of the classical abnormal gaits (see p. 170), particularly ataxic (cerebellar or sensory), spastic, steppage (Charcot–Marie–Tooth) or Parkinsonian (?pill-rolling tremor). As the patient walks make sure you note specifically

4 the **arm swing** (Parkinson's) and

5   any *clumsiness* on **the turns** (ataxia, Parkinson's). Next test
6   **heel to toe** gait (demonstrate as you ask the patient to do this) which will *exacerbate* ataxia (note the side to which the patient tends to fall). Ask the patient to walk
7   **on his toes** (S1) and then
8   **on his heels** (L5; foot drop—lateral popliteal nerve palsy, Charcot–Marie–Tooth disease). If he has a spastic gait or a hemiparesis he may find both these tests difficult to perform.
9   Now ask him to stand with his *feet together, arms out* in front; when you are satisfied with the degree of steadiness with the eyes open, ask him to *close* his *eyes* (you should be standing nearby to catch him if he shows a tendency to fall). **Romberg's test** is only positive (*sensory ataxia*) if the patient is more unsteady with the eyes closed than with them open (dorsal column disease, e.g. subacute combined degeneration, tabes dorsalis, etc.).
10   If you suspect sensory ataxia a further test is to ask the patient to **close his eyes while walking** (he will become *more* ataxic). Again you should be ready to catch the patient should he fall. As always be ready to look for
11   **additional features** of the conditions on the list if appropriate (see individual short cases, and consider what you would do with each).

For *checklist* see p. 360.

17 / 'Examine this patient's rash'

Frequency of instruction:

4% of candidates in our survey were asked to do this

Variations of instruction:

Examine the skin rash.

Diagnoses from survey in order of frequency:

1   Psoriasis 20%
2   Purpura 10%
3   Vasculitis 10%
4   Neurofibromatosis 10%
5   Juvenile chronic arthritis (Still's disease) 10%
6   Xanthomata 5%
7   Necrobiosis lipoidica diabeticorum 5%
8   Radiation burn on the chest 5%

Examination *routine*

This *routine* is generally the same as that discussed under 'Examine this patient's skin'.
1   You should quickly conduct a ***visual survey*** as described under 'skin' and note if there are any similar or related lesions elsewhere. Look at the

2 **distribution** of the lesions, whether confined to a single area (morphoea, erythema nodosum, rodent ulcer, melanoma, alopecia areata, etc.) or present in other areas such as psoriasis, neurofibromatosis, acanthosis nigricans, dermatomyositis, etc. While concentrating on the lesion in question, it is important to look at the

3 **surrounding skin** for any helpful clues such as *scratch marks* as evidence of itching,* *radiotherapy field markings* on the skin in the vicinity of a radiation burn, or *paper-thin skin* with purpura (corticosteroid therapy), etc. You should now

4 **examine the lesion** in detail. To determine the *extent* of the lesion you may have to ask the patient to undress, a procedure which will provide you with a little more time to survey other areas. Decide if the rash is *pleomorphic* or *monomorphic* (all the lesions are similar). If so examine one typical lesion carefully in terms of:

(a) *Colour*, e.g. erythematous or pigmented

(b) *Size*

(c) *Shape*, e.g. oval, circular, annular, etc.

(d) *Surface*, e.g. scaling or eroded

(e) *Character*, e.g. macule, papule, vesicle, pustule, ulcer, etc.

It is advisable to be familiar with the correct use of the terms to describe rashes (especially if you do not recognize the lesion!). To say 'skin lesion' or 'skin rash' conveys no diagnostic meaning. In your presentation you should be able to describe the lesion with respect to the above five features, especially if you do not know the diagnosis. The following are some of the useful terms employed in describing skin lesions:

Macules = Flat, circumscribed lesions, not raised above the skin—size and shape varies

Papules = Raised, circumscribed, firm lesions up to 1 cm in size

Nodules = Like papules but larger; usually lie deeper in skin

Tumours = Larger than nodules, elevated or very deeply placed in the skin

Wheals = Circumscribed elevations associated with itching and tingling

Vesicles = Small well-defined collections of fluid

Bullae = Large vesicles

Pustules = Circumscribed elevations containing purulent fluid which may, in some cases, be sterile (e.g. Behçet's)

Scales = Dead tissue from the horny layer which may be dry (e.g. psoriasis) or greasy (e.g. seborrhoeic dermatitis)

Crusts = These consist of dried exudate

Ulcers = Excavations in the skin of irregular shape; remember that every ulcer has a shape, an edge, a floor, a base and a secretion, and it forms a scar on healing

Scars = The result of healing of a damaged dermis.

5 Finally, if indicated, look for **additional features** (arthropathy in psoriasis or Still's disease, Cushingoid facies if purpura is due to steroids, clubbing with radiation burns on the chest, etc.).

For *checklist* see p. 360.

---

*Some causes of itching:
(a) Dermatological—scabies, dermatitis herpetiformis, lichen planus, eczema.

(b) Medical—cholestasis, chronic renal failure, lymphoma, polycythaemia rubra vera.

18 / 'Examine this patient's legs and arms'

Frequency of instruction:

3% of candidates in our survey were asked to do this

Variations of instruction:

Examine the limbs neurologically—motor function only

Diagnoses from survey in order of frequency:

1. Motor neurone disease 29%
2. Cervical myelopathy 14%
3. Syringomyelia 14%
4. Friedreich's ataxia 14%
5. Parkinson's disease 7%

Examination *routine*

As appropriate from 'Examine this patient's arms' (p. 39) and 'Examine this patient's legs' (p. 25).

19 / 'Examine this patient's cranial nerves'

Frequency of instruction:

3% of candidates in our survey were asked to do this

Variations of instruction:

Look at this patient's cranial nerves

Diagnoses from survey:

Bulbar palsy
Cerebello-pontine angle syndrome
Myasthenia gravis
Ocular palsy and dysarthria
Unilateral VIth, VIIth nerve palsies and nystagmus and possibly a XIIth nerve palsy*
Unilateral IXth, Xth, XIth and XIIth nerve lesions (suggesting jugular foramen syndrome†)

*The candidate diagnosed a XIIth nerve palsy and passed   †This diagnosis was not made by the candidate.
(experience 1, p. 327) but see footnote, p. 56.

Examination *routine*

Perhaps surprisingly this instruction was comparatively rare in our survey. It is one of the most feared instructions but at the same time it can provide an opportunity to score highly. More than in any other system, the well rehearsed candidate can appear competent and professional compared to the unrehearsed. Detailed examination of the individual nerves is not usually required but rather a quick and efficient screen like that used by neurologists at the bedside or in out-patients (it is well worth attending neurology out-patients to watch quick and efficient examination techniques, if for nothing else). Not only can you look good but also the abnormalities are usually easy to detect. Although it is to be hoped that your practised *routine* will not miss out any nerves, it is preferable to perform a smooth, professional examination, which accidentally misses out a nerve, than to test your examiner's patience through a hesitant and meditative examination which takes a long time to start and may never finish! Since the examination is most easily carried out face to face with the patient it is best, if possible, to get him to sit on the edge of the bed facing you. First

1 take a good general and *quick* **look** at the patient; in particular his face, for any obvious abnormality. Next ask him about

2 his sense of **smell** and **taste**:

'Do you have any difficulty with your sense of smell?' (I). Although you should have the ability to formally examine taste and smell if equipment is provided, usually questioning (or possibly the judicious use of a bedside orange) is all that is required. All the examination referable to the eyes is best performed next. Unless there is a Snellen's chart available ask the patient to look at the clock on the wall or some newspaper print to give you a good idea of his

3 **visual acuity:**

'Do you have any difficulty with your vision?'

'Can you see the clock on the wall?' (if he has glasses for long sight he should put them on).

'Can you tell me what time it says?' (II)

A portable Snellen's chart will enable you to perform a more formal test (see Appendix 5). Now test

4 **visual fields** (see p. 48), including for *central scotoma*, with a red-headed hat pin. Follow this by examining

5 **eye movements:**

'Look at my finger; follow it with your eyes' (III, IV, VI),

asking the patient at the extremes of gaze whether he sees one or two fingers. If he has diplopia establish the extent and ask him to describe the 'false' image. As you test eye movements note at the same time any

6 **nystagmus** (VIII, cerebellum or cerebellar connections—see Fig. 3.48, p. 157) or

7 **ptosis** (III, sympathetic).

Remember that either extreme abduction of the eyes or gazing at a finger that is too near can cause nystagmus in normal eyes (optikokinetic). Now examine

8 the **pupils** for the direct and consensual *light reflex* (II—optic tract—lateral geniculate ganglion—Edinger–Westphal nucleus of III—fibres to ciliary muscle) and for the *accommodation–convergence* reflex (cortex—III) with your finger just in front of his nose:

'Look into the distance'.

'Now look at my finger'.

Finally examine the optic discs (II) by

9 **fundoscopy** (this can be left until last if you prefer). Having finished examining the eyes examine

10 **facial movements:**
     'Raise your eyebrows'.
     'Screw your eyes up tight'.
     'Puff your cheeks out'.   } VII
     'Whistle'.
     'Show me your teeth'.
     'Clench your teeth'—feel masseters and temporalis
     'Open your mouth; stop me closing it' } motor V

11 then **palatal movement:**
     'Keep your mouth open; say aah' (IX, X).

12 and **gag reflex**—touch the back of the pharynx on both sides with an orange stick (IX, X). Look at

13 the **tongue** as it lies in the floor of the mouth for *wasting* or *fasciculation* (XII):
     'Open your mouth again'
then get the patient to:
     'Put your tongue out'—note any deviation*—'waggle it from side to side' (XII).

14 Test the **accessory nerve**:
     'Shrug your shoulders; keep them shrugged'—push down on the shoulders (XI).
     'Turn your head to the left side—now to the right'—feel for the sternomastoid muscle on the side opposite to the turned head.

Finally test

15 **hearing:**
     'Any problem with the hearing in either ear?'
     'Can you hear that?'—rub finger and thumb together in front of each ear in turn (VIII—

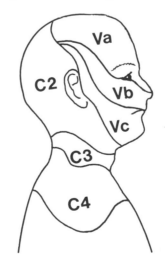

Fig. 2.4. Dermatomes in the head and neck.

*In unilateral facial paralysis the protruded tongue, though otherwise normal, may deviate so that unilateral hypoglossal paralysis is suspected (see p. 184). In unilateral lower motor neurone XIIth nerve palsy there is wasting (?fasciculation) on the side of the lesion and the tongue curves to that side.

proceed to the Rinné and Weber tests* if there is any abnormality, and look in the ears if you suspect disease of the external ear, perforated drum, wax, etc.)

16   and test **facial sensation** including *corneal reflex* (sensory V—Fig. 2.4).

For *checklist* see p. 360.

20 / 'Examine this patient's thyroid status'

Frequency of instruction:

2% of candidates in our survey were asked to do this

Variations of instruction:

Assess thyroid status clinically
Examine this patient's neck; do you think she is euthyroid?
Do you think this lady is thyrotoxic now just looking at her?

Diagnoses from survey in order of frequency:

1   Euthyroid Graves' disease 42%
2   Hyperthyroidism 17%
3   Euthyroid simple goitre 8%

Examination *routine*

Although the patient usually has signs of thyroid disease (exophthalmos, goitre), you are not being asked to examine these, but rather to assess whether the patient is clinically hypo-, eu- or hyperthyroid. Perform a speedy

1   *visual survey* looking specifically for *signs* of *thyroid disease* (exophthalmos, goitre, thyroid acropachy, pretibial myxoedema—all can occur in association with *any* thyroid status), and ask yourself if the facies are in any way myxoedematous. Observe the patient's

2   **composure**, whether *hyperactive, fidgety* and *restless* (hyperthyroid); normal, composed demeanour (euthyroid); or if she is somewhat *immobile* and *uninterested* in the people around her (hypothyroid).

3   Take the **pulse** and *count* it for 15 seconds, noting the presence or absence of *atrial fibrillation* (slow, normal rate, or fast). If the pulse is slow (less than 60), or if you suspect hypothyroidism, proceed immediately to test

---

*Weber test: sound from a vibrating tuning fork held on the centre of the forehead is conducted towards the ear if it has a conductive defect (e.g. wax or otitis media) and away from the ear if it has a nerve deafness.

Rinné test: a positive test (normal) is when the sound of the tuning fork is louder by air conduction (prongs by external auditory meatus) than by bone conduction (base of fork on mastoid process). Negative is abnormal.

4   for **slow relaxation** of the ankle,* supinator or other jerks. To test the reflexes you will require the patient's cooperation and the ensuing conversation may provide you with helpful clues (slow hesitant speech, slow movements, etc.). Otherwise

5   feel the **palms**, whether *warm* and *sweaty* or cold and sweaty (anxiety) and then

6   ask the patient to stretch out his hands to full extension of the wrist and elbow. If the **tremor** is not obvious, place your palm against his outstretched fingers to feel for it. Alternatively, you can place a piece of paper on the dorsum of his outstretched hands—it will oscillate if a fine tremor is present.

7   Look at the **eyes**, noting exophthalmos (sclera visible above the lower lid—a sign not related to thyroid status) but looking specifically for *lid retraction* (sclera visible above the cornea). Test for lid lag (lid lag and retraction may diminish as the hyperthyroid patient becomes euthyroid).

8   Examine the **thyroid** as described under 'Examine this patient's neck', remembering the steps are (i) look, (ii) palpate, (iii) auscultate.†

Putting the above findings together it should be possible to provide a definite conclusion about thyroid status; this is considered a very basic skill and it will not be taken lightly if, in your state of nerves, you make fundamental errors. Though the examiner may put you under pressure to test your confidence, keep calm and be particularly wary of being led to diagnose hypo- or hyperthyroidism in the presence of a normal pulse rate (see experience 72, p. 340).

9   Be prepared with the **standard questions** for assessment of thyroid status (temperature preference, weight change, appetite, bowel habits, palpitations, change of temper, etc.—see pp. 108 and 138) should the examiner wish you to question the patient. Indeed, if there is any doubt about the thyroid status after the above examination, offer to ask the patient these questions.

For *checklist* see p. 360.

*The slow relaxing ankle jerk in hypothyroidism is best demonstrated with the patient kneeling on a chair or bed with the feet hanging over the edge, and the examiner standing behind the patient. However this manoeuvre is not necessary unless the jerk cannot be elicited by the usual procedure.

†A thyroid bruit is good evidence of thyroid overactivity; if present it can be heard over the isthmus and lateral lobe of the thyroid; it will not be obliterated by occluding the internal jugular vein (venous hum) or by rotation of the head and it will not be influenced by pressure of the stethoscope (use light pressure to avoid causing non-thyroid bruits).

Section 3
150 Short Case *Records*

*'Be professional in presentation. I agree it's an easy exam—it's easy to fail.'**

* p. 349.

In this section we present *aides-memoire* (clinical descriptions for presentation to the examiner) for 150 short cases. We have called these aides-memoire *records*. The order has been determined by the frequency with which, according to our survey, these short cases have appeared in the examination. Thus Short Case No. 1 occurred most commonly, followed by Short Case No. 2 and so on. The percentages given represent your chance of meeting a particular short case in any one attempt at the MRCP short cases examination. They range from diabetic retinopathy (34%) to pyoderma gangrenosum (0.1%) which means that on average you will see a diabetic fundus in one out of every three attempts at the examination, but you may have to go through a thousand attempts before you meet pyoderma gangrenosum! Sometimes in the survey a particular short case was an additional feature of another short case. For example, a case of Graves' disease could also have a goitre, exophthalmos or pretibial myxoedema. With each short case we pinpointed what was the main focus of that case. In the previous example, if the examiner asked for examination of the eyes, and all the attention was on the eyes, the main focus would be exophthalmos. If additional features (e.g. in this case goitre and pretibial myxoedema) were present, these were counted separately and the percentages for them are also given.* It cannot be overstressed that the first short cases we have dealt with occurred very commonly and the last very rarely, with all grades in between. The implications for your priorities are obvious.

The style of each *record* imagines you to be in the examination situation with the patient displaying the typical features of a particular condition; you are 'churning out' these to the examiner along with the answers to various anticipated questions. Thus, you play the *record* of the condition to the examiner. Of course the cases in the actual examination will only have some of the features (the *record* tends to describe the 'full house' case) and it is hoped that by becoming familiar with the whole *record* you will be well equipped:

1 To pick up all the features present in the cases you meet on the day by scanning through the *records* in your mind and

2 To adapt the *record* for the purpose of presenting those features which are present.

To facilitate quick revision, the main points of each short case are highlighted in italics. The small print is a mixed bag of additional features and facts, lists of differential diagnoses and answers to some of the questions that might be asked.† With the lists of differential diagnoses we have tended to put the most important ones (which you should consider first) in large print with longer lists in the small print. The lists are not necessarily meant to be comprehensive. Next to the diagnoses on these lists we have used brackets to give some of

---

* We believe that candidates did not always mention all the additional features in their reports to us. As an extreme example, not every candidate who reported meeting a case of mitral stenosis mentioned whether or not the pulse was irregular. Thus our appraisal of when 'irregular pulse' was an additional feature is likely to be an underestimate of its real frequency. Similarly ptosis was not always mentioned as being present in cases of Horner's syndrome or in association with a IIIrd nerve palsy. Consequently we believe that these 'additional features' figures tend to be underestimates.

† As already mentioned, questions and discussion of cases are only a very minor feature of the short cases examination. Obviously the questions that could be asked are legion and a comprehensive coverage is beyond the scope of this book. However, where our survey did point to the possibility of certain questions we have included the answers in the small print.

the features of the conditions concerned, or perhaps one or two features you could look for (indicated by ?). The ? is put there as a cue for you to look for important diagnostic features. We make no apology for repeating some of the features often, in the hope that by constant reinforcement they will become more firmly embedded in your memory. When unilateral signs could affect either side we have not usually specified the side in the *record* but have indicated this by R/L. In these cases, however, each R/L in the *record* refers to the same side. Also . . . is occasionally used for a sign in the lung fields or retina which could occur in any zone or to indicate the size of an organ or sign where the size is unspecified.

Presentation to the examiner

Becoming familiar with the short case *records* will arm you for the examination, though obviously it will not always be necessary, or desirable, for you to use them. Sometimes it may be appropriate just to give the diagnosis—even so it may still be possible to enrich it with some of the well-known features from the *record*. If the examiner's question is: *'What is the diagnosis?'* you could answer 'mitral stenosis' and await his reaction. On the other hand, if you are certain of your diagnosis, it would be better to say: 'The diagnosis is mitral stenosis because there is a rough, rumbling mid-diastolic murmur localized to the apex of the heart, there is a sharp opening snap and a loud first heart sound, a tapping impulse, an impalpable left ventricular apex, a left parasternal heave and a small volume pulse. Furthermore, the chaotic rhythm suggests atrial fibrillation and the patient has a malar flush.'

If you enlarge your response to 'What is the diagnosis?' by giving the features in this way, it is best to give the evidence in order of its importance to the diagnosis (as shown in the example). However, if the question is: *'What are your findings?'* it is best to give them in the order they are elicited: 'The patient has a malar flush and is slightly breathless at rest. The pulse is irregular in rate and volume. The jugular venous pressure is not elevated and the cardiac apex is not palpable but there is a tapping impulse parasternally on the left side and there is a left parasternal heave. The first heart sound is loud and there is an opening snap followed closely by a mid-diastolic rumble which is localized to the apex. These signs suggest that the patient has mitral stenosis.'

Remember, if you are talking in front of the patient, to avoid using words like 'cancer' and 'multiple sclerosis'. Use euphemisms such as 'neoplastic disease' and 'demyelinating disease'.

Remember that you can influence any discussion that follows by what you say. For example, the words: 'The diagnosis is aortic incompetence' may produce an interrogation by the examiner, or you may just be moved on to the next case. However, if you say: 'He has aortic incompetence for which there are several causes', this invites the examiner to ask you the causes. It is, therefore, a good answer—as long as you know them!

1 / Diabetic retinopathy

Frequency in survey: 34% of attempts at MRCP short cases.

Survey note: This is the commonest short case; it is also one of the easiest to fail. Some candidates who saw haemorrhages failed to note whether there were also microaneurysms. The uninitiated failed to recognize photocoagulation scars. The commonest forms reported in the survey were background diabetic retinopathy (40%) and proliferative retinopathy treated with photocoagulation (40%). Most of the rest were fundi with untreated proliferative retinopathy. Advanced diabetic eye disease was only rarely reported.

Record 1

There are *microaneurysms*, *blot haemorrhages*, and *hard exudates* (due to lipid deposition in the retina). The lesions are most numerous in the macular area, especially just temporal to it.

The patient has background diabetic retinopathy.

Record 2

The above plus: there are *soft exudates* (cotton wool spots) and *flame-shaped haemorrhages* (both indicating ischaemia), *circinate rings* of *hard exudates* (indicating oedema), and leashes of *new vessels* (say where). *Photocoagulation scars* are seen (say where).

The patient has proliferative diabetic retinopathy treated by photocoagulation.

Record 3

Any of the above plus: *vitreous haemorrhage/vitreous scar/retinal detachment* (widespread and impairing vision) indicate advanced diabetic eye disease.

NB With diabetic retinopathy there may also be:
(i) Cataracts (p. 232);
(ii) a-v nipping (indicating either coexistent hypertension or arteriosclerosis).

Indications for photocoagulation are the sight-threatening forms of retinopathy:
(i) *Maculopathy* (primarily type 2 = non-insulin-dependent diabetes): Warning signs are hard exudates often in rings (indicating oedema) encroaching on the macula, sometimes with multiple haemorrhages (indicating ischaemia). Macular oedema itself is difficult to recognize though signs of an abnormal greyish reflection or discolouration at the macula are suggestive. Even slight visual deterioration is highly significant if there is any suspicion of maculopathy.

(ii) *Preproliferative and proliferative retinopathy* (commonly type 1 = insulin-dependent diabetes): Preproliferative lesions suggesting that neovascularization is imminent are:

  Multiple cotton wool spots
  Multiple large blot haemorrhages
  Venous beading
  Venous loops
  Arterial sheathing
  Atrophic looking retina

For colour photographs see pp. 371–2.

Fig. 3.1. (*opposite*) (a) Background retinopathy (note microaneurysms, blot haemorrhages and punctate hard exudates). (b) More extensive background changes and soft exudate two-and-a-half disc diameters inferior to the disc. (c) A circinate above the macula with a soft exudate in its centre. (d) A circinate with the macula at its centre (maculopathy). (e) Two circinates near the macula (maculopathy now or imminent). (f) Photocoagulation scars in the superior temporal region.

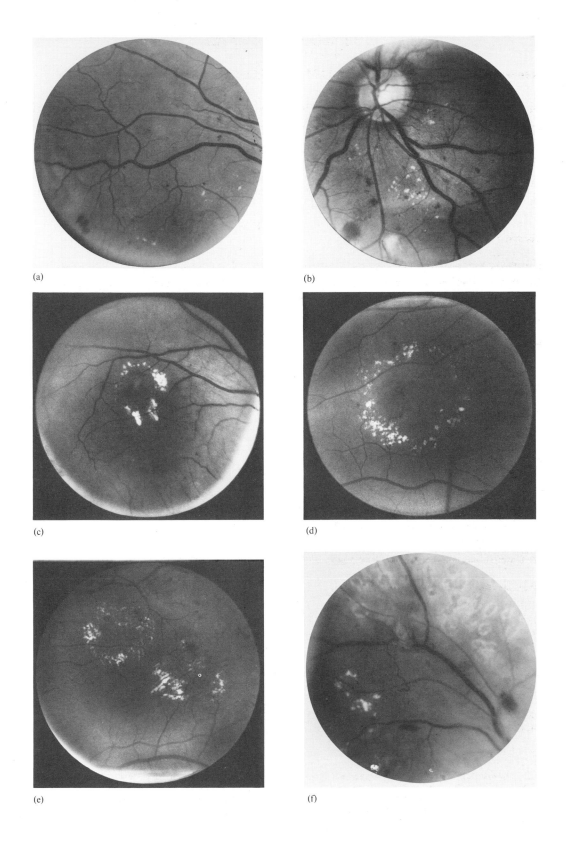

(a)

(b)

(c)

(d)

(e)

(f)

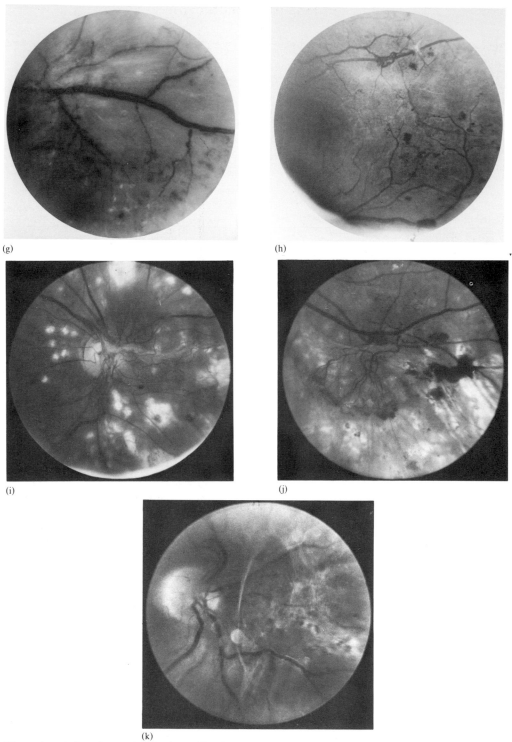

(g)

(h)

(i)

(j)

(k)

(g) Venous irregularity and venous beading (preproliferative signs). (h) Venous reduplication is seen in the upper part of this picture (a preproliferative sign). (i) Leashes of new vessels with a leash of fibrous tissue (healing following haemorrhage of some of the new vessels into the vitreous) projecting into the vitreous and photocoagulation scars in the background (same patient as front cover). (j) Leashes of peripheral new vessels which are haemorrhaging. Photocoagulation scars in the background (same patient as (i)). (k) Advanced diabetic eye disease (note vitreous scar).

2 / Hepatosplenomegaly

Frequency in survey: Main focus of a short case in 24% of attempts at MRCP short cases. Additional feature in a further 8%.

Record

There is hepatosplenomegaly, the *spleen* is enlarged . . . cm below the left costal margin. The *liver* is palpable at . . . cm below the right costal margin; it is non-tender, firm and smooth (now look for clinical *anaemia*, *lymphadenopathy* and signs of *chronic liver disease*).
   Likely causes to be considered are:

No other signs or clinical anaemia only
1   Myeloproliferative disorders. (p. 74)
2   Lymphoproliferative disorders. (p. 74)
3   Cirrhosis of the liver with portal hypertension (less likely if there are no other signs of chronic liver disease).

Hepatosplenomegaly plus palpable lymph nodes*
1   Chronic lymphatic leukaemia.
2   Lymphoma such as Hodgkin's disease.
Other conditions to be considered would include infectious mononucleosis (?throat), infective hepatitis (?icterus) and sarcoidosis.

Signs of chronic liver disease
Cirrhosis of the liver with portal hypertension (p. 78).

Other causes of hepatosplenomegaly

Hepatitis B† (?icterus, tattoo marks)
Brucellosis ('examine this farmer's abdomen')
Weil's disease (?icterus, sewerage worker or fell into canal)
Toxoplasmosis (glandular fever-like illness)
Cytomegalovirus infection (glandular fever-like illness)
Pernicious anaemia and other megaloblastic anaemias (NB SACD—p. 273. NB Associated organ-specific autoimmune disease—p. 254)
Storage disorders (e.g. Gaucher's—spleen is often huge; glycogen storage disease)

Amyloidosis (?underlying chronic disease)‡
Other causes of portal hypertension (e.g. Budd–Chiari syndrome = hepatic vein thrombosis—see pp. 78 and 176)
Infantile polycystic disease (in some variants of this, children have relatively mild renal involvement but hepatosplenomegaly and portal hypertension)

Common causes on a world-wide basis

Malaria
Kala-azar
Schistosomiasis

---

*These conditions can also occur without palpable lymph nodes.
† NB Australia antigen heads the list of investigations of icterus of uncertain cause.
‡Though hepatosplenomegaly can occur in primary and myeloma associated amyloidosis, it is commoner in the secondary form. Other organs particularly involved in secondary amyloidosis are kidneys (nephrotic syndrome), adrenals (clinical adrenocortical failure may occur) and alimentary tract (rectal biopsy). Conditions associated with secondary amyloidosis include rheumatoid arthritis (including juvenile type), tuberculosis, leprosy, chronic sepsis, Crohn's disease, ulcerative colitis, ankylosing spondylitis, paraplegia (bedsores and urinary infection), malignant lymphoma and carcinoma. See also footnote on p. 126.

3 / Mitral stenosis (lone)

Frequency in survey: 20% of attempts at MRCP short cases.

Record

There is a *malar flush* and a *left thoracotomy scar*. The pulse is *irregularly irregular* (give rate) in rate and volume (if sinus rhythm the volume is usually small). The venous pressure is not raised, and there is no ankle or sacral oedema (unless in cardiac failure). The cardiac impulse is *tapping* (palpable first heart sound) and the apex is not displaced. There is a *left parasternal heave*. The *first heart sound* is *loud*, there is a loud pulmonary second sound and an *opening snap* followed by a *mid-diastolic rumbling murmur* (with *presystolic accentuation* if the patient is in sinus rhythm) *localized* to the apex and heard most loudly with the patient in the *left lateral* position.*

The diagnosis is mitral stenosis. The patient has had a valvotomy in the past.

Other signs which may be present

Giant *v* waves (tricuspid incompetence—usually secondary; may be primary—see p. 201)

Graham–Steell murmur—rare (secondary pulmonary incompetence; a high-pitched, brief, early diastolic whiff in the presence of marked signs of pulmonary hypertension and a pulse which is not collapsing)

The opening snap soon after the second sound† in tight mitral stenosis (<0.09 seconds—mean left atrial pressure above 20 mmHg); longer after the second sound in mild mitral stenosis (>0.1 seconds—mean left atrial pressure below 15 mmHg); absent if the mitral valve is calcified (first heart sound soft).

For colour photograph see p. 373.

Indications for surgery

Significant symptoms which limit normal activity

An episode of pulmonary oedema without a precipitating cause

Recurrent emboli

Pulmonary oedema in pregnancy (emergency valvotomy)

Deterioration due to atrial fibrillation which does not respond to medical treatment

Criteria for closed valvotomy

Mobile valve (loud first heart sound, opening snap, absence of calcium on X-ray screening and thin mobile cusps on echocardiography)

Absence of mitral incompetence

---

*If unsure about the presence of the murmur, it can be accentuated by exercise—get the patient to touch her toes and then recline ten times.

†The interval from the second sound to the opening snap varies with heart rate. If the interval is ≤0.07 seconds with the heart rate <100, the mitral stenosis is usually of haemodynamic significance.

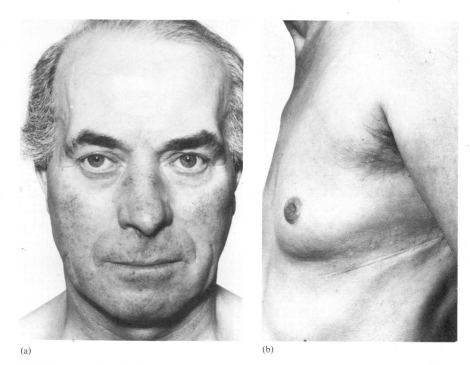

(a)   (b)

Fig. 3.3. (a) Mitral facies. (b) Thoracotomy scar for mitral valvotomy.

4 / Rheumatoid hands

Frequency in survey: Main focus of a short case in 17% of attempts at MRCP short cases. Additional feature in a further 7%.

Record

There is a *symmetrical deforming arthropathy*. There is *spindling* of the fingers due to soft tissue swelling at the *proximal interphalangeal* joints and *metacarpophalangeal joints*. There is generalized *wasting* of the *small muscles* of the hand and use is restricted by weakness, deformity and pain. There are *nodules* at the elbow, over the extensor tendons, and in the palm. There is *ulnar deviation* of the fingers (consequent upon subluxation and dislocation at the metacarpophalangeal joints). The *terminal interphalangeal joints* are *spared*. There are arteritic lesions* in the nail folds.

The patient has rheumatoid arthritis.

Males: Females = 1:3

Other features which may occur

'Swan-neck' deformity (*hyperextension of proximal interphalangeal* joint with fixed flexion of metacarpophalangeal and terminal interphalangeal joints)

Boutonnière deformity (flexion deformity of proximal interphalangeal joint with *extension contracture of terminal interphalangeal* and metacarpophalangeal joints)

Z deformity of the thumb

Triggering of the finger (flexor tendon nodule)

Palmar erythema

Iatrogenic Cushing's (?facies, thin atrophic skin, purpura)

Swollen or deformed knees (p. 264)

Cervical spine disease (upper cervical spine, especially atlanto-axial joint—subluxation can occur with *spinal cord compression*; a lateral X-ray centred on the odontoid peg with the neck in full flexion, shows the distance from the odontoid to the anterior arch of the atlas as abnormal at more than 3 mm—general anaesthesia is dangerous and requires extreme care in neck handling)

Anaemia (five causes†)

Chest signs (?pleural effusions; fibrosing alveolitis‡)

Neurological signs (?peripheral neuropathy, mononeuritis multiplex, carpal tunnel syndrome)

Eye signs (episcleritis, scleromalacia perforans, cataracts due to chloroquine or steroids)

Sjögren's syndrome (?dry eyes, dry mouth)

Felty's syndrome (?spleen—p. 317)

Leg ulceration (vasculitic)*

Cardiac signs (pericarditis is present in up to 40% of patients at autopsy but is rarely apparent clinically; myocarditis, conduction defects and valvular incompetence are rare consequences of granulomatous infiltration)

Secondary amyloidosis (?proteinuria, hepatosplenomegaly, etc.—see footnote to p. 65)

Other autoimmune disorders (see pp. 138, 246, 254)

For colour photographs see pp. 378–9.

---

* As well as causing nail fold infarcts and chronic leg ulceration, the vasculitis (p. 226) which is immune complex-induced and may affect small, medium or large vessels, may also lead to digital gangrene. A purpuric rash may occur due to capillaritis. Raynaud's phenomenon (p. 300) may occur. Pyoderma gangrenosum (p. 314) is a rare cause of ulceration.

† Five causes of anaemia in rheumatoid arthritis are:
1 Anaemia of chronic disease (normochromic normocytic)
2 Gastrointestinal bleeding related to nonsteroidal anti-inflammatory agents
3 Bone marrow suppression (gold, phenylbutazone, indomethacin, penicillamine)
4 Megaloblastic anaemia (folic acid deficiency or associated pernicious anaemia)
5 Felty's syndrome (p. 317)

‡ The lungs may also be affected in other ways. Rheumatoid nodules may occur in the lung fields on chest X-ray and in patients exposed to certain dusts—especially coal miners—nodules may be accompanied by massive fibrotic reactions (Caplan's syndrome). Obliterative bronchiolitis is a recently recognized severe but rare complication which may be associated with penicillamine therapy.

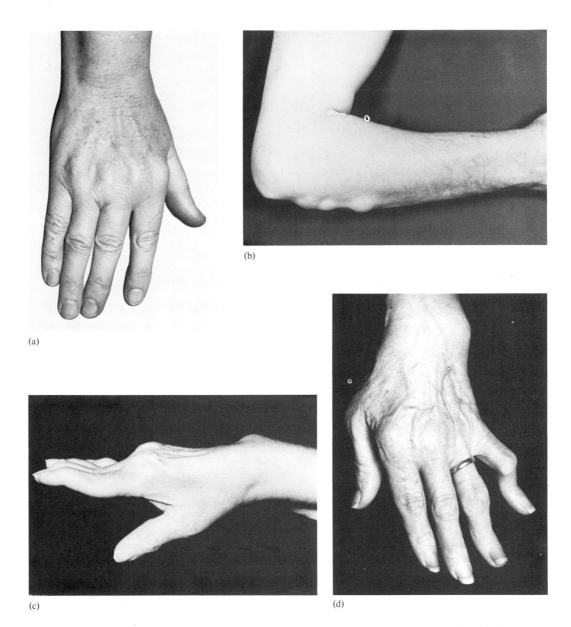

(a)

(b)

(c)

(d)

Fig. 3.4. (a) Early changes—swelling of the metacarpophalangeal joints, slight ulnar deviation. (b) Rheumatoid nodules. (c) 'Swan-neck' deformity. (d) Boutonnière deformity.

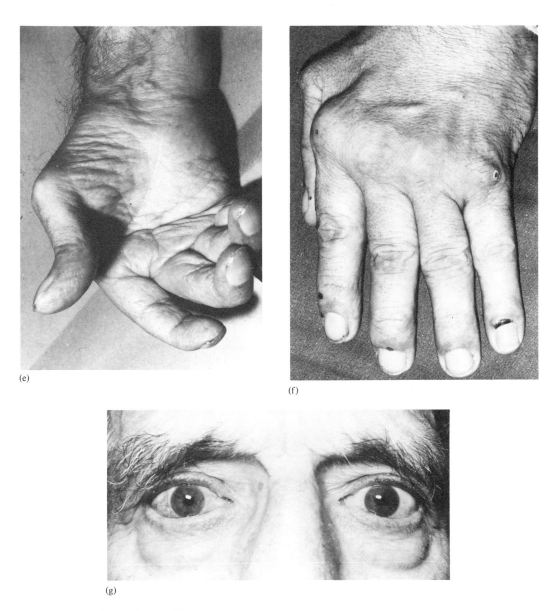

(e)

(f)

(g)

Fig. 3.4 (*continued*) (e) Z-shaped thumb. (f) Vasculitis. (g) Episcleritis.

5 / Mixed mitral valve disease

Frequency in survey: 16% of attempts at MRCP short cases.

Record 1

There is a *malar flush* and a *left thoracotomy scar*. The pulse is irregularly irregular (give rate) in rate and volume and the venous pressure is not raised. The cardiac impulse is *tapping* and the apex beat is *not displaced*. There is a *left parasternal heave*. On auscultation there is a *loud* first heart sound, a *pansystolic murmur** radiating to the axilla, a loud pulmonary second sound, and an *opening snap* followed by a *mid-diastolic rumbling murmur* localized to the apex.

The patient has mixed mitral valve disease. In view of the tapping cardiac impulse, the loud first heart sound and the undisplaced apex, I think this is predominant mitral stenosis.

Record 2

There is a left thoracotomy scar. The pulse is irregularly irregular (give rate) in rate and volume and the venous pressure is not raised. The apex beat is *thrusting* and *displaced* to the sixth intercostal space in the anterior axillary line and there is a *left parasternal heave*. On auscultation the first heart sound is *soft* and there is a loud *pansystolic murmur* at the left sternal edge and/or apex radiating to the axilla. There is a loud pulmonary second sound and with the patient in the left lateral position I could hear a *mid-diastolic rumbling murmur* following an opening snap.†

The patient has mixed mitral valve disease. In view of the soft first heart sound and displaced and vigorous apex beat, I think this is predominant mitral incompetence.

If it is not clear clinically which lesion is predominant (e.g. loud first heart sound but enlarged left ventricle) and the examiners wish your opinion, point out the factors in favour of each (Table 3.5) then come down in favour of the one you think most likely, but point out that in this case cardiac catheter studies would be required to be certain, e.g. 'It is difficult in this case. The loud first heart sound would suggest predominant mitral stenosis; however the enlarged left ventricle suggests mitral incompetence as the more important lesion. I think cardiac catheter studies would be required to resolve the issue.'

Table 3.5 The factors pointing to a predominant lesion in mixed mitral valve disease

	Mitral stenosis	Mitral incompetence
Pulse	Small volume	Sharp and abbreviated
Apex	Not displaced; tapping impulse present	Displaced, thrusting
First heart sound	Loud	Soft
Third heart sound	Absent	Present

*In the patient with severe pulmonary hypertension when a very large right ventricle displaces the left ventricle posteriorly, the murmur of tricuspid incompetence (p. 201) can mimic that of mitral incompetence. The murmur of tricuspid incompetence is ordinarily heard best at the lower left sternal border, increases with inspiration and is not heard in the axilla or over the spine posteriorly. In tricuspid incompetence giant *v* waves will be present.

†In severe mitral incompetence without mitral stenosis a mid-diastolic flow murmur may be heard without an opening snap. The presence of a third heart sound is incompatible with any significant degree of mitral stenosis.

6 / Dullness at the lung base

Frequency in survey: Main focus of a short case in 14% of attempts at MRCP short cases. Additional feature in a further 4%.

Record

The pulse is regular and the venous pressure is not elevated. The trachea is central,* the expansion is normal, but the percussion note is *stony dull* at the R/L base(s), with *diminished* tactile *fremitus* and vocal *resonance*, and *diminished breath sounds*. There is (may be) an area of bronchial breathing above the area of dullness.

The diagnosis is R/L pleural effusion.

Causes of pleural effusion

Exudate (protein content > 30g l⁻¹)

Bronchial carcinoma (?nicotine staining, clubbing, radiation burns on chest, lymph nodes).
Secondary malignancy (?evidence of primary especially breast, lymph nodes, radiation burns).
Pulmonary embolus and infarction (?DVT; bloodstained fluid will be found at aspiration).
Pneumonia (bronchial breathing/crepitations, fever, etc.).
Tuberculosis.
Rheumatoid arthritis (?hands and nodules).
Systemic lupus erythematosus (?typical rash).
Lymphoma (?nodes and spleen).
Mesothelioma (asbestos worker, ?clubbing).

Transudate (protein content < 30 g l⁻¹)

Cardiac failure (?JVP ↑, ankle and sacral oedema, large heart, tachycardia, *S3* or signs of a valvular lesion).
Nephrotic syndrome (?generalized oedema, patient may be young—p. 275).
Cirrhosis (?ascites, generalized oedema, signs of chronic liver disease—p. 78).

Other causes of pleural effusion

Meigs' syndrome (ovarian fibroma)
Subphrenic abscess (?recent abdominal disease or surgery)
Peritoneal dialysis
Hypothyroidism (?facies, pulse, ankle jerks)
Pancreatitis (more common on the left; fluid has high amylase)
Dressler's syndrome (recent myocardial infarction, ?pericardial friction rub)
Trauma
Asbestos exposure
Yellow nail syndrome (yellow beaked nails usually associated with lymphatic hypoplasia)

Chylothorax (trauma or blockage of a major intra-thoracic lymphatic—usually by a neoplastic process)

Other causes of dullness at a lung base

Raised hemidiaphragm (e.g. hepatomegaly)
Basal collapse
Collapse/consolidation (if the airway is blocked by, for example, a carcinoma there may be no bronchial breathing)
Pleural thickening (e.g. old tuberculosis or old empyema)

*The trachea may be deviated if the effusion is very large. A large effusion without any mediastinal shift (clinically and on chest X-ray) raises the possibility of collapse as well as effusion.

7 / Splenomegaly (without hepatomegaly)

Frequency in survey: Main focus of a short case in 14% of attempts at MRCP short cases. Additional feature in a further 2%.

Record

The spleen is palpable at . . . cm.

or

There is a *mass* in the *left hypochondrium*. On palpation I *cannot get above* the mass, it has a *notch*, and on inspiration moves diagonally across the abdomen. The *percussion note* is *dull* over the left lower lateral chest wall and over the mass.

I think this is the spleen enlarged at . . . cm. Likely causes* to be considered are:

Very large spleen†
1 Chronic myeloid leukaemia (Philadelphia chromosome positive in 90%).
2 Myelofibrosis.
and in other parts of the world.
3 Chronic malaria.
4 Kala-azar.

Spleen enlarged 4–8 cm (2–4 finger breadths)
1 Myeloproliferative disorders‡ (e.g. chronic myeloid leukaemia and myelofibrosis).
2 Lymphoproliferative disorders§ (e.g. lymphoma and chronic lymphatic leukaemia).
3 Cirrhosis of the liver with portal hypertension (spider naevi, icterus, etc.—p. 78).

Spleen just tipped or enlarged 2–4 cm (1–2 finger breadths)
1 Myeloproliferative disorders.‡
2 Lymphoproliferative disorders§ (?palpable lymph nodes).
3 Cirrhosis of the liver with portal hypertension.
4 Infections such as:
>   Glandular fever (?throat, lymph nodes)
>   Infectious hepatitis (?icterus)
>   Subacute bacterial endocarditis (?heart murmur, splinter haemorrhages, etc.).

---

*To help you remember some common causes to mention in the examination we have given the three or four most common causes of a spleen of a particular size. An alternative way of dividing up splenomegaly which can be found in many text books is:
1 Infectious and inflammatory splenomegaly (e.g. SBE, infectious mononucleosis, sarcoidosis)
2 Infiltrative splenomegaly
>   Benign (e.g. Gaucher's, amyloidosis)
>   Neoplastic (e.g. leukaemias, lymphoma)
3 Congestive splenomegaly (e.g. cirrhosis, hepatic vein thrombosis)
4 Splenomegaly due to reticuloendothelial hyperplasia (e.g. haemolytic anaemias, immune thrombocytopenias)
†*Gaucher's* disease and *rapidly progressive lymphoma* (especially reticulosarcoma) may also cause a huge spleen. *Chronic congestive splenomegaly* (Banti's syndrome = splenomegaly, pancytopenia, portal hypertension and gastrointestinal bleeding) may also cause massive splenomegaly. A huge spleen

developing in a patient with *polycythaemia rubra vera* is usually due to the development of myelofibrosis.
‡When listing the causes of splenomegaly or hepatosplenomegaly in the limited time of the examination, to use the term 'myeloproliferative disorders' in its broadest interpretation is a useful way of covering several conditions in one phrase. If asked to explain it (unlikely), one strict definition covers a group of related disorders of haemopoietic stem cell proliferation: chronic myeloid leukaemia (CML), myelofibrosis, polycythaemia rubra vera and essential thrombocythaemia. The term can be used more broadly to cover acute myeloid leukaemia as well. A small spleen is more likely to be due to acute leukaemia than CML or myelofibrosis because splenic enlargement in the latter conditions is often already marked at the time of presentation.
§The lymphoproliferative disorders are chronic lymphatic leukaemia, lymphoma, myelomatosis, Waldenstrom's macroglobulinaemia and acute lymphatic leukaemia.

Other causes of splenomegaly

Polycythaemia rubra vera (?plethoric, middle-aged man)

Brucellosis ('examine this farmer's abdomen')

Sarcoidosis (?erythema nodosum or history of, lupus pernio, chest signs)

Haemolytic anaemia (?icterus)

Pernicious anaemia and other megaloblastic anaemias (?pallor; NB SACD—p. 273; NB Associated organspecific autoimmune diseases, especially autoimmune thyroid disease, diabetes, Addison's, vitiligo, hypoparathyroidism—see p. 254)

Idiopathic thrombocytopenic purpura (?young female, purpura)

Felty's syndrome (?hands, nodules)

Amyloidosis (?underlying chronic disease, other organ involvement—see p. 65)

Systemic lupus erythematosus (?typical rash)

Lipid storage disease (spleen may be enormous—e.g. Gaucher's)

Myelomatosis

Chronic iron deficiency anaemia

Thyrotoxicosis

Other infections (subacute septicaemia, typhoid, disseminated tuberculosis, trypanosomiasis, echinococcosis)

Other causes of congestive splenomegaly* (hepatic vein thrombosis, portal vein obstruction, schistosomiasis, congestive heart failure)

8 / Optic atrophy

Frequency in survey: Main focus of a short case in 14% of attempts at MRCP short cases. Additional feature in a further 4%.

Record

The disc is *pale* and *clearly delineated* and (in the severe case) the *pupil reacts consensually* to light but *not directly.** Field testing with the head of a pin (maybe) reveals a *central scotoma*.

The diagnosis is optic atrophy. The well-defined disc edge suggests that it is not secondary to papilloedema† (yellow/grey disc with blurred margins). Common causes of primary optic atrophy are:

1 Multiple sclerosis (may be temporal pallor only; ?nystagmus, scanning speech, cerebellar ataxia. etc.—p. 316).
2 Compression of the optic nerve by:
      Tumour (e.g. pituitary—?bitemporal hemianopia)
      Aneurysm.
3 Glaucoma (?pathological cupping).

Other causes

Ischaemic optic neuropathy (abrupt onset of visual loss in an elderly patient; may be painful; thrombosis or embolus of posterior ciliary artery; temporal arteritis is sometimes the cause)
Leber's optic atrophy (males:females = 6:1)
Retinal artery occlusion (p. 252)
Toxic amblyopia (lead, methyl alcohol, arsenic, insecticides, quinine)

Nutritional amblyopia (famine etc., tobacco-alcohol amblyopia, vitamin B_{12} deficiency, diabetes mellitus‡)
Freidreich's ataxia (?cerebellar signs, pes cavus, scoliosis, etc.—p. 220)
Tabes dorsalis (?Argyll Robertson pupils, etc.—p. 281)
Paget's disease (?large skull, bowed tibia, etc.—p. 82)
Consecutive optic atrophy†

For colour photograph see p. 372.

---

* In early unilateral optic neuritis before the direct reflex is lost, it may simply become more sluggish than the consensual reflex. In this situation it may be possible to demonstrate the *Marcus Gunn* phenomenon. In this the direct reflex may at first appear to be brisk. However, when the light is alternated from one side to the other, the pupil on the affected side may be seen to dilate slowly when exposed to the light. The mechanism is as follows: When the light shines in the healthy eye a rapid constriction occurs in both eyes. As the light then moves to the affected eye, this fails to transmit the message to continue constriction as quickly as normal. As a result the pupils have time to recover and dilate, despite the light shining on the abnormal eye.

†Optic atrophy can be divided into primary, secondary and consecutive. Consecutive optic atrophy follows damage to the parent ganglion cells of the retina as in widespread choroidoretinitis, retinitis pigmentosa, and retinal artery occlusion.

‡Optic atrophy in diabetes mellitus may also occur in the DIDMOAD syndrome—with diabetes insipidus, diabetes mellitus, and deafness. It is a rare, recessively inherited disorder.

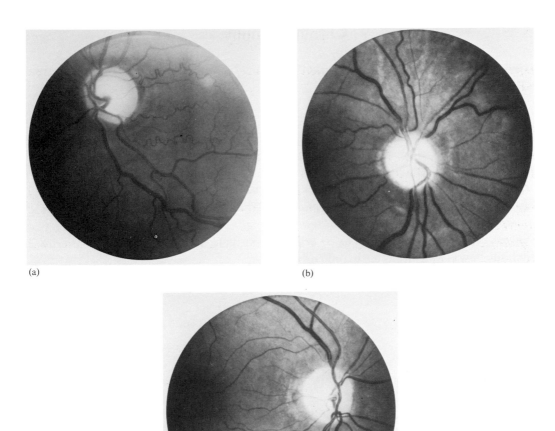

(a)

(b)

(c)

Fig. 3.8. (a), (b), (c) Optic atrophy.

9 / Chronic liver disease

Frequency in survey: Main focus of a short case in 13% of attempts at MRCP short cases. Additional feature in a further 3%.

Record

The patient is *icteric, pigmented* and *cyanosed* (due to pulmonary venous shunts). He has *clubbing, leuconychia, palmar erythema, Dupuytren's contracture** and there are several *spider naevi.* He has a flapping tremor of the hands (suggesting some portosystemic encephalopathy). There are scratch marks on the forearms and back, and there is purpura. There is *gynaecomastia, scanty body hair* and his *testes* are *small.* There is 5 cm *hepatomegaly* and 3 cm *splenomegaly.* He has *ascites* and *ankle oedema,* and there are *distended abdominal veins* in which the flow is away from the umbilicus.

The diagnosis is likely to be cirrhosis of the liver with portal hypertension.

Possible causes

1   Alcohol.
2   Viral hepatitis—B (male; HBsAg positive)
                —Non-A Non-B.
3   Lupoid hepatitis (pubertal or menopausal female, steroid responsive; associated with diabetes, inflammatory bowel disease, thyroiditis and pulmonary infiltrates; ?smooth muscle antibodies).
4   Primary biliary cirrhosis (middle-aged female, scratch marks, xanthelasma; ?antimitochondrial antibody—p. 208).
5   Haemochromatosis (male, slate-grey pigmentation—p. 233).
6   Cryptogenic.

Other causes

Cardiac failure (?JVP ↑, *v* waves, *S3* or a valvular lesion, tender pulsatile liver if tricuspid incompetence)

Constrictive pericarditis† (JVP raised, abrupt *x* and *y* descent, loud early *S3* ['pericardial knock'—a valuable sign but only present in <40% of cases] though heart sounds often normal, slight 'paradoxical pulse', *no signs in lung fields,* chest X-ray may show calcified pericardium, rare but important cause of ascites as reponse to treatment may be dramatic)

Budd–Chiari syndrome (in the acute phase ascites develops rapidly with pain, there are no cutaneous signs of chronic liver disease and the liver is smoothly enlarged and tender; if the inferior vena cava is involved there is no hepatojugular reflux)

Biliary cholestasis (bile obstruction with or without infection)

Toxins and drugs (methotrexate, methyldopa, isoniazid, carbon tetrachloride)

Wilson's disease (?Kayser–Fleischer rings, tremor, rigidity, dysarthria)

Alpha$_1$ antitrypsin deficiency (?lower zone emphysema)

Other metabolic causes (galactosaemia, tyrosinaemia, type IV glycogenosis)

---

*Nineteen signs which may be present in the hands of the patient with chronic liver disease are clubbing, Dupuytren's contracture, palmar erythema, spider naevi, flapping tremor, leuconychia, scratch marks, icterus, pallor, pigmentation, cyanosis, xanthomata, purpura, koilonychia, paronychia, abscesses, oedema, muscle wasting, tattoos (?Australia-antigenaemia).

†The spleen may be palpable. In the absence of evidence of *bacterial endocarditis* or *tricuspid valve disease,* the presence of splenomegaly in a patient with congestive heart failure should arouse suspicion of *constrictive pericarditis* or *pericardial effusion with tamponade.*

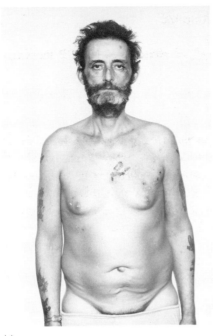

(a)

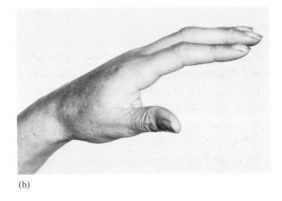

(b)

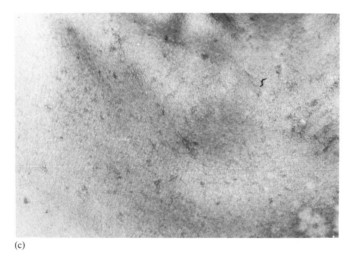

(c)

Fig. 3.9. (a) Note from above downwards: spider naevi, herpes zoster (debilitated patient), gynaecomastia, tattoo marks, everted umbilicus, swelling of the flanks, abdominal wall veins and paucity of hair. (b) Clubbing of the fingers and leuconychia (same patient as (a)). (c) Spider naevi (close up).

10 / Polycystic kidneys

Frequency in survey: Main focus of a short case in 12% of attempts at MRCP short cases. Additional feature in a further 2%.

Record

There are *bilateral masses* in the *flanks* which are *bimanually ballotable*. I can *get above* them and the percussion note is *resonant* over them.* I suspect, therefore, that they are renal masses and a likely diagnosis is polycystic kidneys (*?uraemic facies*; the *blood pressure* may be raised). The *arterio-venous fistula/shunt* on his arm indicates that the patient is being treated with haemodialysis (about 5% develop renal failure).

Other causes of bilateral renal enlargement include:
1   Bilateral hydronephrosis.
2   Amyloidosis (?underlying chronic disease, hepatosplenomegaly, etc.—see p. 65).

Polycystic disease of the liver in adults may cause a nodular liver enlargement (liver function may be normal despite massive hepatomegaly). About 50% have renal involvement. Cystic liver is a major feature of infantile polycystic disease (autosomal recessive) but a minor feature of adult polycystic kidney disease (autosomal dominant).

Other features of adult polycystic kidney disease

Cysts may also occur in other organs—most important are sacular aneurysms of the cerebral arteries (10%) which, in combination with the hypertension, leads to serious risk of intracranial haemorrhage (cause of death in 10% of cases according to some authorities)

It may present with flank pains, bleeding, urinary tract infection, nephrolithiasis or obstructive uropathy

---

*Look for abdominal scars from previous peritoneal dialysis or cyst aspiration. The latter is performed to relieve obstruction of the outflow tract by the cyst, intractable pain or haematuria.

11 / Paget's disease

Frequency in survey: Main focus of a short case in 12% of attempts at MRCP short cases. Additional feature in a further 1%.

Survey note: Candidates were often asked follow-up questions on investigation, complications, treatment, etc.—NB experience 61, p. 338.

Record

There is (in this elderly patient) *enlargement* of the *skull*. There is also *bowing* of the R/L *tibia* (or femur) which is *warmer* (due to increased vascularity) than the other and the patient is (may be) *kyphotic* (vertebral involvement leads to *loss of height* and kyphosis from disc degeneration and vertebral collapse).

The diagnosis is Paget's disease. (There may be evidence of complications, e.g. a *hearing aid*—see below.)

Paget's disease occurs in 3% (autopsy series) of the population over the age of 40, rising to 10% over the age of 70, though it is not clinically important in the vast majority of these. Though it is often asymptomatic, patients may have symptoms such as bone pain, headaches, tinnitus and vertigo. Serum *alkaline phosphatase* and *urinary hydroxyproline* are elevated except sometimes in very early disease. Serum calcium and phosphate concentrations are usually normal in mobilized patients but may be increased or decreased. Urinary calcium and hydroxyproline rise in immobilized patients. High serum uric acid and erythrocyte sedimentation rate may also occur. Specific therapies which can be considered if indicated* include calcitonin, diphosphonates and mithramycin.

Complications

Progressive closure of skull foramina may lead to:
  Deafness (also results from Pagetic involvement of the ossicles†)
  Optic atrophy‡
  Basilar invagination (platybasia causing brainstem signs)

Other complications include:
  High output cardiac failure (?bounding pulse—occurs when more than 30–40% of the skeleton is involved)
  Pathological fractures
  Urolithiasis
  Sarcoma (incidence is probably <1%; increase in pain and swelling may occur; 'explosive rise' in alkaline phosphatase occurs only occasionally)

Causes of 'bowed tibia'

True bowing due to soft bone:
  Paget's disease
  Rickets
Apparent bowing due to thickening of the anterior surface of the tibia secondary to periostitis:
  Congenital syphilis (?saddle nose, bulldog jaw, rhagades, Hutchinson's teeth, Moon's molars, etc.—p. 282)
  Yaws

---

*Indications for specific therapy in Paget's disease are: bone pain; osteolytic lesions in weight-bearing bones; neurological complications (except deafness); delayed or non-union of fractures; immobilization hypercalcaemia; before and after orthopaedic surgery.
†Although hearing loss is frequently attributed to compression

of the eighth cranial nerve in the canal in the temporal bone, this is unlikely to be the major cause because the facial nerve, which follows the same course, is rarely affected.
‡The other ophthalmological finding which may occur in Paget's disease is angioid streaks in the retina.

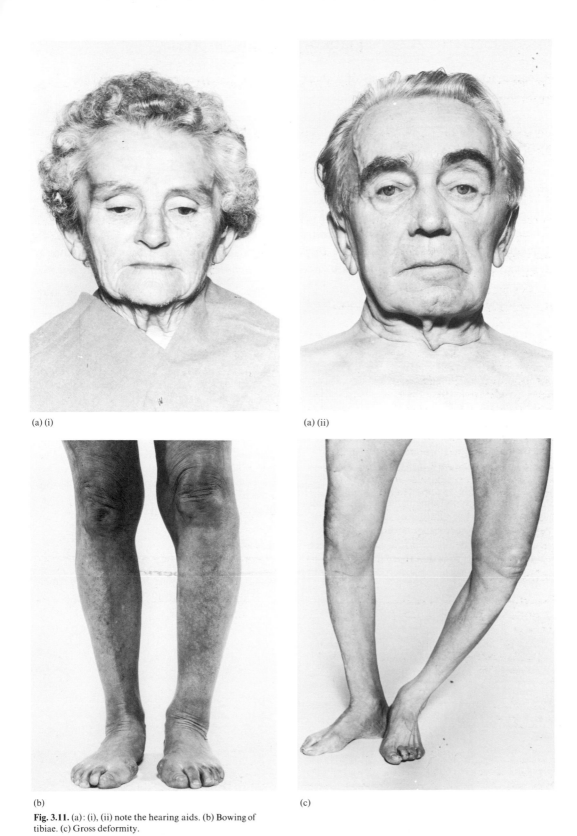

(a) (i)

(a) (ii)

(b)

(c)

Fig. 3.11. (a): (i), (ii) note the hearing aids. (b) Bowing of tibiae. (c) Gross deformity.

12 / Psoriatic arthropathy/psoriasis

Frequency in survey: Main focus of a short case in 11% of attempts at MRCP short cases. Additional feature in a further 1%.

Survey note: Patients had arthropathy and/or skin lesions. Questions such as treatment only occasionally asked.

Record

There is an *asymmetrical arthropathy* involving mainly the *terminal interphalangeal joints*. There is *pitting* of the finger nails and *onycholysis*. Some of the nail plates (say which) are thickened and there is a thick scale (*hyperkeratosis*) under them. There are patches of psoriasis at the *elbows*. The plaques are circular with well-defined edges and they are *red* with a *silvery scaly* surface.

   The patient has psoriatic arthropathy.

Psoriatic arthropathy (even if severe) can occur with minimal skin involvement. If there is no obvious psoriasis at the elbows the following areas should particularly be checked for skin lesions:
   The extensor aspects
   The scalp
   Behind the ears
   In the navel

Other forms of psoriatic arthropathy

Arthritis mutilans
Arthritis clinically indistinguishable from rheuma-
   toid arthritis but consistently seronegative
Asymmetrical oligo- or mono-arthropathy
Ankylosing spondylitis occurring alone or in con-
   junction with any of the other forms

Treatment

Treatments of the skin lesions include sunlight, u.v. light, coal tar, dithranol, local steroids, PUVA (psoralen and u.v. light). Systemic treatment with corticosteroids, ceromatic retinoid ($\pm$PUVA) or antimetabolites (methotrexate, hydroxyurea, razo-zane) are not often used. Analgesic anti-inflamma-tory agents are used for the pain of the arthropathy. Gold and penicillamine are not particularly effec-tive. Choroquine is contraindicated as it may exacerbate the skin lesions (exfoliative dermatitis). Intra-articular steroids are useful for a single inflamed troublesome joint.

Incidence

1–5% of Caucasians in north-western Europe and USA. Uncommon among Japanese, North Ameri-can Indians and American Negroes.

For colour photograph see p. 373.

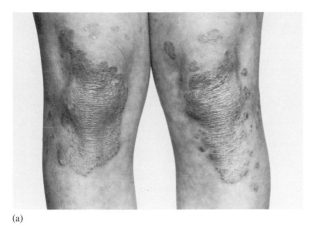

(a)

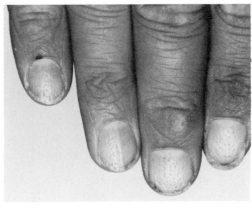

(b)

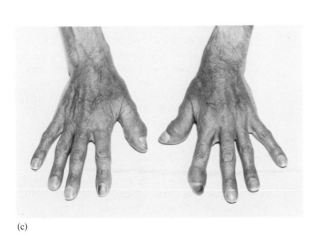

(c)

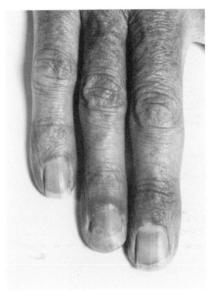

(d)

Fig. 3.12. (a) Typical plaques. (b) Nail pitting. (c) Terminal interphalangeal arthropathy and nail changes. (d) Onycholysis.

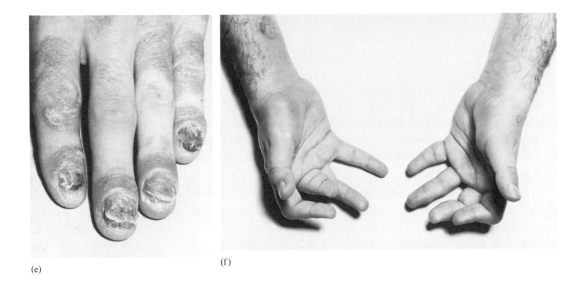

(e)

(f)

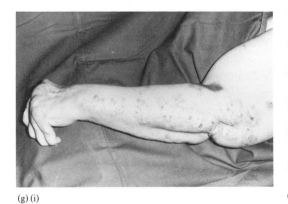

(g) (i)

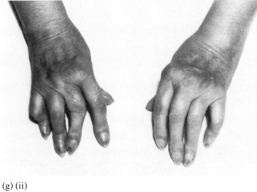

(g) (ii)

Fig. 3.12 (*continued*) (e) Advanced nail changes (note the psoriatic plaques and hyperkeratosis of the nail beds). (f) Note the typical plaque on the forearm and telescopic middle finger.

(g): (i), (ii) indistinguishable from rheumatoid arthritis. Note plaques in (i) and nails in (ii).

13 / Other combinations of mitral and aortic valve disease

Frequency in survey: 11% of attempts at MRCP short cases.

Survey note: Patients with any combination of aortic and mitral valve disease may be found in the examination (including, very rarely, lesions of one valve in combination with a prosthetic valve—see p. 214). Whenever you are examining the heart it is essential that, having found some obvious murmurs, you go in search of the others which may be present and less obvious, before presenting your findings (see experience 64, p. 339, and anecdote 20, p. 343).

If the examiner seeks an opinion as to which are the main lesions, or if you feel confident to offer, the criteria used are the same as those described under mixed mitral valve disease (p. 72) and mixed aortic valve disease (p. 89). The example here is of a *record* of mixed mitral and aortic valve disease.

Record

There is a left thoracotomy scar, and the patient has a malar flush. The pulse is irregularly irregular (give rate) and *slow rising* in character. The venous pressure is not elevated. The apex is .... (give appropriate word on the basis of what you find; e.g. thrusting, heaving, lifting, etc.) in the anterior axillary line and there is a *left parasternal heave*. There is a *systolic thrill* at the apex, in the aortic area and in the neck. The first heart sound is *loud*, there is a harsh *ejection systolic murmur* in the aortic area radiating into the neck, a *pansystolic murmur* at the lower left sternal edge radiating to the *apex* and to the *axilla*, an *early diastolic murmur* just audible in the aortic area and down the *left sternal edge* with the patient *sitting forward* in *expiration*, and an *opening snap* followed by a *mid-diastolic rumbling murmur* localized to the apex.

The findings suggest mixed aortic and mitral valve disease. The slow rising pulse suggests aortic stenosis is the dominant aortic valve lesion. It is not possible to ascertain clinically which is the major mitral valve lesion.* Cardiac catheterization with left ventricular angiography would be required to assess the haemodynamic significance of each lesion.

---

*In the case of severe mitral stenosis the signs of significant aortic stenosis may be underestimated. A displaced apex in the above setting would tend to suggest that mitral incompetence is haemodynamically dominant.

14 / Mixed aortic valve disease

Frequency in survey: 11% of attempts at MRCP short cases.

Record 1

The pulse is regular (give rate) and *slow rising* (may have a *bisferiens* character). The venous pressure is not raised. The apex beat is palpable 1 cm to the left of the midclavicular line as a *forceful, sustained heave.* There is a *systolic thrill* palpable at the apex, in the aortic area and also in the carotid. There is a *harsh ejection systolic murmur* in the aortic area radiating into the neck, the *aortic component* of the second sound is *soft*, and there is an *early diastolic murmur* down the *left sternal edge* audible when the patient is sitting forward in expiration.

The diagnosis is mixed aortic valve disease. Since the pulse is slow rising rather than collapsing, there is a systolic thrill, the second sound is soft and the apex has a forceful heaving quality, I think this is predominant aortic stenosis. (Systolic blood pressure will be low with a low pulse pressure.)

Record 2

The pulse is regular (give rate), of *large volume* and *collapsing* (may have a *bisferiens* character). The venous pressure is not raised. The apex beat is *thrusting* in the *anterior axillary line* in the sixth intercostal space. There is a harsh *ejection systolic murmur* in the aortic area radiating into the neck and an *early diastolic murmur* down the *left sternal edge* (loudest with the patient sitting forward in expiration).

The diagnosis is mixed aortic valve disease. Since the pulse is collapsing rather than plateau in character and the apex is displaced and thrusting, I think the predominant lesion is aortic incompetence. (Blood pressure will show a wide pulse pressure.)

Often mixed aortic murmurs will be due to either aortic stenosis with incidental aortic incompetence or severe aortic incompetence with a systolic flow murmur.* In such cases commenting on dominance is easy. If it is not clear clinically which lesion is predominant and the examiners wish your opinion, point out the factors in favour of each (Table 3.14), stress that you would like to measure the blood pressure and how this would help and lean towards or, if possible, come down in favour of the one you think most likely, giving the reasons; but point out that in this case cardiac catheter studies with left ventricular angiography would be required to be certain. (see p. 72 for an example of how this might be done in the case of mixed mitral valve disease.)

Table 3.14 The factors pointing to a predominant lesion in mixed aortic valve disease

	Aortic incompetence	Aortic stenosis
Pulse	Mainly collapsing	Mainly slow rising
Apex	Thrusting, displaced	Heaving, not displaced much
Systolic thrill	Absent	Present
Systolic murmur	Not loud, not harsh	Loud, harsh
Blood pressure		
Systolic	High	Low
Pulse pressure	Wide	Narrow

* NB The causes of aortic incompetence in this latter case—see p. 98.

15 / Systemic sclerosis/CRST syndrome

Frequency in survey: Main focus of a short case in 11% of attempts at MRCP short cases. Additional feature in a further 1%.

Record

The *skin* over the *fingers* and *face* (of this middle-aged female) is *smooth, shiny* and *tight*. There is *sclerodactyly*, the *nails* are *atrophic* and there is evidence of *Raynaud's phenomenon* (p. 300). There is atrophy of the soft tissues at the ends of the fingers. There is *telangiectasia* of the face and pigmentation. There are nodules of *calcinosis** palpable in some of the fingers.

The diagnosis is systemic sclerosis or CRST† syndrome.

Other signs which may be present

Skin ulcers

Vitiligo (p. 254)

Dry eyes and dry mouth (Sjögren's syndrome—see p. 207)

Dyspnoea or inspiratory crackles (diffuse interstitial fibrosis‡—decreased pulmonary diffusion capacity is the first sign; overspill pneumonitis may also occur)

Other systems which may be involved

Oesophagus (dysphagia or other oesophageal symptoms are present in 45–60%; oesophageal manometry is abnormal and shows diminished peristalsis in 90%)

Kidney (renal failure occurs in 20%—it is late but often fatal; it may be associated with malignant hypertension which is resistant to therapy)

Heart (pericardial effusion is not an uncommon finding if careful echocardiography is performed; cardiomyopathy may occur but is rare)

Musculoskeletal (inflammatory arthritis or myositis—their presence raises the possibility of mixed connective tissue disease§ and therefore increased likelihood of improvement with steroid therapy)

Intestine (rarely hypomotility with a dilated second part of the duodenum leads to bacterial overgrowth, which in turn leads to steatorrhoea and malabsorption; wide-mouthed colonic diverticuli, and the rare pneumatosis cystoides are other abnormalities which may occur)

Liver (may be associated with primary biliary cirrhosis—p. 208)

For colour photograph see p. 375.

---

* If there is diffuse deposition of calcium in subcutaneous tissue in the presence of acrosclerosis this is termed the Thibierge–Weissenbach syndrome.

† CRST or CREST is the association of Calcinosis, Raynaud's, oesophageal involvement, Sclerodactyly and Telangiectasia. It may be a variant of systemic sclerosis associated with a more benign prognosis.

‡ Pulmonary hypertension may develop independent of parenchymal changes, suggesting primary pulmonary vessel disease which may respond to steroids.

§ Mixed connective tissue disease is a clinical overlap between systemic sclerosis, SLE and polymyositis. The serum has a high titre of antiribonuclear protein antibody. The fluorescent antinuclear antibodies are typically distributed in a speckled pattern.

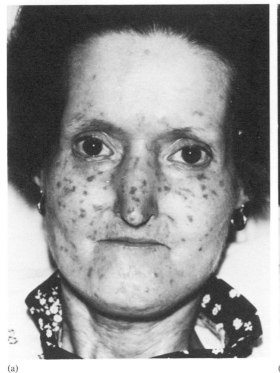

(a)

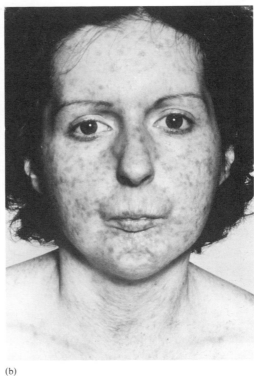

(b)

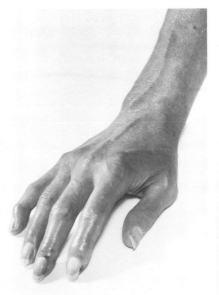

(c)

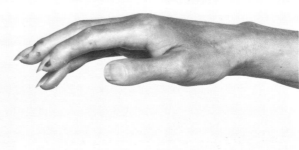

(d)

Fig. 3.15. (a) Note telangiectasia, pinched nose and adherent skin. (b) Perioral tethering with pseudorhagades. (c) Tight, shiny, adherent skin and vasculitis. (d) Atrophy of the finger pulps.

16 / Exophthalmos

Frequency in survey: Main focus of a short case in 11% of attempts at MRCP short cases. Additional feature in a further 8%.

Record 1

There is (may be) bilateral *swelling* of the *medial caruncle* and *vascular congestion of the lateral canthus* with exophthalmos (protrusion of the eye revealing the *sclera above the lower lid* in the position of forward gaze) which is greater on the R/L side. Likely causes include:

1   Hyperthyroid Graves' disease (?lid retraction or lag, tachycardia, bruit over the goitre; exophthalmos usually symmetrical).
2   Euthyroid Graves' disease (?no lid lag, *normal* pulse rate, no sweating or tremor, etc.).
3   Hypothyroid Graves' disease (?facies, scar of thyroidectomy, hoarse voice, slow pulse, ankle jerks, etc.).

Record 2

There is severe exophthalmos, *chemosis, corneal ulceration* and *ophthalmoplegia** which is reducing the upward and lateral gaze most and which is responsible for the *diplopia*. Convergence (check for this) is also impaired. Testing the eye movements caused the patient discomfort (or pain).

The diagnosis is Graves' malignant exophthalmos (patient may be hyper-, eu- or hypothyroid).

Graves' malignant exophthalmos (congestive ophthalmopathy) can cause severe pain and the patient is at risk of blindness due to pressure on the optic nerve, if not treated. The condition may require large doses of systemic steroids and sometimes *tarsorrhaphy* (which may be in evidence in the examination patient) or even orbital decompression may be necessary.

Other causes of exophthalmos

Bilateral (though asymmetrical) with conjunctival oedema:

Cavernous sinus thrombosis (follows infection of the orbit, nose and face; eyeball is painful and there is extreme venous congestion)
Carotico-cavernous fistula (pulsating exophthalmos)

Unilateral:

Retro-orbital tumour (the protrusion measured with the Hertel exophthalmometer is usually > 5 mm more than the unaffected eye by the time of presentation, whereas Graves' eyes rarely achieve a difference of 5 mm†)
Orbital cellulitis

---

*The ophthalmoplegia is due to infiltration, oedema and subsequent fibrosis of the external ocular muscles. It may occur with oedema of the lids and conjunctivae and precede the exophthalmos. For this reason the term 'congestive ophthalmopathy' may be preferable to 'malignant exophthalmos'.

†Unless the diagnosis is unquestionably Graves' disease, the possibility of a retro-orbital tumour should always be investigated with CT scan, etc., regardless of the Hertel exophthalmometer measurement.

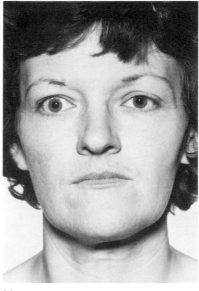

(a)

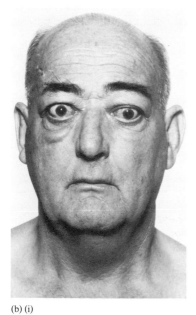

(b) (i)

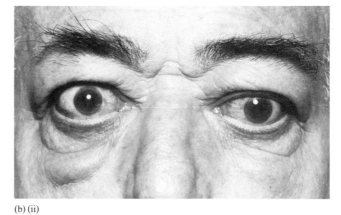

(b) (ii)

Fig. 3.16. (a) Unilateral exophthalmos. (b): (i), (ii) Bilateral exophthalmos (note proptosis, ophthalmoplegia, conjunctival congestion, swelling of the medial caruncle and periorbital swelling).

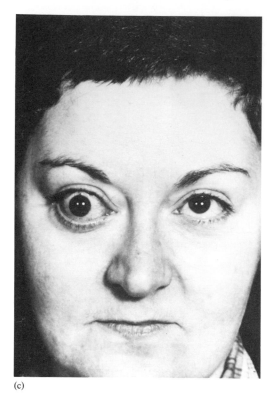

(c)

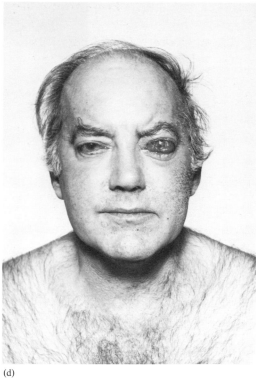

(d)

Fig. 3.16 (*continued*) (c) Ophthalmoplegia of the right eye. (d) Severe congestive ophthalmopathy, chemosis and corneal ulceration.

17 / Hepatomegaly (without splenomegaly)

Frequency in survey: Main focus of a short case in 10% of attempts at MRCP short cases. Additional feature in at least a further 9%.

Record

The liver is palpable at ... cm below the right costal margin (*?icterus, ascites,* signs of *cirrhosis* [don't miss gynaecomastia], *pigmentation, lymph nodes*).

Common causes

$3 C's$.

Cirrhosis—usually alcoholic (?spider naevi, gynaecomastia, etc.—p. 78).
Secondary carcinoma (?hard and knobbly, cachexia, evidence of primary).
Congestive cardiac failure (?JVP ↑, ankle oedema, *S3* or cardiac murmur; tender pulsatile liver with giant *v* waves in the JVP in tricuspid incompetence).

Other causes of hepatomegaly

Infections such as hepatitis A, glandular fever, Weil's disease and hepatitis B (remember Australia antigen heads list of investigations in icterus of uncertain cause)

Primary tumours both malignant (hepatoma may complicate cirrhosis) and benign (liver cell adenoma is associated with oral contraceptive use)

Lymphoproliferative disorders (?lymph nodes)

Primary biliary cirrhosis (?middle-aged female, scratch marks, xanthelasma, etc.—p. 208)

Haemochromatosis (?male, slate-grey pigmentation, etc.—p. 233)

Sarcoidosis (?erythema nodosum or history of, lupus pernio, chest signs)

Amyloidosis (?rheumatoid arthritis or other underlying chronic disease—see footnote to p. 65)

Hydatid cyst (?Welsh connection—NB patient's name)

Amoebic abscess (?tropical connection—name, appearance)

Budd–Chiari syndrome (?icterus, ascites, tender hepatomegaly)

Riedel's lobe

Emphysema (apparent hepatomegaly)

Hard and knobbly hepatomegaly—possible causes

Malignancy—primary or secondary

Polycystic liver disease (?kidneys)

Macronodular cirrhosis (following hepatitis B with widespread necrosis)

Hydatid cysts (may be eosinophilia; rupture may be associated with anaphylaxis)

Syphilitic gummas (late benign syphilis; there is usually hepatosplenomegaly and anaemia; rapid response to penicillin)

18 / Spastic paraparesis

Frequency in survey: Main focus of a short case in 10% of attempts at MRCP short cases. Additional feature in a further 2%.

Record

The *tone* in the legs is *increased* and they are *weak* (in chronic immobilized cases there may be some disuse atrophy, and in severe cases there may be contractures). There is bilateral *ankle clonus*, patellar clonus and the *plantar* responses are *extensor*. (?Abdominal reflexes.)

    The patient has a spastic paraparesis.* The most likely causes are:

1   Multiple sclerosis (?impaired rapid alternate motion of arms—p. 316).

2   Cord compression (?sensory level; root pain; no signs above level of lesion. NB Cervical spondylosis—see p. 198).

3   Trauma (?scar or deformity in back).

4   Birth injury (cerebral palsy—Little's disease).

5   Motor neurone disease (?no sensory signs, muscle fasciculation, etc.—p. 116).

Other causes

Subacute combined degeneration of the cord† (?posterior column loss, absent ankle jerks,‡ peripheral neuropathy, anaemia—p. 273)

Parasagittal cranial meningioma

General paralysis of the insane (?dementia, vacant expression, trombone tremor of the tongue, etc.—see p. 310)

Taboparesis (?Argyll Robertson pupils, posterior column loss, etc.—p. 310)

Syringomyelia (?kyphoscoliosis, wasted hands, dissociated sensory loss, Horner's syndrome, etc.—p. 268)

Anterior spinal artery thrombosis (sudden onset, ?dissociated sensory loss up to the level of the lesion)

Friedreich's ataxia (?pes cavus, cerebellar signs, kyphoscoliosis, etc.—p. 220)

Hereditary spastic paraplegia

---

*A clue to the underlying cause of spastic paraparesis may be:
   Cerebellar signs: Multiple sclerosis
                    Friedreich's ataxia (?pes cavus)
   Wasted hands: Cervical spondylosis (?inverted reflexes)
                    Syringomyelia (?Horner's)
                    Motor neurone disease (?prominent fasciculation)

†Stocking sensory loss (with or without absent ankle jerks) in association with a spastic paraplegia is strongly suggestive of subacute combined degeneration of the cord.
‡Absent ankle jerks and upgoing plantars—p. 290.

19 / Fibrosing alveolitis

Frequency in survey: Main focus of a short case in 10% of attempts at MRCP short cases. Additional feature in a further 1%.

Record

There is *clubbing* of the fingers, (may be) *cyanosis*, and there are *fine inspiratory crackles* (or crepitations—whichever term you prefer) at both bases.

The likely diagnosis is (cryptogenic*) fibrosing alveolitis.

Conditions which may be associated with cryptogenic fibrosing alveolitis

Rheumatoid arthritis (?hands, nodules)
Systemic lupus erythematosus (?typical rash)
Systemic sclerosis (?typical mask-like facies, telangiectasia, sclerodactyly—p. 90)
Sjögren's syndrome (?dry eyes and dry mouth)
Polymyositis (?proximal muscle weakness and tenderness—p. 280)
Dermatomyositis (?heliotrope rash on eyes/hands and polymyositis—p. 252)
Ulcerative colitis (?colostomy)
Chronic active hepatitis (?icterus, hepatosplenomegaly)
Raynaud's phenomenon
Digital vasculitis

Conditions in which alveolitis and pulmonary fibrosis occur

Sarcoidosis (?erythema nodosum or history of, lupus pernio)
Extrinsic allergic alveolitis (?farmer, pigeon racer, etc.)
Asbestosis (?lagger, etc.)
Silicosis (?slate worker or granite quarrier, etc.)
Drug reactions (e.g. bleomycin, busulphan, nitrofurantoin)
Chemical inhalation (e.g. beryllium, mercury)
Poison ingestion (e.g. paraquat)
Radiation fibrosis
Mitral valve disease
Uraemia
Adult respiratory distress syndrome (complicating acute severe illness often with septicaemia)

*In the absence of an identifiable causal agent the fibrosing alveolitis is termed 'cryptogenic'.

20 / Aortic incompetence (lone)

Frequency in survey: Main focus of a short case in 9% of attempts at MRCP short cases. Additional feature in a further 1% (not counting where additional to other valve lesions).

Record

The pulse is regular* (give rate), of large volume and *collapsing* in character. The venous pressure is not raised but *vigorous arterial pulsations* can be seen in the neck (Corrigan's sign†). The apex beat is *thrusting* in the anterior axillary line, in the sixth intercostal space. There is an *early diastolic murmur* audible down the left sternal edge and in the aortic area; it is *louder* in *expiration* with the patient *sitting forward*. (The blood pressure may be wide with a high systolic and low diastolic. In severe cases it may be 250–300/30–50.)

The diagnosis is aortic incompetence (now consider looking for *Argyll Robertson pupils*, *high-arched palate* or *Marfanoid* appearance, or obvious features of an arthropathy especially *ankylosing spondylitis*. If these are not present the aortic incompetence is likely to be rheumatic in origin—rheumatic fever and infective endocarditis are the commonest identifiable causes).

The early diastolic murmur can be difficult to hear and is easily overlooked (see anecdote 20, p. 343). It should be specifically sought with the patient sitting forward in expiration. Listen for the 'absence of silence' in the early part of diastole. The murmur is usually best heard over the mid-sternal region or at the lower left sternal edge. In some cases, particularly syphilitic aortitis, it is loudest in the aortic area. There is often an accompanying systolic murmur due to increased flow which does not necessarily indicate coexistent aortic stenosis (see p. 89).

If there is a mid-diastolic murmur at the apex it may be an Austin Flint murmur‡ or it may represent some associated mitral valve disease. These two may be clinically indistinguishable, though the presence of a loud first heart sound and an opening snap suggest the latter. Though the first heart sound in the Austin Flint may be loud, it is never palpable (i.e. no tapping impulse).

Causes of aortic incompetence

Rheumatic fever
Infective endocarditis (usually occurs on a deformed valve)
Syphilitic aortitis (?Argyll Robertson pupils; there may be an aneurysm of the ascending aorta)
Ankylosing spondylitis (?male with fixed kyphosis and stooped 'question mark' posture—p. 168; aortic incompetence may also occur in the other seronegative arthropathies—psoriatic, ulcerative colitic and Reiter's syndrome)
Rheumatoid arthritis (?hands, nodules)
Marfan's syndrome (?tall with long extremities, arachnodactyly and high-arched palate, etc.—p. 244)
Hurler's syndrome
Severe hypertension (by causing aortic dilatation; complications of hypertension such as ascending aortic aneurysm or dissecting aneurysm may also cause aortic incompetence)
Associated ventricular septal defect (loss of support for valve)

---

*The pulse is usually regular unless there is associated mitral valve disease.

†Other physical signs which result from a large pulse volume and peripheral vasodilatation include de Musset's sign (the head nods with each pulsation) and Quincke's sign (capillary pulsation visible in the nail beds). Of greater clinical value is Duroziez's sign—the femoral artery is compressed and auscultated proximally with a stethoscope; a diastolic murmur implies retrograde flow and aortic incompetence of at least moderate severity.

‡The Austin Flint murmur occurs in severe aortic incompetence. It is probably attributable to (i) the regurgitant jet interfering with the opening of the anterior mitral valve leaflet and (ii) the left ventricular diastolic pressure rising more rapidly than the left atrial diastolic pressure.

Indications for surgery

Although patients tolerate aortic incompetence longer than aortic stenosis (p. 106), the clinician's aim is to replace the valve *before* serious left ventricular dysfunction occurs. Every effort should be made to recognize any reduction in left ventricular function or reserve as early as possible. Serial chest X-rays, echocardiograms and radionuclear angiography will show a gradual increase in cardiac size.

The last-mentioned technique can be particularly useful in showing evidence of early left ventricular dysfunction in asymptomatic patients. The left ventricular ejection fraction, though normal at rest, may show a subnormal rise during exercise. Aortic valve replacement may have to be undertaken as a matter of urgency in patients with infective endocarditis in whom the leaking valve causes rapidly progressive left ventricular dilatation.

21 / Hemiplegia

Frequency in survey: Main focus of a short case in 9% of attempts at MRCP short cases. Additional feature in a further 3%.

Record

There is a R/L *upper motor neurone VIIth* nerve lesion.* The R/L *arm* and *leg* are *weak* (without wasting) with *increased tone* and *hyperreflexia*. The R/L plantar is *extensor* and the *abdominal reflexes* are *diminished* on the R/L side.

This is a R/L hemiplegia.

There is also (may be) *hemisensory loss* on the R/L side. Visual field testing reveals (may be) a R/L homonymous hemianopia. The most likely causes are:

1 Cerebrovascular accident due to cerebral
  thrombosis (?hypertension)
  haemorrhage (?hypertension)
  embolism (?atrial fibrillation, murmurs, bruits).
2 Brain tumour (?insidious onset, papilloedema, headaches; ?evidence of primary e.g. clubbing).

A right-sided hemiplegia associated with dysphasia would suggest that the patient is right-handed and that the causative lesion is affecting the speech centres in the dominant hemisphere (see p. 239) as well as the motor cortex (precentral gyrus) and if there are sensory signs, the sensory cortex (postcentral gyrus). If cerebrovascular in origin the causative lesion is likely to be in the *carotid* distribution.

The presence of signs such as nystagmus, ocular palsy, dysphagia (?nasogastric feeding tube) and cerebellar signs would suggest that the hemiparesis is due to a brain-stem lesion. If cerebrovascular in origin the lesion is likely to be in the *vertebrobasilar* distribution (see p. 320 for the eponymous syndromes).

Parietal lobe and related signs†

Agnosia Though peripheral sensation is intact (tactile, visual, auditory) the patient fails to appreciate the significance of the sensory stimulus without the aid of other senses.

Tactile agnosia or *astereognosis* (contralateral posterior parietal lobe)—inability to recognize a familiar object placed in the hand (e.g. pen, keys) with the eyes closed. Opening the eyes or hearing the keys rattle may allow recognition.

Visual agnosia (parieto-occipital lesions—especially in the left hemisphere of right-handed patients)—the patient is not able to identify the familiar object by sight (e.g. a pen, surroundings) but may do at once when he is allowed to handle it.

Auditory agnosia (temporal lobe of dominant hemisphere)—the patient may only be able to recognize the sound of a voice, telephone or music when he is allowed to use the senses of vision or touch.

Autotopagnosia (usually a left hemiplegia in a right-handed person)—difficulty in perceiving or identifying the various parts of the body; the patient may be unaware of the left side of his body. It may be associated with anosognosia in which case there is no appreciation of a disability (e.g. hemiplegia, blindness) on the same side.

---

* In an upper motor neurone VIIth nerve lesion, the lower face is much weaker than the upper because the muscles frontalis, orbicularis oculi and corrugator superficialis ('raise your eyebrows', 'screw your eyes up tight', 'frown') are bilaterally innervated and are all only minimally impaired.
† These did not occur in our survey of MRCP short cases.

Apraxia Whereas in agnosia the difficulty is in recognition, in apraxia it is in execution. Though power, sensation and coordination are all normal, the patient is unable to perform certain familiar activities. It may affect:

The upper limbs—e.g. difficulty using a pen, comb or toothbrush, winding a watch, dressing or undressing ('dressing apraxia').

The lower limbs—may mimic ataxia or weakness*—the patient may appear unable to lift one foot in front of the other.

The trunk—the patient may have difficulty seating himself on a chair or lavatory seat, getting on to his bed, or in turning over in bed.

The face—the patient may be unable to whistle, put out his tongue or close his eyes.

The lesions (tumours or atrophy) tend to be in the corpus callosum, parietal lobes and premotor areas. Dominant lobe lesions may produce bilateral apraxia. Unilateral left-sided apraxia may be caused by a lesion in the right posterior parietal region or in the corpus collosum of a right-handed patient. The lesion in 'dressing apraxia' is usually in the right parieto-occipital region. In 'constructional apraxia' (most often seen in patients with hepatic encephalopathy) the patient is unable to construct simple figures such as triangles, squares or crosses from matchsticks.

Dyslexia (impairment of reading ability), **dysgraphia** (impairment of writing ability) and **dyscalculia** (difficulty with calculating) usually represent lesions in the posterior parietal lobe.

---

*A parietal lobe lesion may cause ataxia, hemiparesis or marked astereognosis. In hemiparesis of parietal origin, the limbs are often hypotonic with an absent plantar response, rather than spastic. The limb muscles may even waste (like a lower motor neurone lesion). Often the patient is disinclined to move the limb rather than actually paralysed.

22 / Old tuberculosis

Frequency in survey: 8% of attempts at MRCP short cases.

Record 1

The trachea is *deviated* to the R/L. The R/L upper chest shows *deformity* with *decreased expansion*, *dull percussion* note, *bronchial breathing* and *crepitations*. The apex beat is (may be) *displaced* to the R/L. There is a *thoracotomy scar* posteriorly with evidence of rib resections.

The patient has had a R/L thoracoplasty for treatment of tuberculosis before the days of chemotherapy.

Record 2

The tracheal deviation to the R/L and the diminished expansion and crackles at the R/L apex suggest R/L apical fibrosis.

Old tuberculosis is the likely cause.

Record 3

Expansion is diminished on the R/L and there is a R/L supraclavicular scar (there may also be crepitations).

The patient has had a phrenic nerve crush for tuberculosis before the days of chemotherapy.

23 / Acromegaly

Frequency in survey: Main focus of a short case in 8% of attempts at MRCP short cases. Additional feature in a further 1%.

Survey note: Candidates were sometimes asked questions on subjects such as presentation, investigation and complications.

Record

The patient has prominent *supraorbital ridges* and a *large lower jaw*. The facial wrinkles are exaggerated and the lips are full. There is *poor occlusion* of the teeth, the *lower teeth overbiting* in front of the upper. The *nose, tongue* and *ears* are enlarged and the patient is *kyphotic*. The *hands* are *large*, doughy and spade-shaped,* and the *skin* over the back of them is *thickened* (shake hands and examine the dorsum). There is (may be) loss of the thenar eminence bilaterally with impaired sensation in the median nerve distribution (*carpal tunnel syndrome*). The patient is *sweating* excessively and is *hirsute*. The *voice* is husky and cavernous. There is a *bitemporal peripheral visual field defect*.

   The diagnosis is acromegaly.

Other physical signs which may be present

Bowed legs
Rolling gait
Goitre
Gynaecomastia
Galactorrhoea
Small gonads
Greasy skin
Acne
Prominent superficial veins of extremities
Proximal muscle weakness
Cardiomegaly (hypertension and cardiomyopathy)
Third nerve palsy

Other features

Diabetes mellitus (glycosuria, glucose intolerance or frank diabetes may occur; it is usually mild and ketoacidosis is rare; it is somewhat resistant to insulin)
Hypertension (20–50%)

Hypercalciuria (common)
Hypercalcaemia† (occasionally)
Diabetes insipidus (normally due to hypothalamic pressure effect; if there is impaired cortisol secretion symptoms may be masked)
Hypopituitarism (p. 262)
Osteoporosis

Symptoms before presentation‡

Excessive sweating
Increasing size of shoes, gloves, hats, dentures and rings
Paraesthesiae of hands and feet
Digital pain and stiffness (of slowly expanding fingers and toes)
Arthralgia
Hypogonadism (amenorrhoea, loss of libido)
Headache (may be severe; may occur without clinically detectable enlargement of the pituitary tumour; the mechanism is not clear)
Visual field or acuity disturbance

*Shaking hands with the patient may give the impression of losing one's hands in a mass of dough.
†In some this disappears when the acromegaly is successfully treated. In others it is due to associated hyperparathyroidism as part of *multiple endocrine adenopathy Type 1* (Werner's syndrome) which is two or more of:
   Pituitary tumour (eosinophil or chromophobe)
   Islet-cell tumour (gastrin or insulin)
   Primary hyperparathyroidism (adenoma or hyperplasia)
   Adrenocortical adenoma (see also p. 218 and footnote)

MEA Type 1 should probably be regarded as a complex of separate genetic abnormalities rather than as a consequence of a single primary disease. It should not be confused with MEA Type II which is usually an autosomal dominant trait with a high degree of penetrance (see footnote p. 120).
‡The mean age of onset has been estimated at about twenty-seven years whereas the mean age of presentation is over forty years, i.e. there is an average pre-presentation lapse of thirteen to fourteen years.

Investigations: comparative study of old photographs of the patient; skull X-ray; X-ray for heel pad thickness (increased); visual fields; glucose tolerance test with growth hormone response (lack of suppression; sometimes a paradoxical rise); tests of anterior pituitary function (insulin tolerance test, TRH, LHRH).

Treatments: (i) trans-sphenoidal hypophysectomy; (ii) transfrontal hypophysectomy in some cases with large extensive adenomas; (iii) external irradiation (especially if surgery fails; takes 1–2 years to take effect); (iv) radioactive gold or yttrium implants (very restricted in terms of availability); (v) bromocriptine (50% respond but the size of the tumour is not reduced; useful for GH hypersecretion after surgery).

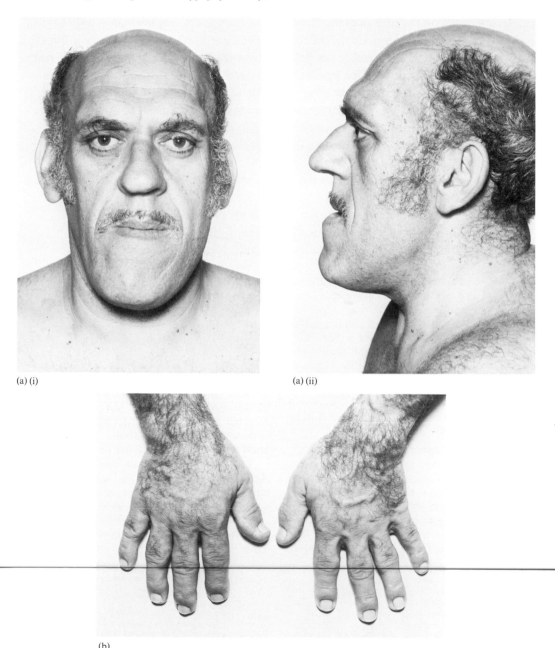

(a) (i)

(a) (ii)

(b)

Fig. 3.23. (a): (i), (ii) acromegalic facies. (b) Large hands with thickened skin.

24 / Aortic stenosis (lone)

Frequency in survey: 8% of attempts at MRCP short cases.

Record 1

The *pulse* is regular (give rate), of *small volume* and *slow rising*. The venous pressure is not raised (unless there is cardiac failure). The apex beat is palpable 1 cm to the left of the midclavicular line in the fifth intercostal space (the apex position is normal or only slightly displaced in pure aortic stenosis unless the left ventricle is starting to fail) as a forceful *sustained heave*.* There is a *systolic thrill* palpable over the aortic area and the carotids (may be felt over the apex). Auscultation reveals a *harsh ejection systolic murmur* in the aortic area *radiating* into the *neck*, and the *aortic second sound* is *soft* (or absent). (The blood pressure is usually low normal with a decreased difference between systole and diastole—pulse pressure.)

The diagnosis is aortic stenosis.

Possible causes

1   Rheumatic heart disease (mitral valve is usually involved as well and aortic incompetence is often present).
2   Bicuspid aortic valve (commoner in males; typically presents in the sixth decade).
3   Degenerative calcification (in the elderly; the stenosis is usually relatively mild).
4   Congenital (may worsen during childhood and adolescence due to calcification).

In the late stages of aortic stenosis when cardiac failure with low cardiac output supervenes, the murmur may become markedly diminished in intensity. The murmur of associated mitral stenosis should be carefully sought, particularly in the female patient, because the association of these two obstructive lesions tends to diminish the physical findings of each. Mitral stenosis is easily missed and the severity of aortic stenosis underestimated.

Indications for surgery

In the adult patient valve replacement is indicated for symptoms or a systolic pressure gradient greater than 50–60 mmHg, as without operation the outlook for these patients is poor. Critical coronary lesions can be bypassed at the same time. Asymptomatic children and young adults can be treated with valvotomy if the obstruction is severe, as the operative risk appears to be less than the risk of sudden death. This is only temporary but may postpone the need for valve replacement for many years.

Record 2

The *carotid pulses* are *normal*, the apical impulse is just palpable and not displaced. There are *no thrills*. There is an *ejection systolic murmur* which is not (usually) harsh or loud and is audible in the aortic area but only faintly in the neck. The aortic component of the second sound is well heard. The blood pressure is normal (or may be hypertensive).

These findings suggest aortic sclerosis (or minimal aortic stenosis) rather than significant aortic stenosis. (NB The differentiation of this from the other causes of a short systolic murmur: prolapsing mitral valve, p. 196; trivial mitral incompetence and hypertrophic obstructive cardiomyopathy, p. 318.)

---

* There may also be a presystolic impulse due to left atrial overactivity (this is also felt in moderately severe cases of HOCM). The result is a double apical impulse best felt in the left lateral recumbent position. Other signs which may be present include: a fourth heart sound; a single second sound or even paradoxical splitting of the second sound which are both due to prolonged left ventricular ejection.

25 / Graves' disease

Frequency in survey: Main focus of a short case in 8% of attempts at MRCP short cases. Additional feature in a further 8%.

Record 1

The patient (usually female) is *thin*, has *sweaty palms*, a *fine tremor* of the outstretched hands, a *tachycardia*,* and she is *fidgety* and nervous. There is a small diffuse *goitre* with a *bruit*, and she has *exophthalmos* (p. 92) with *lid lag*.

This patient is *thyrotoxic* and has Graves' disease.

Record 2

There is *exophthalmos* (?chemosis, ophthalmoplegia, diplopia, lateral tarsorrhaphy), *thyroid acropachy*,† and the lesions on the front of the shins are *pretibial myxoedema* (p. 252). The pulse is regular* and the *pulse rate* is *normal* (give rate), the palms are *not sweaty*, and there is *no hand tremor* or *lid lag*. There is a *thyroidectomy scar*.

The diagnosis is *euthyroid* Graves' disease,‡ the patient having been treated by thyroidectomy in the past.

Male : Female = 1 : 5

Record 3

This patient with *exophthalmos* (?chemosis, ophthalmoplegia, diplopia, lateral tarsorrhaphy, goitre, thyroidectomy scar, pretibial myxoedema, thyroid acropachy) has *hypothyroid facies*, a *hoarse voice*, *slow pulse** and *slowly relaxing reflexes*.

The patient has Graves' disease and is clinically *hypothyroid*. It is likely that she had hyperthyroidism treated in the past (?thyroidectomy or radio-active iodine) and is probably now on inadequate thyroxine replacement. (Because of the close links between the autoimmune thyroid diseases—see below—patients with Graves' disease occasionally go on to develop hypothyroidism spontaneously.)

Other signs which may occur
Fever (rarely hyperpyrexia)
Systolic hypertension with wide pulse pressure

Cutaneous vasodilatation
Systolic murmur due to increased blood flow
Proximal muscle weakness (thyrotoxic myopathy)
Hyperactive reflexes
Choreoathetoid movements (in children)
Fine thin hair (females may show temporal recession of the hairline)
Onycholysis (Plummer's nails, typically found bilaterally on the fourth finger)
Palmar erythema
Spider naevi
Splenomegaly (minimal)
Hepatomegaly (minimal)
Palpable lymph nodes (especially axillae)
Thyrotoxic osteoporosis (only rarely causes kyphosis or loss of height)

Important symptoms of hyperthyroidism (if asked to ask the patient some questions) are heat intolerance, weight loss, increased appetite, diarrhoea, exertional

---

*The pulse may be regular or irregular—the patient may have sinus rhythm or atrial fibrillation whatever the thyroid status (hyperthyroid; eu- or hypothyroid due to treatment).
†Thyroid acropachy may resemble finger clubbing in hypertrophic pulmonary osteoarthropathy (HPOA). However, in thyroid acropachy new bone formation seen on X-ray has the appearance of soap bubbles on the bone surface with coarse spicules. In HPOA new bone is formed in a linear distribution. Sometimes the new bone formation in acropachy is both visible and palpable along the phalanges.
‡Graves' exophthalmos is due to increased retro-orbital fat and enlarged intra-orbital muscles infiltrated with lymphocytes and

containing increased water and mucopolysaccharide. It may develop in the absence of hyperthyroidism and remit, persist or develop further despite successful treatment of hyperthyroidism. Pretibial myxoedema tends to develop after the hyperthyroidism has been treated—especially with radioactive iodine.
§Graves' disease is one of the three closely related autoimmune thyroid diseases—the others being Hashimoto's thyroiditis and its atrophic variant, myxoedema. Among patients with one of these three it is typical to find relatives with one of the other two. Some patients appear to have a combination which has been termed 'Hashitoxicosis'.

dyspnoea, undue fatiguability, 'can't keep still', irritability and nervousness.

The other organ-specific autoimmune diseases of which autoimmune thyroid disease§ is an example include

    Pernicious anaemia
    Atrophic gastritis with iron deficiency anaemia
    Diabetes mellitus
    Addison's disease
    Idiopathic hypoparathyroidism
    Premature ovarian failure
    Renal tubular acidosis
    Fibrosing alveolitis
    Chronic active hepatitis
    Primary biliary cirrhosis

All of these diseases show a *marked female preponderance*. Premature greying of the hair, alopecia areata and vitiligo (see also p. 254) are all associated with this group of diseases. Autoimmune thyroiditis is also associated with

    Sjögren's syndrome
    Myasthenia gravis
    Systemic sclerosis
    Mixed connective tissue disease
    Cranial arteritis
    Polymyalgia rheumatica

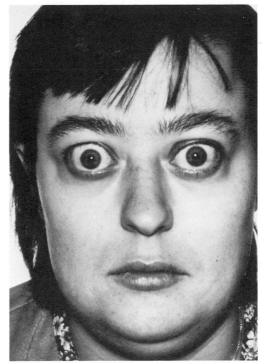

(a)

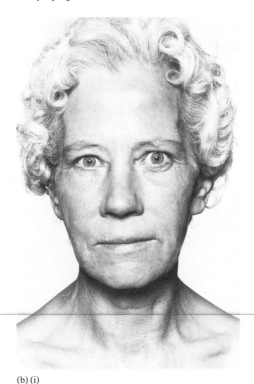

(b) (i)

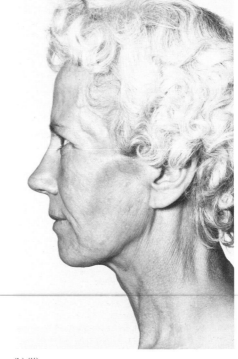

(b) (ii)

Fig. 3.25. (a) Graves' disease. (b): (i), (ii) hyperthyroidism in a patient who presented with the complaint that she had noticed a staring appearance of her left eye (note thinning of the hair in the temporal region).

26 / Ocular palsy

Frequency in survey: Main focus of a short case in 8% of attempts at MRCP short cases. Additional feature in a further 3%.

Record 1

The patient has a *convergent strabismus* at rest. There is *impairment* of the *lateral movement* of the R/L eye and *diplopia* is worse on looking to the R/L (the outermost image comes from the affected eye).

The patient has a *sixth nerve palsy*.

Possible causes
1   The causes of mononeuritis multiplex.*
2   Multiple sclerosis (?ipsilateral facial palsy because the VIth and VIIth nuclei are very close in the pons; ?nystagmus, cerebellar signs, pyramidal signs, pale discs, etc.—p. 316).
3   Raised intracranial pressure (?papilloedema) causing stretching of the nerve (a false localizing sign) during its long intracranial course.
4   Neoplasm (?papilloedema; associated ipsilateral facial palsy if pontine tumour).
5   Encephalitis.
6   Brain-stem vascular lesions (probably common as a cause of 'idiopathic' VIth nerve palsy).
7   Compression by aneurysm (uncommon).
8   Meningovascular syphilis (see p. 310).

Record 2

There is *ptosis*. Lifting the eyelids reveals *divergent strabismus* and a *dilated pupil*. The eye is fixed in a *down and out position* (and there is *angulated diplopia*).

The diagnosis is complete (NB the condition is often partial) *third nerve palsy*.

Possible causes
1   Unruptured aneurysm of posterior communicating (or internal carotid) artery (painful).
2   The causes of mononeuritis multiplex.*
3   Midbrain vascular lesion (if there is a contralateral hemiplegia the diagnosis is Weber's syndrome).
4   Midbrain demyelinating lesion (?cerebellar signs, staccato speech, pale discs, etc.—p. 316).

Other causes of a third nerve palsy

Meningovascular syphilis (at one time the commonest cause)
Ophthalmoplegic migraine (similar to posterior communicating artery aneurysm except that it begins in childhood or adolescence, recovery is more rapid and is always complete; recovery is never complete with an aneurysm)
Encephalitis
Parasellar neoplasms
Sphenoidal wing meningiomas
Carcinomatous lesions of the skull base

*The causes of mononeuritis multiplex include diabetes mellitus, polyarteritis nodosa and Churg–Strauss syndrome, rheumatoid disease, SLE, Wegener's granulomatosis, sarcoidosis, carcinoma and amyloidosis.

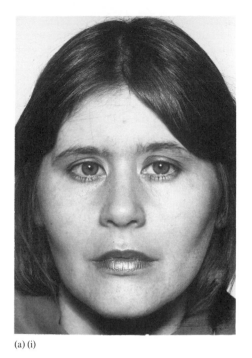

(a) (i)

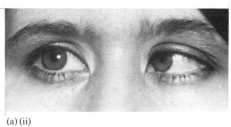

(a) (ii)

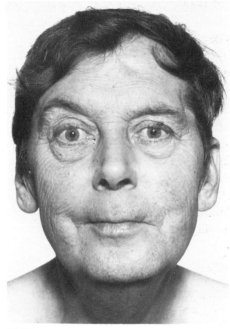

(b) (ii)

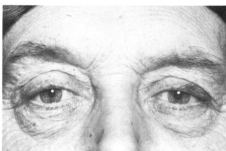

(b) (i)

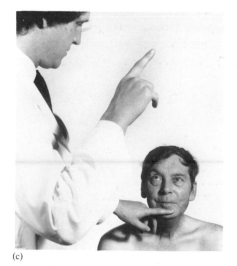

(c)

Fig. 3.26. (a) Right sixth nerve palsy—diabetic mononeuritis.
(i) Patient looking straight ahead (note convergent
strabismus); (ii) looking to the right. (b): (i), (ii) left third
nerve palsy (note ptosis and mydriasis of the left pupil). The
patient had had surgery for a prolactinoma (note scar on upper
forehead and left frontal alopecia). (c) Upward gaze being
tested (note the failure of the left eye to follow the examiner's
finger).

Other causes of ocular palsy

Internuclear ophthalmoplegia (adduction impaired bilaterally but abduction normal or vice versa; ataxic nystagmus is present and distinguishes it from bilateral VIth nerve palsy—see p. 156; ?cerebellar signs)

Exophthalmic ophthalmoplegia (exophthalmos and diplopia —upward and outward gaze most often reduced)

Myasthenia gravis (?ptosis, variable strabismus, facial weakness with a snarling smile, proximal muscle weakness, weak nasal voice, all of which worsen with repetition—p. 246. NB It may superficially resemble IIIrd or even VIth nerve palsy)

Cavernous sinus and superior orbital fissure syndromes (total or subtotal ophthalmoplegia which is often painful, together with sensory loss over the first division of the Vth nerve—absent corneal reflex; it is due to a tumour or carotid aneurysm affecting the IIIrd, IVth, Vth and VIth nerves as they travel together through the cavernous sinus into the superior orbital fissure— see Fig. 3.29d, p. 121)

Fourth nerve palsy (adducted eye cannot look downwards—the patient experiences 'one above the other' diplopia when attempting to do this; angulated diplopia occurs when looking down and out; the diplopia is worse when reading and going down stairs)

Ocular myopathy (see p. 212 and footnote p. 296)

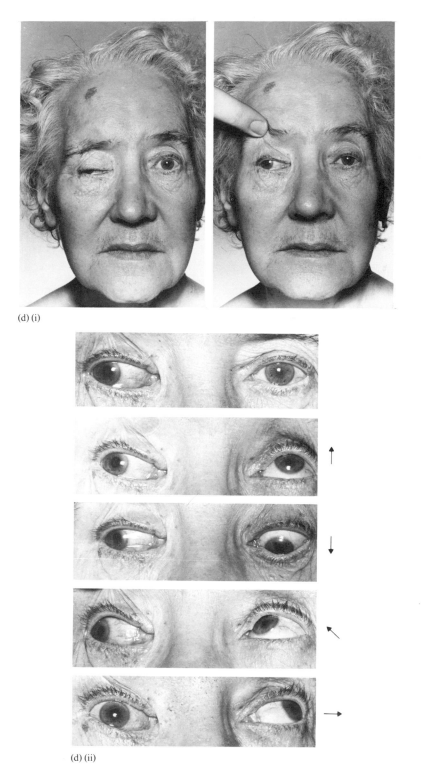

(d) (i)

(d) (ii)

Fig. 3.26 (*continued*) (d) Complete right third nerve palsy: (i) note mydriasis of the right pupil and the down and outward deviation of the right eye (due to the unopposed action of the superior oblique and lateral rectus muscles innervated by the fourth and sixth nerves respectively); (ii) testing eye movements (note the failure of the right eye to look straight, upwards, downwards, upwards and laterally, and medially).

Frequency in survey: 7% of attempts at MRCP short cases.

Record

The pulse is regular (give rate). The venous pressure is not raised and there is no ankle or sacral oedema (unless in cardiac failure). The apex beat is *thrusting* in the sixth intercostal space in the anterior axillary line, and there is (may be) a systolic thrill. There is a left *parasternal heave*. The *first heart sound* is *soft*, and there is a *third heart sound* (both suggest severe mitral incompetence). There is a loud *pansystolic murmur* at the apex, *radiating* to the *axilla*.

   The diagnosis is mitral incompetence.

Causes* of mitral incompetence

1   Rheumatic heart disease (males more commonly than females; contrast with mitral stenosis which affects females more commonly than males).
2   Previous mitral valvotomy for mitral stenosis (left thoracotomy scar).
3   Papillary muscle dysfunction (ischaemia, infarction or other disease of papillary muscles or adjacent myocardium).
4   Severe left ventricular dilatation (due to any cause—lateral displacement of the papillary muscles and sometimes possibly dilatation of the mitral annulus† interfere with coaptation of the valve leaflets).
5   Mitral valve prolapse (p. 196).

Other physical signs *which may occur in severe mitral incompetence*

Mid-diastolic rumbling murmur‡ (brief)
Sharp and abbreviated peripheral pulse (lack of sustained forward stroke volume because of the regurgitant leak)
Wide splitting of the second sound (early closure of the aortic valve because the regurgitant loss shortens the left ventricular ejection time)
Fourth heart sound (acute severe regurgitation with sinus rhythm)

Other causes* of mitral incompetence

Infective endocarditis (fever, splenomegaly, petechiae, splinter haemorrhages, clubbing, Osler's nodes, Janeway's lesions, Roth spots, etc.)
Annular calcification (especially in the elderly female)
Hypertrophic obstructive cardiomyopathy (see p. 318)
Rupture of the chordae tendinae§ (usually causes acute severe mitral incompetence; causes include

---

* Regardless of the aetiology, mitral incompetence is a condition which gradually worsens spontaneously ('mitral incompetence begets mitral incompetence')—enlargement of the left atrium and left ventricle both worsen the incompetence and a vicious circle is set up.
† Left ventricular dilatation is common but the frequency of dilatation of the mitral valve annulus is an uncertain and controversial point. The mitral valve ring is a thick fibrous structure, so that if significant dilatation does occur, it probably indicates severe left ventricular disease.
‡ A short mid-diastolic murmur in the context of mitral incompetence could indicate associated mitral stenosis, or it

could represent a flow (LA to LV) murmur. The presence of an opening snap in such cases indicates mitral stenosis. In the absence of an opening snap the mid-diastolic murmur has two possible causes: (i) severe mitral incompetence with an increased flow murmur; (ii) associated mitral stenosis and a calcified mitral valve. In the former there is often a third heart sound. In the latter the murmur is usually longer.
§ If the posterior leaflet is predominantly involved the systolic murmur is best heard at the left sternal edge whereas if the anterior leaflet is involved the murmur is best heard over the spine.

infective endocarditis, rheumatic mitral valve disease, mitral valve prolapse, trauma)

Connective tissue disorders

Systemic lupus erythematosus (Libman–Sachs endocarditis—p. 222)

Rheumatoid arthritis (?hands, ?nodules).

Ankylosing spondylitis (?male with fixed kyphosis and stooped posture; aortic valve more commonly affected—p. 168)

Congenital with or without other abnormalities

Ostium primum atrial septal defect

Marfan's syndrome (?tall with long extremities, arachnodactyly, high-arched palate, etc.—p. 244)

Ehlers–Danlos syndrome (?hyperextensible skin and joints, thin scars, etc.—p. 240)

Pseudoxanthoma elasticum (?loose skin or 'chicken-skin' appearance in anticubital fossae, inguinal regions, neck, etc.—p. 270)

Osteogenesis imperfecta (?blue sclerae, deformity from old fractures, etc.—p. 298)

Endomyocardial fibrosis (10% of cardiac admissions in East Africa; also occurs in West Africa, Southern India and Sri Lanka; the aetiology is unknown)

Indications for surgery

Improvements in surgical techniques and artificial valves, and the reduction in operative mortality, have reduced the threshold of physicians for considering surgery in moderately disabled patients (i.e. breathlessness caused by normal activity)—particularly if cardiomegaly and an elevated endsystolic left ventricular volume ($\geqslant 30$ ml m^{-2} BSA) persist despite medical therapy (digoxin, diuretics, vasodilators). Asymptomatic patients should not be considered for surgery since the condition progresses slowly;* they may live for many years with little noticeable deterioration in their condition. Acute severe mitral incompetence (e.g. infective endocarditis, ruptured chordae tendinae) may require emergency valve replacement.

28 / Motor neurone disease

Frequency in survey: Main focus of a short case in 7% of attempts at MRCP short cases. Additional feature in a further 1%.

Record

This patient has *weakness*, *wasting* and *fasciculation* of the muscles of the hand (p. 148), arms and shoulder girdle (*progressive muscular atrophy* in its pure form is characterized by minimal pyramidal signs), but the upper limb reflexes are exaggerated (reflexes in MND may be increased, decreased, or absent depending on which lesion is predominant). There is upper motor neurone *spastic weakness* with *exaggerated reflexes* in the legs (*amyotrophic lateral sclerosis*). There is ankle clonus and the patient has bilateral *extensor plantar* responses. The patient also has (may have) indistinct *nasal speech*, a *wasted fasciculating tongue* and *palatal paralysis* (*progressive bulbar palsy*—p. 236). There are *no sensory signs*.

The diagnosis is motor neurone disease.

Other conditions in which fasciculation may occur

Cervical spondylosis (see below)

Syringomyelia (fasciculation less apparent, dissociated sensory loss, etc.—p. 268)

Charcot–Marie–Tooth disease (fasciculation less apparent, atrophy which stops abruptly part of the way up the legs, pes cavus, sometimes palpable lateral popliteal and ulnar nerves, etc.—p. 230)

Acute stages of poliomyelitis (and rarely also in old polio; see below)

Neuralgic amyotrophy (pain, wasting and weakness of a group of muscles in a limb, sometimes following a viral infection; usually C5, C6 innervated muscles—shoulder)

Thyrotoxic myopathy (tachycardia, tremor, sweating, goitre with bruit, lid lag, etc.—p. 108)

Syphilitic amyotrophy (see below)

Chronic asymmetrical spinal muscular atrophy (see below)

Differential diagnosis of motor neurone disease

Cervical cord compression (p. 198) is the most important condition to be excluded in the diagnosis of motor neurone disease. Bulbar palsy and sensory signs should be carefully sought but a myelogram is often required to exclude it. *Syphilitic amyotrophy* (slowly progressing wasting of the muscles of the shoulder girdle and upper arm with loss of reflexes and no sensory loss; fasciculation of the tongue may occur) should always be excluded in the investigation of motor neurone disease as it is amenable to treatment. Occasionally patients with *old polio*, after many years, develop a progressive wasting disease (with prominent fasciculation) which is indistinguishable from progressive muscular atrophy motor neurone disease. Also, in immunologically incompetent patients (carcinoma, lymphoma, steroid therapy) a pure amyotrophy may develop that progresses over several months and is found at autopsy to be chronic poliomyelitis. The diagnosis of *chronic asymmetrical spinal muscular atrophy* (CASMA), a condition which appears to be distinct from classical motor neurone disease, is favoured by age of onset under 40 years, absence of pyramidal or bulbar involvement after three or more years of symptoms, and depressed or absent reflexes. CASMA is only slowly progressive and carries a considerably better prognosis than classical MND. Patients with CASMA sometimes have relatives with Werdnig–Hoffmann disease.

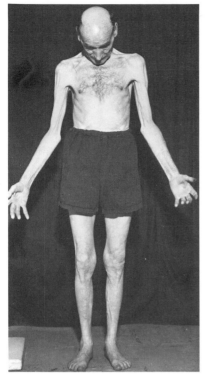

(a) (i)

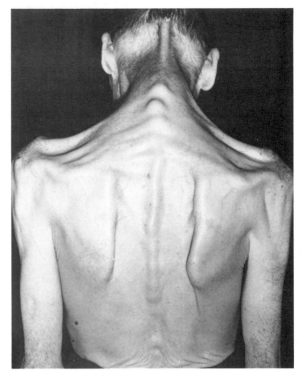

(a) (ii)

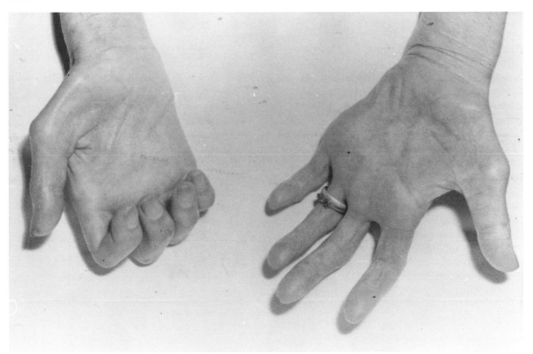

(b)

Fig. 3.28. (a): (i), (ii) generalized muscle wasting (note weakness of the extensors of the neck). (b) Wasting of the small muscles of the hand.

29 / Goitre

Frequency in survey: Main focus of a short case in 7% of attempts at MRCP short cases. Additional feature in a further 6%.

Record 1

There is a *multinodular* goitre, the R/L lobe being enlarged more than the R/L. There are *no lymph nodes* palpable, there is *no retrosternal* extension, there is *no bruit* and the patient is clinically *euthyroid* (having checked pulse, palms, tremor, lid lag, tendon reflexes).

The diagnosis (in this middle-aged or elderly patient) is likely to be simple multinodular goitre.

Simple multinodular goitre is due to relative iodine deficiency in a susceptible person. The multinodular nature suggests that it is long-standing. If there has been no recent rapid increase in size and if the gland is not causing symptoms or worrying the patient then no further investigation or treatment is required. The patient should be observed in six months or a year to confirm that there is still no change.

Record 2

There is a *firm, diffusely enlarged* goitre without retrosternal extension (check for bruit and if allowed feel the pulse and assess thyroid status).

Possible causes

Simple goitre (euthyroid, no bruit, relative iodine deficiency, especially females, ?puberty, ?pregnancy)

Treated Graves' disease* (?exophthalmos ± bruit, patient is euthyroid—normal pulse, no tremor or sweatiness—or even hypothyroid—slow pulse, facies, ankle jerks)

Hyperthyroid Graves' disease* (?bruit, tachycardia, exophthalmos, tremor, sweatiness, etc.)

Hashimoto's disease* (goitre usually, but not always, finely micronodular, firm and symmetrical; ?hypothyroid facies, pulse, ankle jerks, etc.)

De Quervain's (viral) thyroiditis (thyroid tender ± constitutional upset; flat radioactive iodine uptake on scan though the serum thyroxine may be elevated)

Goitrogens (e.g. lithium, iodide in large doses, phenylbutazone, PAS, amiodarone and others are all rare causes)

Dyshormonogenesis (six different types of congenital enzyme defect, all rare)

Record 3

There is a *solitary nodule* in the thyroid (check for lymphadenopathy).

Possible causes

Only one palpable nodule in a multinodular goitre

Thyroid adenoma (scan may show decreased, normal or increased [subclinical toxic nodule] uptake)

Toxic adenoma (hot nodule on scan, tachycardia, sweaty palms, lid lag, etc.)

Thyroid cyst

Thyroid carcinoma (?hard, lymph nodes, recent change, cold on scan)

The nodule should be scanned and thyroid function checked. If the nodule is hot it is not malignant but if it is cold it may be. In an older patient in whom the nodule has been present without changing for a long time, observation only (perhaps with full dose thyroxine therapy which will reduce many nodules) may sometimes be justified initially. Otherwise exploration of the neck and biopsy of the nodule are indicated, proceeding to subtotal lobectomy if the nodule is benign.

---

* NB The possibility of associated autoimmune disease adding extra interest to the case of goitre in the Membership (see experience 19, p. 332; e.g. diabetes mellitus, rheumatoid arthritis, Addison's disease, pernicious anaemia. About 7% of patients with Graves' disease have vitiligo. About 5% of patients with myasthenia gravis have thyrotoxicosis at some time. (See also pp. 108, 138, 254.)

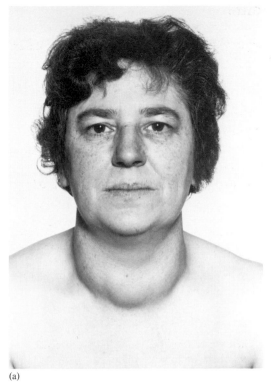

(a)

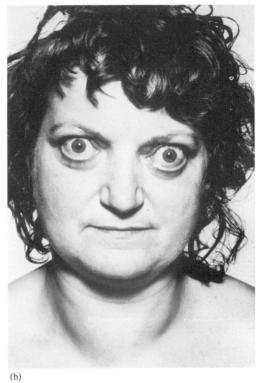

(b)

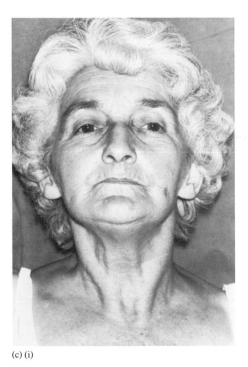

(c) (i)

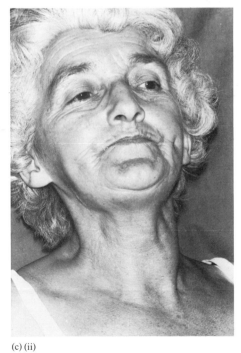

(c) (ii)

Fig. 3.29. (a) Multinodular goitre. (b) Diffusely enlarged thyroid (Graves' disease). (c): (i), (ii) solitary nodule only made obvious by swallowing (right).

Types of thyroid carcinoma

Papillary carcinoma is often TSH-dependent and responds to thyroxine

Follicular carcinoma (and its secondaries) often takes up and responds to radioactive iodine

Anaplastic carcinoma is highly malignant

Medullary carcinoma* is rare, secretes calcitonin and sometimes ACTH, but usually carries a good prognosis

*Multiple endocrine adenopathy (MEA) Type IIa (Sipple's syndrome) describes the association of
    Medullary cell carcinoma of the thyroid
    Phaeochromocytoma
    Parathyroid hyperplasia (50%)
In MEA Type IIb, medullary cell carcinoma of the thyroid and sometimes phaeochromocytoma are associated with a variety of neurological abnormalities including mucosal neuromas (lumpy, bumpy lips and eyelids), Marfanoid habitus, hyper- plastic corneal nerves, skin pigmentation, proximal myopathy and intestinal disorders such as megacolon and ganglioneuro- matosis. Parathyroid hyperplasia is less common. In MEA Type IIa medullary carcinoma may occasionally secrete other substances such as ACTH, histaminase, VIP, prostaglandins and serotonin whereas in MEA Type IIb production of hormones other than calcitonin is rare. Both are autosomal dominant.

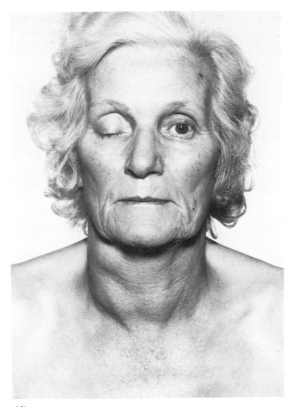

(d)

Fig. 3.29 (*continued*) (d) Follicular carcinoma of the thyroid with secondaries in the cavernous sinus (total ophthalmoplegia and absent corneal reflex on the right).

30 / Ulnar nerve palsy

Frequency in survey: 7% of attempts at MRCP short cases.

Record

The hand shows *generalized muscle wasting** and *weakness* which *spares* the *thenar eminence*. There is sensory loss over the *fifth finger*, the *adjacent half* of the *fourth finger* and the dorsal and palmar aspects of the *medial side* of the *hand*.† (Look for hyperextension at the metacarpophalangeal joints with flexion of the interphalangeal joints in the fourth and fifth fingers—the *ulnar claw hand*.‡)

The patient has an ulnar nerve lesion. (Now examine the elbow for a cause.)

Likely causes

1　Fracture or dislocation at the elbow (?scar or deformity; history of injury).
2　Osteoarthrosis at the elbow with osteophytic encroachment on the ulnar nerve in the cubital tunnel ('filling in' of the ulnar groove due to palpable enlargement of nerve; limitation of elbow movement is often seen; certain occupations predispose to osteoarthrosis at the elbow—see below).

Other causes

Occupations with constant leaning on elbows (clerks, secretaries on telephone, etc.)

Occupations with constant flexion and extension at the elbow (bricklayer, painter/decorator, carpenter, roofer—shallow ulnar groove will predispose; these occupations may also lead to osteoarthrosis—see above)

Excessive carrying angle at elbow (malunited fracture of the humerus or disturbance of growth leading to cubitus valgus and, over the years, 'tardy ulnar nerve palsy')

Injuries at the wrist or in the palm (different degrees of the syndrome depending on which branches of the nerve are damaged; e.g. occupations using screwdrivers, drills, etc.)

The causes of mononeuritis multiplex (diabetes, polyarteritis nodosa and Churg–Strauss syndrome, rheumatoid, SLE, Wegener's, sarcoid, carcinoma, amyloid, leprosy)

NB Other causes of wasting of the small muscles of the hand (p. 148) may sometimes resemble ulnar nerve palsy. The major features pointing to ulnar nerve palsy as the cause are sparing of the thenar eminence and the characteristic sensory loss pattern. The main distinguishing features of the differential diagnoses which may mimic the muscle wasting of ulnar paralysis are:

Syringomyelia—dissociated sensory loss extending beyond the ulnar zone; loss of arm reflexes; ?Horner's

C8 lesion—sensory loss involves radial side of fourth finger, ?Horner's

Cervical rib—objective sensory disturbances are usually slight or absent and without characteristic ulnar distribution

---

*(i) The *hypothenar eminence wastes*, though in the manual worker with thickened skin the hand contour may be preserved and the wasting may only be detected on palpation. Loss of the other small muscles is seen from (ii) *loss of the first dorsal interosseous* in the dorsal space between the first and second metacarpals and (iii) *guttering of the dorsum* of the hand—which becomes more prominent as the lesion advances.

†*Record* (continuation): There is *weakness* of *abduction* and *adduction* of the *fingers*, and *adduction* of the *extended thumb* against the palm (inability to grip a piece of paper between thumb and index finger without flexing the affected thumb—

Froment's 'thumb sign'). Flexion of the fourth and fifth fingers is weak. When the proximal portions of these fingers are held immobilized, flexion of the terminal phalanges is not possible. There is also *wasting* of the *medial aspect* of the *forearm* (flexor carpi ulnaris and half of the flexor digitorum profundus). When the hand is flexed to the ulnar side against resistance the tendon of flexor carpi ulnaris is not palpable.

‡The ulnar claw hand or partial *main-en-griffe* is due to the unopposed action of the long extensors and is only seen in the fourth and fifth fingers because the radial lumbricals are supplied by the median nerve.

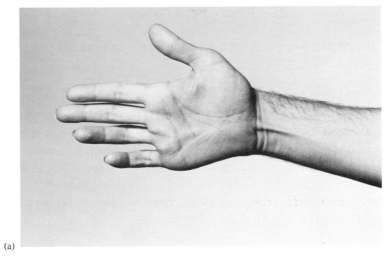

(a)

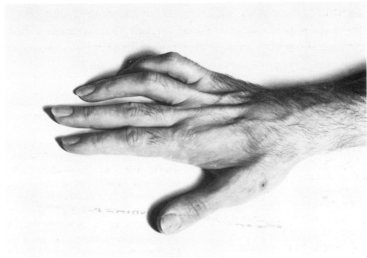

(b)

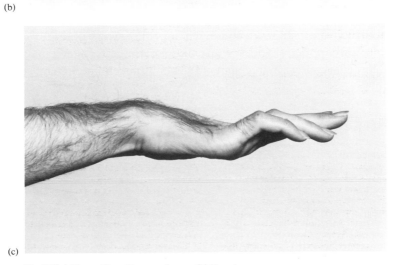

(c)

Fig. 3.30. (a) Loss of hypothenar eminence. (b) Dorsal guttering. (c) Typical ulnar claw hand.

31 / Visual field defect

Frequency in survey: Main focus of a short case in 6% of attempts at MRCP short cases. Additional feature in a further 3%.

Record 1

There is an *homonymous hemianopia*. This suggests a lesion of the *optic tract* behind the optic chiasma (with sparing of the macula and hence normal visual acuity).

Likely causes
1 CVA (?ipsilateral hemiplegia, atrial fibrillation, heart murmurs or bruits, hypertension).
2 Tumour (?ipsilateral pyramidal signs, papilloedema).

Record 2

There is a *bitemporal* visual field defect worse on R/L side. This suggests a lesion at the *optic chiasma*. (NB There may be optic atrophy, sometimes with a central scotoma, on the R/L side due to simultaneous compression of the optic nerve by the lesion.)

Possible causes
1 Pituitary tumour (?acromegaly, hypopituitarism, gynaecomastia, galactorrhoea, menstrual disturbance, etc.).
2 Craniopharyngioma (?calcification on skull X-ray).
3 Suprasellar meningioma.
4 Aneurysm.
Rarer causes are glioma, granuloma and metastasis.

Record 3

The visual fields are considerably constricted, the central field of vision being spared. This is *tunnel vision*. I would like to examine the fundi, looking for evidence of retinitis pigmentosa, glaucoma (pathological cupping) or widespread choroidoretinitis. (Hysteria may occasionally be a cause; papilloedema causes enlargement of the blind spot and peripheral constriction.)

Record 4

There is a *central scotoma*. (NB The discs may be pale [atrophy], swollen and pink [papillitis], or normal [retrobulbar neuritis].)

Causes to be considered

Demyelinating diseases (?nystagmus, cerebellar signs, etc.; however multiple sclerosis frequently causes retrobulbar neuritis without other signs)
Compression*

---

*There may be clues as to the site of the compression. (i) A lesion compressing the optic nerve in the frontal lobe may cause dementia. (ii) It may also cause contralateral papilloedema (the *Foster–Kennedy syndrome* due to a frontal tumour or aneurysm, e.g. olfactory groove meningioma). (iii) A lesion in front of the chiasma involving crossing fibres that loop forward into the opposite optic nerve may cause a contralateral upper temporal quadrantic field defect. (iv) A lesion at the chiasma may cause a bitemporal field defect. (v) A lesion at the lateral chiasma (pituitary tumour, aneurysm, meningioma) involving the terminal optic tract as well as the optic nerve may cause an homonymous hemianopia.

Ischaemia
Leber's optic atrophy (males:females = 6:1)
Toxins (e.g. methyl alcohol)
Macular disease
Nutritional (famine etc., tobacco-alcohol ambly-
    opia, Vitamin B$_{12}$ deficiency, diabetes mellitus)

Record 5

There is *homonymous upper quadrantic visual field
loss*. This suggests a lesion in the temporal cortex.

NB Field defects may sometimes originate from
retinal damage, e.g. occlusion of a branch of the
retinal artery or a large area of choroidoretinitis

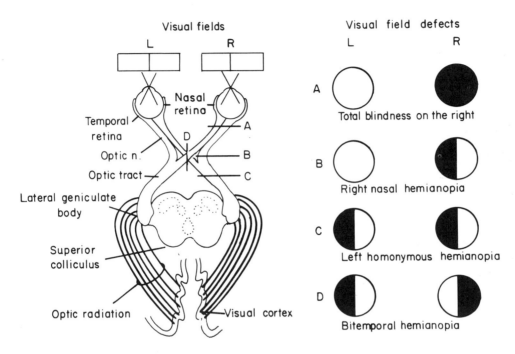

Fig. 3.31. The visual pathways and visual field defects
resulting from different lesions.

32 / Peripheral neuropathy

Frequency in survey: Main focus of a short case in 6% of attempts at MRCP short cases. Additional feature in a further 5%.

Record

There is *impairment* of *sensation* to light touch, vibration sense, joint position sense and pinprick over a *stocking* and, to a lesser extent, a *glove distribution* (much less common).
   The patient has a peripheral neuropathy.

Most likely causes

1   Diabetes mellitus (?fundi, amyotrophy).
2   Carcinomatous neuropathy (?evidence of primary, cachexia, clubbing).
3   Vitamin B_{12} deficiency (SACD not always present; ?plantars).
4   Vitamin B deficiency (alcoholics*).
5   Drugs (e.g. isoniazid, vincristine, nitrofurantoin, gold).
6   Idiopathic (50%).
There are many rare causes (see below).

Leprosy is a cause of major importance world-wide.

Important rare causes

Guillain–Barré syndrome (also motor involvement, absent reflexes, ?bilateral LMN VII n. palsy; ?peak flow rate)
Polyarteritis nodosa (?arteritic lesions)
Rheumatoid arthritis and other collagen disease (hands, facies)
Amyloidosis (? thick nerves, autonomic involvement)†

Causes of predominantly motor neuropathy

Carcinomatous neuropathy (?evidence of primary, cachexia)
Lead (wrists mainly)
Porphyria

Other rare causes of peripheral neuropathy

Myxoedema (?facies, pulse, reflexes, etc.—p. 138)

Acromegaly (?facies, hands, etc.—p. 104)
Sarcoidosis (?lupus pernio, chest signs)
Uraemia (?pale brownish yellow complexion)
Diphtheria
Tetanus
Botulism (can be mistaken for Guillain–Barré, encephalitis, stroke or myasthenia gravis; EMG resembles Eaton–Lambert)
Paraproteinaemia
Hereditary ataxias
Charcot–Marie–Tooth disease (?atrophy of peronei, pes cavus, etc.—p. 230)
Refsum's disease (cerebellar ataxia, pupillary abnormalities, optic atrophy, deafness, retinitis pigmentosa, cardiomyopathy, ichthyosis)
Arsenic poisoning (e.g. pesticides; Mee's transverse white lines may occur on the finger nails and raindrop pigmentation may occur on the skin)
Other chemical poisoning (e.g. tri-ortho-cresyl phosphate)

---

*Can also occur with nutritional deficiencies from other causes, e.g. dialysis for chronic renal failure, prison camp victims.
†Neuropathy is a feature of primary and myeloma-associated amyloidosis (it is exceptional in secondary amyloidosis). Carpal tunnel syndrome is not uncommon. Sensory or mixed sensory and motor neuropathy are commonest. Signs of autonomic involvement would be orthostatic hypotension, impotence, impairment of sweating and diarrhoea. The other organs mainly involved in primary and myeloma-associated amyloidosis include heart (cardiomyopathy), tongue (dysarthria), skeletal and visceral muscle and alimentary tract (rectal biopsy). See also footnote on p. 65.

33 / Hypertensive retinopathy

Frequency in survey: Main focus of a short case in 6% of attempts at MRCP short cases. Additional feature in a further 1%.

Record

The retinal arterioles are *narrow* (normal ratio of vein to artery is 1.1 : 1), they are (may be) tortuous and (may) vary in calibre (localized constriction followed by segments of arteriolar dilatation) with increased light reflex (copper or *silver wiring*) and *a-v nipping* (these changes all occurring with ageing and arteriosclerosis as well as with hypertension). There are *flame-shaped* and (less frequently) *blot haemorrhages*, and *cotton wool exudates* (all indicating grade 3 retinopathy and a diagnosis of malignant [accelerated] hypertension *even without* papilloedema), and there is *papilloedema* (indicating cerebral oedema; papilloedema may occur in malignant hypertension even without haemorrhages and exudates).

This is grade 4 hypertensive retinopathy.

The causes of hypertension

Essential—94% (cause unknown)

Renal—4% (renal artery stenosis—?*bruit*, acute nephritis, pyelonephritis, glomerulonephritis, polycystic disease, systemic sclerosis, SLE, hydronephrosis, renin secreting tumour, and renoprival—after bilateral nephrectomy)

Endocrine—1%* (Cushing's, Conns, phaeochromocytoma, acromegaly, hyperparathyroidism, hypothyroidism and oral contraceptive use)

Miscellaneous—< 1% (coarctation of the aorta—?*radio-femoral delay*, polycythaemia, acute porphyria, pre-eclampsia)

NB Cerebral tumour or raised intracranial pressure from any cause may lead to secondary hypertension (Cushing's reflex).

For colour photographs see p. 372.

---

*The figure 1% does not include hypertension due to oral contraceptive use.

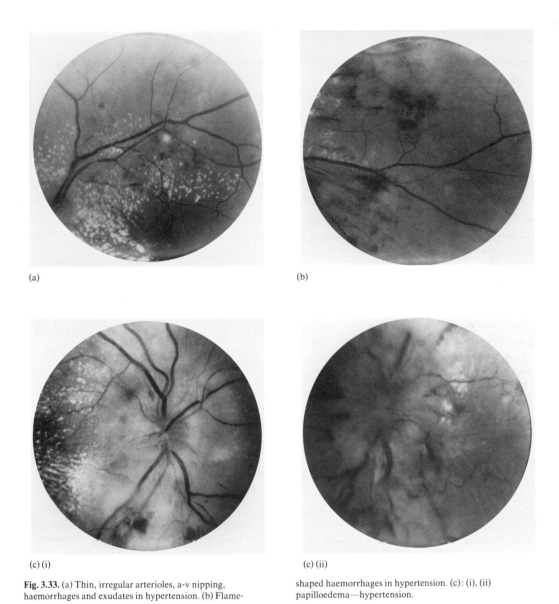

(a)

(b)

(c) (i)

(c) (ii)

Fig. 3.33. (a) Thin, irregular arterioles, a-v nipping, haemorrhages and exudates in hypertension. (b) Flame-shaped haemorrhages in hypertension. (c): (i), (ii) papilloedema—hypertension.

Frequency in survey: Main focus of a short case in 6% of attempts at MRCP short cases. Additional feature in a further 6%.

Record 1

There is nystagmus to the R/L and there is ataxia with the eyes open as shown by impairment of rapid alternate motion on the same side (*dysdiadochokinesis*). The *finger–nose test* is impaired on the R/L with *past pointing* to that side and an *intention tremor*. The *heel–shin test* is *impaired* on the R/L and the *gait* is *ataxic* with a tendency to fall to the R/L. There is *ataxic dysarthria* with explosive speech (staccato).

    The patient has a R/L cerebellar lesion.

Causes

1   Multiple sclerosis (?internuclear ophthalmoplegia, optic neuritis or atrophy, etc.—p. 316).

2   Brain-stem vascular lesion.

3   Posterior fossa space occupying lesion (?papilloedema; e.g. tumour or abscess*).

4   Cerebellar syndrome of malignancy (?clubbing, cachexia, etc.).

5   Alcoholic cerebellar degeneration (nutritional†).

6   Friedreich's ataxia (?scoliosis, pes cavus, pyramidal and dorsal column signs, absent ankle jerks, etc.—p. 220).

7   Other cerebellar degeneration syndromes.‡

Other cerebellar signs

Ipsilateral hypotonia and reduced power
Ipsilateral pendular knee jerk
Skew deviation of the eyes (ipsilateral down and in, contralateral up and out)
Failure of the displaced ipsilateral arm to find its original posture (ask the patient to hold his arms out in front of him and keep them there. If you push the ipsilateral arm down it will fly past the starting point on release without reflex arrest)

Record 2 (Vermis lesion)

There is a wide-based *cerebellar ataxia* (ataxic gait and Rombergism more or less the same with eyes open and closed; cf. sensory ataxia—worse with eyes closed), but there is little or no abnormality of the limbs when tested separately on the bed. This suggests a lesion of the cerebellar vermis.

---

*NB Otitis media may underlie a cerebellar abscess. Intracranial abscesses may result from direct spread from the upper respiratory passages (nasal sinuses, middle ear, mastoid). Less often the cause is haematogenous spread (e.g. intrathoracic suppuration), congenital heart disease or fracture of the base of the skull. Abscesses secondary to otitis occur in the temporal lobe about twice as often as they do in the cerebellum.

†Other causes of nutritional deficiency such as pellagra, amoebiasis and protracted vomiting may cause a similar syndrome.
‡The names associated with these other rare hereditary ataxias apart from Friedreich are Charcot, Marie, Déjèrine, Alajouanine, André Thomas, Gowers and Holmes.

35 / Retinitis pigmentosa

Frequency in survey: 6% of attempts at MRCP short cases.

Record

There is *widespread* scattering of *black pigment* in a pattern resembling *bone corpuscles*. The macula is spared. There is *tunnel vision*.

The diagnosis is retinitis pigmentosa.

The patient may well have presented with night blindness. The condition progresses remorselessly with increasing retinal pigmentation, deepening disc pallor of consecutive optic atrophy as the ganglion cells die, and increasing constriction of visual field. It may occur on its own although it is often associated with other abnormalities such as cataracts,* deaf-mutism and mental deficiency. Pigmentary degeneration of the retina may also occur in many conditions such as

Laurence–Moon–Biedl syndrome (autosomal recessive; ?obesity, hypogonadism, dwarfism, mental retardation and polydactyly)
Refsum's disease (autosomal recessive; ?pupillary abnormalities, cerebellar ataxia, deafness, peripheral neuropathy, cardiomyopathy and icthyosis)

as well as some of the

Hereditary ataxias
Familial neuropathies
Neuronal lipidoses (ceroid lipofuscinosis)

For colour photograph see p. 372.

*Visual acuity may sometimes be considerably improved by cataract removal.

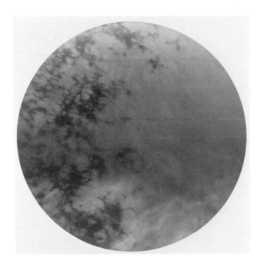

Fig. 3.35. Peripheral pigmentation resembling bone corpuscles.

36 / Carcinoma of the bronchus

Frequency in survey: Main focus of a short case in 5% of attempts at MRCP short cases. Additional feature in a further 4%.

Survey note: Candidates reported a variety of signs. The three *records* given are typical.

Record 1

There is *clubbing* of the fingers which are *nicotine-stained*. There is a hard *lymph node* in the R/L supraclavicular fossa. The pulse is 80/min and regular, and the venous pressure is not raised. The trachea is central, chest expansion normal, but the percussion note is *stony dull* at the R/L base and *tactile fremitus, vocal resonance* and *breath sounds* are all *diminished* over the area of dullness.

The likely diagnosis is carcinoma of the bronchus causing a *pleural effusion*.

Record 2

The patient is *cachectic*. There is a *radiation burn* on the R/L upper chest wall. There is *clubbing* of the fingers which are *nicotine-stained*. The pulse is 80/min, venous pressure not elevated and there are no lymph nodes. The *trachea* is *deviated* to the R/L and *expansion* of the R/L upper chest is *diminished*. *Tactile vocal fremitus* and *resonance* are *increased* over the upper chest where the *percussion note* is *dull* and there is an area of *bronchial breathing*.

It is likely that this patient has had radiotherapy for carcinoma of the bronchus which is causing *collapse* and *consolidation of the* R/L *upper lung*.

Record 3

There is a *radiation burn* on the chest. There are *lymph nodes* palpable in the R/L axilla. The trachea is central. I did not detect an abnormality in expansion, vocal fremitus, vocal resonance or breath sounds, but there is *wasting* of the *small muscles* of the R/L *hand*, and *sensory loss* (plus pain) over the *T1** dermatome. There is a R/L *Horner's syndrome* (p. 164).

The diagnosis is *Pancoast's syndrome* (due to an apical carcinoma of the lung involving the lower brachial plexus and the cervical sympathetic nerves).

Other complications of carcinoma of the bronchus

(i) Other local effects such as:
Superior vena cava obstruction (?oedema of the face and upper extremities, suffusion of eyes, fixed engorgement of neck veins and dilatation of superficial veins, etc.—p. 224)
Stridor (often associated with superior vena cava obstruction; dysphagia may occur)
(ii) Metastases and their effects (pain, ?hepatomegaly, neurological signs, etc.)

(iii) Non-metastatic effects such as:
Hypertrophic pulmonary osteoarthropathy (?clubbing plus pain and swelling of wrists and/or ankles—subperiosteal new bone formation on X-ray)
Neuropathy (peripheral neuropathy—sensory, motor or mixed; cerebellar degeneration and encephalopathy; proximal myopathy, polymyositis, dermatomyositis, reversed myasthenia—Eaton–Lambert syndrome)
Endocrine (inappropriate ADH, ectopic ACTH, ectopic PTH† and carcinoid)

*The weakness, sensory loss and especially pain may be more widespread (C8, T1, T2).

†Hypercalcaemia may also be due to bone secondaries.

Gynaecomastia (if rapidly progressive and painful may be an HCG secreting tumour)

Thrombophlebitis migrans (?DVT)

Non-bacterial thrombotic endocarditis

Anaemia (usually normoblastic; occasionally leucoerythroblastic from bone marrow involvement)

Pruritus

Herpes zoster (p. 278)

Acanthosis nigricans (grey-brown/dark brown areas in the axillae and limb flexures, in which skin becomes thickened, rugose and velvety with warts)

Erythema gyratum perstans (irregular wavy bands with a serpiginous outline and marginal desquamation on the trunk, neck and extremities)

Record 4 (Lobectomy)

There is a R/L *thoracotomy scar*. The *trachea* is *deviated* to the R/L. On the R/L side *chest expansion* is *diminished*, percussion note more resonant and breath sounds are harsher. The patient has had a R/L lobectomy to remove a tumour, resistant lung abscess or localized area of bronchiectasis.

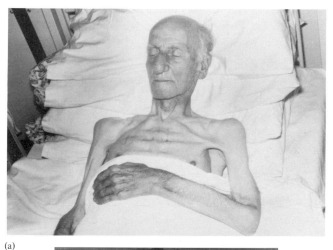

(a)

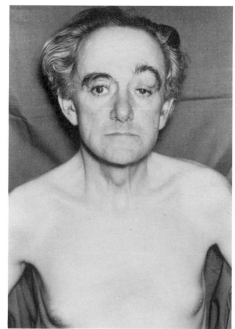

(b)

Fig. 3.36. (a) Cachexia due to carcinoma of the bronchus (note radiotherapy ink marks). (b) Pancoast's tumour (note gynaecomastia and left Horner's syndrome).

37 / Parkinson's disease

Frequency in survey: 5% of attempts at MRCP short cases.

Record

This man has an *expressionless, unblinking face* and slurred *low volume monotonous speech*. He is drooling (due to excessive salivation and some dysphagia) and there is *titubation*. He has difficulty starting to walk ('freezing') but once started, progresses with quick shuffling steps as if trying to keep up with his own centre of gravity. As he walks he is *stooped* and he *does not swing his arms* which show a continuous *pill-rolling tremor*. (He has poor balance and tends to fall, being unable to react quickly enough to stop himself.) His arms show a *lead-pipe rigidity* at the elbow but *cog-wheel rigidity* (combination of lead pipe rigidity and tremor—i.e. worse with anxiety) at the wrist. He has a positive glabellar tap sign (an unreliable sign) and his signs generally are *asymmetrical*—note the greater tremor in the R/L arm. (The tremor is decreased by intention but hand-writing may be small, tremulous and untidy.)

The diagnosis is Parkinson's disease.

Males:Females = 3:1

The features of Parkinson's disease are

Tremor
Rigidity
Bradykinesia
Bradykinesia (the most disabling) can be demonstrated by asking the patient to touch his thumb successively with each finger. He will be slow in the initiation of the response and there will be a progressive reduction in the amplitude of each movement and a peculiar type of fatiguability. He will also have difficulty in performing two different motor acts simultaneously.

Other causes of the Parkinsonian syndrome

Drug-induced (p. 206)
Post-encephalitic (increasingly rare; definite history of encephalitis—encephalitis lethargica pandemic 1916–1928; there may be ophthalmoplegia, pupil abnormalities and dyskinesias; poor response to L-dopa)
Brain damage from anoxia (e.g. cardiac arrest), carbon monoxide or manganese poisoning (dementia and pyramidal signs likely with all)
Neurosyphilis
Cerebral tumours affecting the basal ganglia

Other conditions which may have some Parkinsonian features

Arteriosclerotic Parkinson's (stepwise progression, broad-based gait, pyramidal signs)

Normal pressure hydrocephalus (following head injury, meningitis, or subarachnoid haemorrhage; urinary incontinence, gait apraxia, dementia)
Steele–Richardson–Olszewski syndrome (supranuclear gaze palsy, axial rigidity, a tendency to fall backwards, pyramidal signs, subtle dementia or frontal lobe syndrome)
Shy–Drager syndrome (idiopathic orthostatic hypotension, impotence, urinary incontinence, anhidrosis, cerebellar and pyramidal signs and peripheral neuropathy; L-dopa contraindicated)
Alzheimer's disease (severe dementia, mild extrapyramidal signs)
Olivo-ponto-cerebellar degeneration (sometimes familial; cerebellar and extrapyramidal signs)
Wilson's disease (Kayser–Fleischer rings, cirrhosis, chorea, psychotic behaviour, dysarthria, dystonic spasms and posturing; leading, if untreated, to dementia, severe dysarthria and dysphagia, contractures and immobility)
Jakob–Creutzfeldt disease (slow virus encephalopathy leading to rapidly progressive dementia with myoclonus and multifocal neurological signs including aphasia, cerebellar ataxia, cortical blindness and spasticity)
Hypoparathyroidism (basal ganglia calcification)

NB A condition which is often misdiagnosed as Parkinson's disease in the elderly is *benign essential tremor* (often autosomal dominant, intention tremor worse with stress, no other neurological abnormality; usually improves when alcohol is taken and sometimes with diazepam or propranolol).

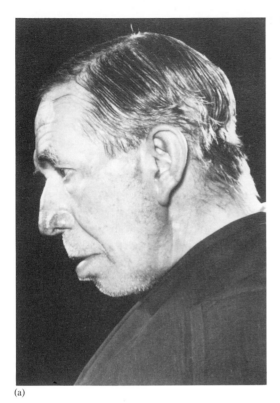

(a)

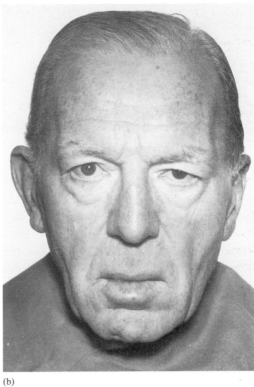

(b)

Fig. 3.37. (a), (b) Parkinson's disease.

38 / Chronic bronchitis and emphysema

Frequency in survey: Main focus of a short case in 5% of attempts at MRCP short cases. Additional feature in a further 1%.

Survey note: Usually the patients in the examination fall between the extremes of the classical *records* below.

Record 1

This thin man (with an anxious, drawn expression) presents the classic 'pink puffer' appearance. He has *nicotine* staining of the fingers. He is tachypnoeic at rest with *lip pursing* during expiration, which is *prolonged*. The suprasternal notch to cricoid distance is reduced (a sign of hyperinflation; normally > 3 finger breadths). His chest is *hyperinflated, expansion* is mainly *vertical* and there is a *tracheal tug*. He uses his *accessory muscles* of respiration at rest and there is *indrawing* of the *lower ribs* on inspiration (due to a flattened diaphragm). The percussion note is hyper-resonant, obliterating cardiac and hepatic dullness, and the breath sounds are quiet (this is so in classical pure emphysema—frequently, though, wheezes are heard due to associated bronchial disease).
These are the physical findings of a patient with emphysema.*

Record 2

This (male) patient (who smokes, lives in a foggy city, works amid dust and fumes, and has probably had frequent respiratory infections) presents the classic 'blue bloater' appearance. He has *nicotine staining* on the fingers. He is stocky and *centrally cyanosed* with suffused conjunctivae. His chest is *hyperinflated*, he uses his *accessory muscles* of respiration; there is *indrawing* of the *intercostal muscles* on inspiration and there is a *tracheal tug* (both signs of hyperinflation). His pulse is 80/min, the venous pressure is not elevated (may be raised with ankle oedema and hepatomegaly if cor pulmonale is present), the trachea is central, but the suprasternal notch to cricoid distance is reduced. *Expansion* is equal but *reduced* to 2 cm and the percussion note is resonant; on auscultation the expiratory phase is prolonged and he has widespread *expiratory rhonchi*. (His forced expiratory time [p. 32] is 8 seconds.) There is no flapping tremor of the hands (unless he is in severe hypercapnoeic respiratory failure in which case ask to examine the fundi—?papilloedema).
These are the physical findings of advanced chronic bronchitis† producing chronic small airways obstruction (and, if ankle oedema, etc., right heart failure due to cor pulmonale).

Causes of emphysema

Smoking (usually associated with chronic bronchitis; mixed centrilobular and panacinar)
Alpha$_1$ antitrypsin deficiency (?young patient; lower zone emphysema, panacinar in type; ?icterus, hepatomegaly, etc. of hepatitis or cirrhosis)
Coal dust (centrilobular emphysema—simple coal worker's pneumoconiosis—only minor abnormalities of gas exchange)

---

*Emphysema is, however, a pathological diagnosis.
†Chronic bronchitis, though, is defined as sputum production (not due to specific disease such as bronchiectasis or tuberculo-sis) on most days for three months of the year on two consecutive years.

Macleod's (Swyer–James) syndrome—rare (unilateral emphysema following childhood bronchitis and bronchiolitis with subsequent impairment of alveolar growth; breath sounds diminished on affected side—more likely to meet this in the slides section of MRCP Part 2)

Record 1 (continuation)

The decreased breath sounds over the . . . zone of the R/L lung of this patient with emphysema raises the possibility of an emphysematous bulla.

39 / Hypothyroidism

Frequency in survey: Main focus of a short case in 5% of attempts at MRCP short cases. Additional feature in a further 1%.

Record 1

The patient is *overweight* with myxoedematous facies (*thickened* and *coarse facial features*, *periorbital puffiness* and pallor). The *skin* is rough, *dry*, *cold* and inelastic with a distinct yellowish tint (due to carotenaemia), and there is generalized *non-pitting swelling* of the subcutaneous tissues. The patient's voice is *hoarse* and *croaking*, she is somewhat hard of hearing and her movements are *slow*. There is *thinning* of the *hair* which is *dry* and *brittle* and there is (may be) loss of the outer third of the eyebrows (not a reliable sign). The pulse is *slow* (give rate). There is no palpable goitre. The relaxation phase of the *ankle jerks* (and other reflexes) is delayed and *slow*.

This patient has *myxoedema* (? evidence of associated autoimmune disease—see below).

Record 2

As appropriate from the above plus: In view of the symmetrical, firm, finely micronodular (the typical features of a Hashimoto's goitre though there are many exceptions) *goitre* the likely diagnosis is hypothyroidism due to *Hashimoto's thyroiditis* (?associated autoimmune disease—see below).

Record 3

As appropriate from the above plus: In view of the *exophthalmos* it is likely that this patient was treated in the past for *Graves' disease* by radioactive iodine (or thyroidectomy, if scar) and is now hypothyroid (occasionally Graves' disease progresses spontaneously to hypothyroidism—see p. 92).

Associated autoimmune diseases

Pernicious anaemia (?spleen, SACD)
Addison's disease (?buccal + scar pigmentation)
Rheumatoid arthritis (?hands, nodules)
Sjögren's syndrome (?dry eyes and mouth)
Ulcerative colitis
Lupoid hepatitis (?icterus, etc.)
Systemic lupus erythematosus (?rash)
Haemolytic anaemia
Diabetes mellitus (?fundi)
Graves' disease
Hypoparathyroidism
Premature ovarian failure

Important symptoms (if asked to ask the patient some questions—NB deafness and hoarse voice):
Cold intolerance
Tiredness and depression
Constipation (may occasionally present to the surgeons with faecal impaction)
Angina (treatment may unmask, therefore start with low doses if age > 50, or if patient has angina)
Menorrhagia (middle-aged ladies)
Primary or secondary amenorrhoea (younger patients)

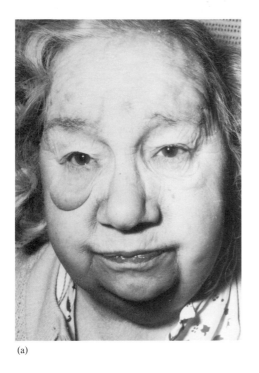

(a)

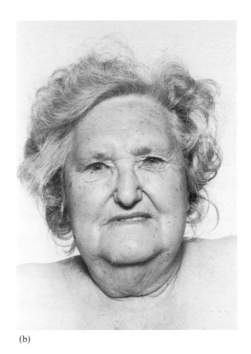

(b)

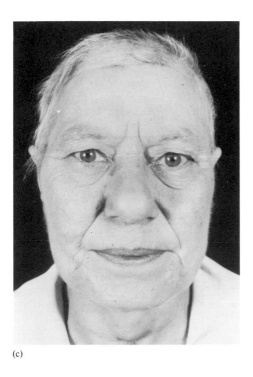

(c)

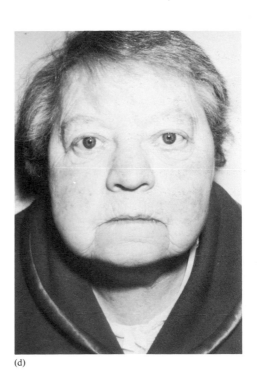

(d)

Fig. 3.39. (a), (b), (c), (d) Note thickened skin, periorbital swelling, sparse eyebrows and alopecia the patient in (d) had a malar flush (see also p. 373).

Other features

Anaemia (normochromic, iron deficient—atrophic gastritis, or megaloblastic—frank PA; slight macrocytosis may occur in hypothyroidism without a megaloblastic change in the marrow)
Carpal tunnel syndrome (p. 284)
Peripheral cyanosis (there may be a malar flush)
Raynaud's phenomenon
Hypertension
Accident proneness (may present to the Casualty Department)

For colour photograph see p. 373.

Hypothermia (especially the elderly living alone)
Hoffman's syndrome (pain, aching and swelling in muscles after exertion together with signs of myotonia)
Psychosis (myxoedematous madness)
Hypothyroid coma

A variety of other central nervous system disorders may occur,* such as peripheral neuropathy, cerebellar ataxia, pseudodementia, drop attacks and epilepsy.

---

*Always exclude concomitant vitamin B_{12} deficiency as the association with PA is strong. If you find peripheral neuropathy think also of concomitant diabetes mellitus before putting it down to the hypothyroidism.

Frequency in survey: 5% of attempts at MRCP short cases.

Record

There is *telangiectasia* on the face, around the *mouth*, on the lips, on the *tongue* (look under the tongue), the buccal and nasal mucosa and on the fingers, of this (?clinically anaemic) patient (who has none of the features of systemic sclerosis—p. 90).

The diagnosis is Osler–Weber–Rendu syndrome (hereditary haemorrhagic telangiectasia). The lesions may occur elsewhere, especially in the gastrointestinal tract, and may bleed. Patients may present with *epistaxis* (the most common and sometimes the only site of bleeding), *gastrointestinal haemorrhage*, chronic iron deficiency *anaemia* and occasionally with haemorrhage elsewhere (e.g. haemoptysis).

Autosomal dominant.

The telangiectasis consists of a localized collection of non-contractile capillaries and shows a prolonged bleeding time if punctured. In some variants (the pattern in individual families tends to be constant) pulmonary arteriovenous aneurysms are common and increase in frequency (as do the telangiectases) with advancing age. These cases may have cyanosis and clubbing, and bruits over the lung fields.

For colour photographs see p. 376.

Treatment

Chronic oral iron therapy may be required. Oestrogens (inducing squamous metaplasia of the nasal mucosa) may be helpful if epistaxis is the main symptom. Individual lesions should not be cauterized.

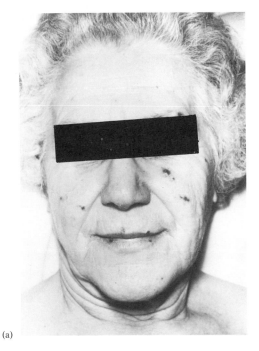

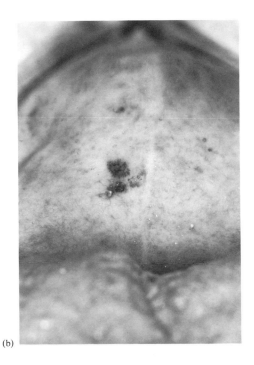

(a)   (b)

Fig. 3.40. (a), (b) Note palatal telangiectasia in (b).

41 / Abdominal mass

Frequency in survey: Main focus of a short case in 4% of attempts at MRCP short cases. Additional feature in a further 3%.

Survey note: Discussion usually concerned differentiation from/of enlarged organs (spleen, kidney, liver) or differential diagnosis.

Record 1

In this young (?somewhat pale-looking) adult patient there is a freely mobile 5×4 cm (measure) firm non-tender mass in the *right iliac fossa*. None of the abdominal organs is enlarged, and there are no fistulae.

The diagnosis could be Crohn's disease (p. 194).

Other causes of a mass in the right iliac fossa
1 Ileocaecal tuberculosis (?ethnic origin, chest signs).
2 Carcinoma of the caecum (?older person, non-tender and hard mass, lymph nodes).
3 Amoebic abscess (?travelled abroad).
4 Lymphoma (?hepatosplenomegaly, lymph nodes elsewhere).
5 Appendicular abscess.
6 Neoplasm of the ovary.
7 Ileal carcinoid (rare).

Record 2

A freely mobile tender 6×5 cm mass is palpable in the *left iliac fossa* in this elderly patient. None of the other organs is palpable.

It is probably a diverticular abscess.

Other causes of a mass in the left iliac fossa
1 Carcinoma of the colon (?non-tender, hepatomegaly).
2 Neoplasm of the left ovary.
3 A faecal mass (no other signs).
4 Amoebic abscess.

Record 3

In this thin and pale patient there is a round, hard 8×6 cm non-tender mass with ill-defined edges in the *epigastrium*. It does not move with respiration. Neither the liver nor the spleen is enlarged (check neck for lymph nodes).

The probable diagnosis is a neoplasm such as:
1 Carcinoma of the stomach (?Troisier's sign).
2 Carcinoma of the pancreas (?icterus. NB Courvoisier's sign).
3 Lymphoma (?generalized lymphadenopathy, spleen).

Record 4

In this elderly patient there is a *pulsatile* (pulsating anteriorly as well as transversely), 6 × 4 cm firm mass* palpable 2 cm above the umbilicus and reaching the epigastrium. Both femoral pulses are palpable just before the radials (no evidence of dissection) and there are no bruits heard either over the mass or over the femorals. (Look for evidence of peripheral vascular insufficiency in the feet.)

This patient has an aneurysm of his abdominal aorta (the commonest cause is arteriosclerosis†).

If you find a mass in either upper quadrant you should define its:

Size
Shape
Consistency
Whether you can get above it
Whether it is bimanually ballotable
Whether it moves with respiration
Whether it is tender.

In either upper quadrant it has to be differentiated from a renal mass (pp. 80 and 175); if in the left hypochondrium it has to be differentiated from a spleen (p. 74) and in the right hypochondrium from a liver (p. 95). Other causes of an upper quadrant mass include

Carcinoma of the colon
Retroperitoneal sarcoma
Lymphoma (?generalized lymphadenopathy, spleen)
Diverticular abscess (?tender)

*Pulsations without a mass may be transmitted from a normal aorta. A mass from a neighbouring structure may overlie the aorta and transmit (only anterior) pulsations.

†Mycotic aneurysms (see anecdote 23, p. 343) are a major complication (2.5% of patients with valvular infections) of infective endocarditis and are most commonly associated with relatively non-invasive organisms such as *Streptococcus viridans*. They may occur at any age, either during the active phase or months (sometimes years) after the endocarditis has been successfully treated. More common sites of mycotic aneurysms are brain (2–6% of all aneurysms in the brain), sinuses of Valsalva, and ligated ductus arteriosus. Clinical manifestations of abdominal aortic aneurysms (e.g. backache) appear after the lesions have started to leak slowly. Surgical treatment is almost always indicated.

42 / Dystrophia myotonica

Frequency in survey: 4% of attempts at MRCP short cases.

Record

The patient has *myopathic facies* (drooping mouth and long, lean, sad, lifeless, somewhat sleepy expression) frontal *balding* (in the male), *ptosis* (may be unilateral) and *wasting* of the *facial muscles*, temporalis, masseter, *sternomastoids*, shoulder girdle and quadriceps. The forearms and legs are involved and the *reflexes* are *lost*. The patient has *cataracts*. After he made a fist he was unable to quickly open it, especially when I asked him to do this repetitively (this gets worse in the cold and with excitement). He has difficulty opening his eyes after firm closure. When I shook hands with him there was a delay before he released his grip* (these are all features of *myotonia*). When dimples and depressions are induced in his muscles by percussion, they fill only slowly (*percussion myotonia*—e.g. tongue and thenar eminence).

The diagnosis is dystrophia myotonica.

Males > females.
Autosomal dominant.

Other features

Cardiomyopathy (?small volume pulse, low blood pressure, splitting of first heart sound in mitral area; low voltage P wave, prolonged PR interval, notched QRS and prolonged QT_c on the ECG; sudden death may occur)

Intellect and personality deterioration

Slurred speech due to combined tongue and pharyngeal myotonia

Testicular atrophy (small soft testicles but secondary sexual characteristics preserved; usually develops after the patient has had children and thus the disease is perpetuated; evidence regarding ovarian atrophy is indefinite)

Diabetes mellitus (end-organ unresponsiveness to insulin)

Nodular thyroid enlargement, small pituitary fossa but normal pituitary function, dysphagia, abdominal pain, hypoventilation, and postanaesthetic respiratory failure may also occur.

The condition may show 'anticipation'—progressively worsening signs and symptoms in succeeding generations; e.g. presenile cataracts may be the sole indication of the disorder in preceding generations.

Myotonia congenita (Thomsen's disease)

There is difficulty in relaxation of a muscle after forceful contraction (myotonia) but none of the other features of dystrophia myotonica (e.g. weakness, cataracts, baldness, gonadal atrophy, etc.). The *reflexes are normal*. Some patients have a 'Herculean' appearance from very developed musculature (?related to repeated involuntary isometric exercise). Myotonia congenita is usually autosomal dominant.

---

*There may be absence of grip myotonia in advanced disease because of progressive muscle wasting. Though myotonia can be relieved by phenytoin, quinine or procainamide, it is weakness (for which there is no treatment) rather than the myotonia which is the main cause of disability in dystrophia myotonica.

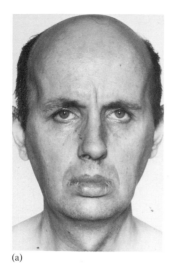
(a)

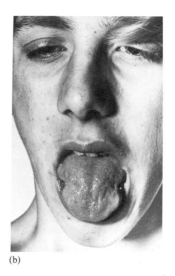
(b)

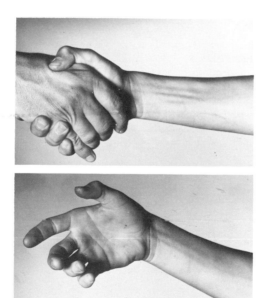
(c)

Fig. 3.42. (a), (b), (c) Note balding, ptosis, myotonia of the tongue and hands.

43 / Bronchiectasis

Frequency in survey: Main focus of a short case in 4% of attempts at MRCP short cases. Additional feature in a further 1%.

Record

This patient (who may be rather *underweight, breathless* and *cyanosed*) has *clubbing* of the fingers (not always present) and a frequent *productive cough* (the patient may cough in your presence; there may be a *sputum pot* by the bed). There are (may be) *inspiratory clicks* heard with the unaided ear. There are *crepitations* over the . . . zone(s) (the area(s) where the bronchiectasis is) and (may be) widespread *rhonchi*.

The diagnosis could well be bronchiectasis. The frequent productive cough and inspiratory clicks are in favour of this. Other possibilities (clubbing and crepitations) are:

Carcinoma of the lung (?heavy nicotine staining, lymph nodes, etc.).

Fibrosing alveolitis (marked sputum production and clicks are against this).

Lung abscess.

Possible causes of bronchiectasis

Respiratory infection in childhood (especially whooping cough, measles, tuberculosis)

Cystic fibrosis (young, thin patient, may have malabsorption and steatorrhoea)

Bronchial obstruction due to foreign body, carcinoma, granuloma (tuberculosis, sarcoidosis) or lymph nodes (e.g. tuberculosis)

Fibrosis (complicating tuberculosis, unresolved or suppurative pneumonia with lung abscess, mycotic infections or sarcoidosis)

Hypogammaglobulinaemia (congenital and acquired)

Allergic bronchopulmonary aspergillosis (proximal airway bronchiectasis)

Congenital disorders such as sequestrated lung segments, bronchial atresia, and Kartagener's syndrome*

---

*The features of Kartagener's syndrome are dextrocardia, situs inversus, infertility, dysplasia of frontal sinuses, sinusitis and otitis media. Patients have ciliary immotility.

44 / Wasting of the small muscles of the hand

Frequency in survey: Main focus of a short case in 4% of attempts at MRCP short cases. Additional feature in a further 11%.

Record

There is *wasting* (and weakness) of the *thenar* and *hypothenar* eminences and of the other small muscles of the hand so that *dorsal guttering* is seen. There is (may be) hyperextension at the metacarpophalangeal joints and flexion at the interphalangeal joints (due to the action of the long extensors of the fingers being unopposed by the lumbricals. In the advanced case a claw hand or *main-en-griffe* is produced).

Generalized wasting of the small muscles of the hand suggests a lesion affecting the lower motor neurones which originate at the level C8, T1 (unless there is arthropathy leading to disuse atrophy).

Causes

A lesion affecting the anterior horn cells at the level C8/T1 such as:

Motor neurone disease (?prominent fasciculation, spastic paraparesis, wasted fibrillating tongue, no sensory signs—p. 116)

Syringomyelia (fasciculation not prominent, ?dissociated sensory loss, burn scars, Horner's, nystagmus—p. 268)

Charcot–Marie–Tooth disease* (?distal wasting of the lower limb, pes cavus, etc.—p. 230)

Other causes are old polio, tumour, meningovascular syphilis, and cord compression

A root lesion at the level C8/T1 such as:

Cervical spondylosis affecting the C8/T1 level (usually affects higher roots—C6/C7, and therefore significant wasting of the small muscles of the hand is uncommon—see p. 198; ?pyramidal signs in the legs, no signs above the level of the lesion, cervical collar)

Tumour at the C8/T1 level (e.g. neurofibroma)

A lesion damaging the brachial plexus (especially lower trunk and medial cord) such as:

Cervical rib (symptoms provoked by a particular posture or movement, e.g. sleeping on the limb, cleaning windows, etc.; ?supraclavicular bruit though Raynaud's and other vascular manifestations are rare in the presence of prominent neurological features)

Pancoast's tumour (?Horner's, clubbing, chest signs, lymph nodes, cachexia, etc.)

Damage caused by violent traction of arm (e.g. the patient who tried to stop himself falling from a tree by grabbing a passing branch; the same damage in obstetric practice produces Klumpke's paralysis)

Combined ulnar and median nerve lesions

Arthritis leading to disuse atrophy† (wasting out of proportion to weakness)

Cachexia

---

*It is not known whether the degenerative process in Charcot–Marie–Tooth disease originates in the distal axons, ventral nerve roots or in the anterior horn cells.

†e.g. Rheumatoid arthritis. The factors which may contribute to small muscle wasting in the hand in rheumatoid arthritis are disuse atrophy, vasculitis, peripheral neuropathy, mononeuritis multiplex and entrapment neuropathy (median nerve at wrist, ulnar at elbow, and branches—e.g. the deep palmar branch of the ulnar nerve damaged by subluxation of the carpal bones on the radius and ulna).

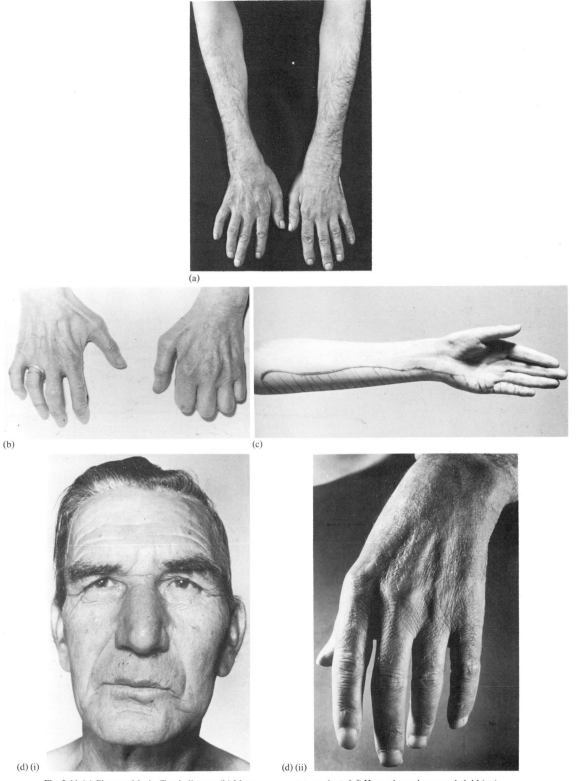

Fig. 3.44. (a) Charcot–Marie–Tooth disease. (b) Motor neurone disease. (c) Cervical rib. (d): (i), (ii) Pancoast's tumour (note left Horner's syndrome and clubbing).

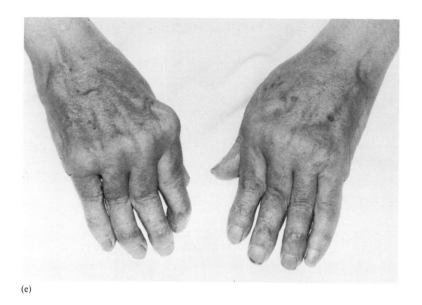

(e)

(f)

Fig. 3.44 (*continued*) (e) Rheumatoid arthritis. (f) Main-en-griffe (cervical rib).

45 / Generalized lymphadenopathy

Frequency in survey: Main focus of a short case in 4% of attempts at MRCP short cases. Additional feature in a further 6%.

Record

There is generalized lymphadenopathy with/without . . . cm *splenomegaly* (or hepatospleno-megaly).

The likeliest causes would be a *lymphoreticular disorder* (Hodgkin's and non-Hodgkin's lymphoma, reticulosarcoma, etc.) or *chronic lymphatic leukaemia*.

Other causes

Infectious mononucleosis (?sore throat)
Sarcoidosis (?erythema nodosum or history of)
Tuberculosis (?ethnic origin, lung signs)

Brucellosis (?farm worker)
Toxoplasmosis (glandular fever-like illness)
Cytomegalovirus (glandular fever-like illness)
Thyrotoxicosis (?exophthalmos, goitre, tachycardia, etc.—p. 108)

46 / Papilloedema

Frequency in survey: Main focus of a short case in 3% of attempts at MRCP short cases. Additional feature in a further 2%.

Record

There is bilateral papilloedema* (search carefully for haemorrhages, exudates and a-v nipping).

Possible causes

1 *An intracranial space-occupying lesion* (?localizing neurological signs†)

Tumour (infratentorial more often than supratentorial)

Abscess (fever not always present, ?underlying middle ear infection, underlying suppuration elsewhere—e.g. bronchiectasis or empyema)

Haematoma.

2 *Malignant hypertension* (check blood pressure—haemorrhages and exudates are not always present; ?narrow tortuous arterioles that vary in calibre, a-v nipping—p. 128).

3 *Benign intracranial hypertension‡* (?obese female aged 15 to 45, no localizing neurological signs).

The first sign of raised intracranial pressure is loss of venous pulsation, but recognition of this sign requires much practice and experience (see p. 21). If there is doubt about the normality of the disc, the presence of venous pulsation makes papilloedema and raised intracranial pressure unlikely.

Other causes of papilloedema

Meningitis (especially tuberculous)

Hypercapnoea (cyanosis, flapping tremor of the hands)

Central retinal vein thrombosis (sight affected, usually unilateral, dilated veins, widespread haemorrhages)

(Graves') Congestive ophthalmopathy (= malignant exophthalmos though exophthalmos is not always present; prominent eyes, eyelids and conjunctivae swollen and inflamed, marked ophthalmoplegia, often pain)

Cavernous sinus thrombosis (usually becomes bilateral, follows infection of orbit, nose and face; eyeball(s) protrudes, is painful, immobile and there is extreme venous congestion)

Hypoparathyroidism (tetany, epilepsy, cataracts, etc.)

Severe anaemia especially due to massive blood loss and leukaemia (there may be haemorrhages and cotton wool spots as well)

Guillain–Barré syndrome (papilloedema possibly due to impaired CSF resorption because of the elevated protein content)

---

*The disc oedema of papillitis (disc usually pink due to hyperaemia) must be differentiated from developing papilloedema due to raised intracranial pressure. Papilloedema causes enlargement of the blindspot and constriction of the peripheral field, but visual acuity is unaffected. Papillitis (optic neuritis affecting the intra-orbital portion of the optic nerve) causes central scotoma, diminished visual acuity, and sometimes tenderness and pain on eye movement during the acute attack. Furthermore, in papillitis there may be a pupillary reflex defect, loss of the central cup and cells may be present in the vitreous over the disc.

†VIth nerve palsy in the presence of papilloedema may be a false localizing sign due to raised intracranial pressure stretching the nerve during its long intracranial course. A localizing sign may occasionally be rapidly apparent in the case of contralateral optic atrophy—*the Foster–Kennedy syndrome* (a frontal tumour pressing on the optic nerve to cause atrophy and at the same time raising intracranial pressure to cause papilloedema in the other eye).

‡This syndrome is known to have occurred following middle ear infection which caused lateral sinus thrombosis. It may be that thrombosis of the venous sinuses is the aetiological factor in many other cases. The condition has been associated with the contraceptive pill, corticosteroids (often reduction in dose during long term therapy), head injury and times of female physiological hormone disturbance such as menarche, pregnancy and puerperium.

Paget's disease (large head, bowed tibiae)
Hurler's syndrome (dwarf, large head, coarse features, hepatosplenomegaly, heart murmurs)

For colour photograph see p. 372.

Poisoning with Vitamin A, lead, tetracyclines or naladixic acid
Ocular toxoplasmosis

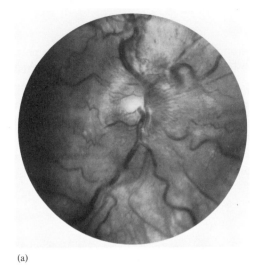

(a)

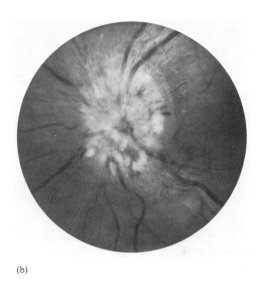

(b)

Fig. 3.46. (a), (b) Papilloedema.

47 / Diabetic foot

Frequency in survey: Main focus of a short case in 3% of attempts at MRCP short cases. Additional feature in a further 2%.

Record 1

There is an *ulcer* on the sole of the R/L foot (most commonly at the site of the pressure point under the head of the first metatarsal) and two of the toes have previously been amputated. There is thick *callous* formation over the pressure points of the feet, and the normal concavity of the transverse arch at the head of the metatarsals is lost. There is *loss* of *sensation* to light touch, vibration and pinprick in a *stocking distribution*. The feet are *cold*, the foot pulses are not palpable* and there is *loss of hair* on the lower legs which are *shiny*.

   This patient has *peripheral neuropathy*, a *neuropathic ulcer* on the sole of his foot and evidence of *peripheral vascular disease*. It is likely that he has underlying diabetes mellitus (?fundi).

Factors which may contribute to the production of the diabetic foot lesions

Injury—always a provocative factor
Neuropathy—trivial injury is not noticed
Consequent formation of callosities at repeatedly traumatized pressure points
Small vessel disease
Large vessel disease producing ischaemia and gangrene of the foot
Increased susceptibility to infection
Maldistributed pressure and foot deformity leading to increased likelihood of friction and trauma

From the list of causes of peripheral neuropathy (p. 126) **neuropathic ulcers** are particularly associated with
   Tabes dorsalis (?facies, pupils, etc.—p. 310)
   Leprosy
   Porphyria
   Amyloidosis
   Progressive sensory neuropathy (both familial and cryptogenic)
and rarely as a late manifestation of
   Charcot–Marie–Tooth disease (distal muscle wasting, pes cavus, etc.—p. 230)

Record 2 (Charcot's joint)

As relevant from *Record* 1 plus: The ankle joint is greatly *deformed* and *swollen*, and there is loud crepitus accompanying *movement* which is of an *abnormal range*.

   This is a Charcot's joint (neuropathic arthropathy—gross osteoarthrosis and new bone formation from repeated minor trauma without the normal protective responses which accompany pain sensation; the joint is painlessly destroyed).

The main causes *of a Charcot's joint*
   Diabetes mellitus (toes—common; ankles—rare)
   Tabes dorsalis (especially hip and knee;—?facies, pupils, etc.)
   Syringomyelia (elbow and shoulder;—?Horner's, wasted hand muscles, dissociated sensory loss, etc.—p. 268)
   Leprosy (important on a worldwide basis)
Other rare causes include yaws, progressive sensory neuropathy (familial and cryptogenic), other hereditary neuropathies (e.g. Charcot–Marie–Tooth), and neurofibromatosis (pressure on sensory nerve roots), though any cause of loss of sensation in a joint may render it liable to the development of a neuropathic arthropathy.

---

*NB In the predominantly neuropathic foot the pulses may be present or even bounding, and the veins may be prominent.

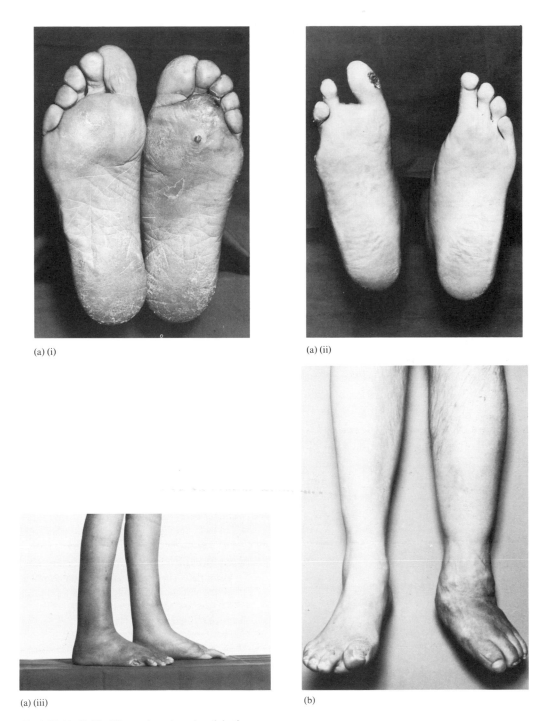

(a) (i)

(a) (ii)

(a) (iii)

(b)

Fig. 3.47. (a): (i), (ii), (iii) note ulcers, hyperkeratinization over pressure areas and loss of arches. (b) Charcot's ankle.

48 / Nystagmus

Frequency in survey: Main focus of a short case in 3% of attempts at MRCP short cases. Additional feature in a further 2%.

Survey note: In most cases nystagmus was cerebellar in origin—usually due to multiple sclerosis.

Record 1

There is nystagmus, greater on the R/L with the fast component to the same side. This suggests:
    an ipsilateral cerebellar lesion (?cerebellar signs—p. 130)
or
    a contralateral vestibular lesion (?vertical nystagmus, ?vertigo—see below).
(Now, if allowed, *look for cerebellar signs*; occasionally there will be signs of a lesion in the brain-stem, e.g. infarction—p. 320, syringobulbia*—p. 268.)

Record 2

The nystagmus is *ataxic* in that the abducting eye has greater nystagmus than the adducting eye. With this there is dissociation of conjugate eye movements. There is (may be) a divergent strabismus at rest. On looking to the right, the right eye abducts normally, but there is impairment of adduction of the left eye. On looking to the left, the left eye abducts normally but there is impairment of adduction of the right eye (occasionally the reverse may occur with weakness of abduction on each side but adduction remains normal). When the abducting eye is covered, however, the medial movement of the other eye occurs normally.

The diagnosis is *internuclear ophthalmoplegia*. It suggests multiple sclerosis† with a lesion in the medial longitudinal bundle. (Now, if allowed, *look for cerebellar signs*, pyramidal signs, pale discs, etc.—pp. 130 and 316.)

Causes and types of nystagmus

A diagramatic representation of conjugate gaze and its various connections is depicted in Figure 3.48. As can be seen from the multiplicity of these pathways a disorder within the end-organs (i.e. eye, labyrinth, semicircular canals), or in the medial longitudinal bundle anywhere through its long course, or in its nuclear connections (i.e. cerebellar, vestibular nuclei, etc.) can cause nystagmus. Nystagmus can be divided into:
    Optikokinetic nystagmus (a few brief jerks can occur in the normal eye at the extreme lateral gaze)

Ocular nystagmus (in patients with a congenital visual defect in one eye a pendular movement of the eye occurs while gazing straight—fixation nystagmus)
Vestibular nystagmus (see below)
Cerebellar nystagmus (*Record* 1)
Ataxic nystagmus (*Record* 2)

Vestibular nystagmus

This may arise in the periphery (labyrinth or vestibular nerve) or in the central vestibular nuclei and its connections.

*As can be seen from the diagram, the medial longitudinal bundle extends into the spinal cord so that syringomyelia confined to the spinal cord, if extending above C5, may also cause nystagmus.
†Internuclear ophthalmoplegia is highly characteristic of multiple sclerosis though rarely it may be caused by brain stem

gliomas or vascular lesions, or Wernicke's encephalopathy (ocular palsy, nystagmus, loss of pupillary reflexes, ataxia, peripheral neuropathy, Korsakoff's psychosis or other disturbance of mentation; dramatic response to thiamine in the early stages).

Peripheral The fast component is towards the contralateral side (except with an early irritative lesion when it can be on the side of the lesion) and the nystagmus is fatiguable—it becomes less and less intense on repetition of the test. The patient tends to be unsteady on the ipsilateral side (contralateral to the fast component) as can be revealed while testing for Rombergism (the patient cannot stand on a narrow base) and gait (tends to reel on the affected side). Cochlear function is usually affected (diminishes leading to deafness—e.g. Menière's syndrome) and the patient may have vertigo. Causes of peripheral vestibular nystagmus:

Labyrinthitis (probably viral and self-limiting; nystagmus may be absent and only positional and provoked by movements of the head—often it can be elicited by bending the head backwards about 45°—the nystagmus, as well as the vertigo, may appear but fades with repeated testing)

*Acute alcohol toxicity may cause nystagmus. Nystagmus is also almost always present in Wernicke's encephalopathy. Paradoxically alcohol may reduce congenital nystagmus—a condition which may be gross but symptomless.

Menière's syndrome (progressive deafness and tinnitus, with recurrent attacks of vertigo)

Acoustic neuroma (progressive tinnitus and nerve deafness; neighbouring nerves—Vth, VIth, VIIth may be involved and there may be cerebellar signs, etc.—p. 285)

Vestibular neuronitis (acute vertigo without deafness or tinnitus which usually improves within 48 hours; full recovery may take weeks or months; may be viral)

Other causes include degenerative middle ear disease, hypertension and head injury.

Central Lesions affecting vestibular nuclei (CVA, multiple sclerosis, encephalitis, tumours, syringobulbia, alcoholism,* anticonvulsants, etc.) cause nystagmus which is spontaneous but may be brought on or increased by head movements. It is not adaptable and usually has a vertical component.

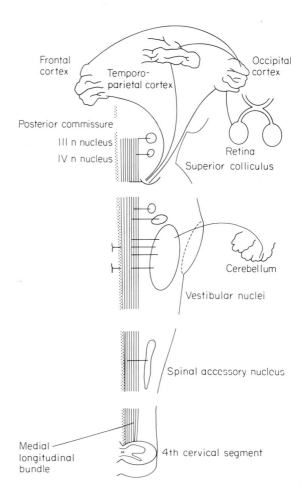

Fig. 3.48. Cortical, brain-stem and peripheral control of conjugate gaze. The medial longitudinal bundle starts just below the posterior commissure and ends in the upper cervical spinal cord. During its long course it receives fibres from various nucleii which are concerned with the control of conjugate gaze. Interruption in the cortical or midbrain connections often produces a disorder of conjugate gaze rather than nystagmus. Lesions in the brain-stem or below result in nystagmus.

49 / Old choroiditis

Frequency in survey: 3% of attempts at MRCP short cases.

Record

There is evidence of old choroiditis in the . . . region of the R/L fundus.
OR
In the . . . region of the R/L fundus there is a *patch of white* (or yellow or grey). It suggests exposed sclera due to atrophy of the choroidoretina secondary to old choroiditis. Together with this there are also scattered *pigmented patches* due to proliferation of the retinal pigment epithelium.

In most cases the cause of the choroiditis is unknown but *toxoplasmosis* is commonly implicated.

Other causes

Sarcoidosis (?lupus pernio, chest signs, etc.)
Tuberculosis (often inactive; ?ethnic origin, chest signs)

Syphilis (?tabetic facies and pupils, posterior column signs, extensor plantars, etc.)
Toxocara

For colour photograph see p. 372.

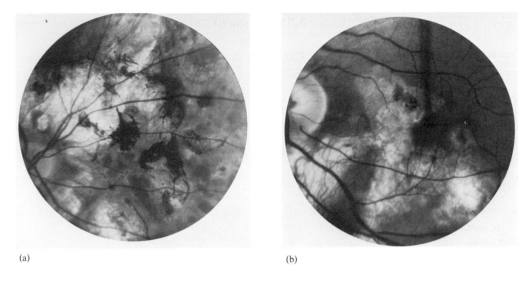

(a)

(b)

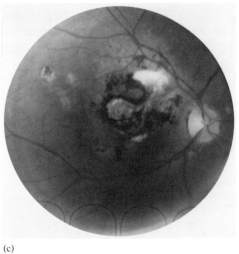

(c)

Fig. 3.49. (a), (b), (c) Three different cases of choroidoretinitis (the artifact on (ii) is the shadow cast by the internal fixation device of the fundus camera).

50 / Neurofibromatosis (von Recklinghausen's disease)

Frequency in survey: Main focus of a short case in 3% of attempts at MRCP short cases. Additional feature in a further 1%.

Survey note: Occurred as either a spot diagnosis, with or without a mention of the associated features, or as a case with an associated nerve pressure effect (such as one with an ulnar nerve/T1 lesion).

Record

There are multiple *neurofibromata* and *café-au-lait spots* (normal person allowed up to five of the latter).
  The diagnosis is neurofibromatosis.

or

There are multiple skin lesions: *sessile* and *pedunculated* cutaneous *fibromata*, as well as neurofibromata which are both *soft* and *firm, single* and *lobulated*, and felt both as mobile subcutaneous lumps* and *nodules* along the course of peripheral nerves. There are *café-au-lait* spots (especially in the axillae).
  The diagnosis is neurofibromatosis.

Autosomal dominant.
The condition is usually asymptomatic.

Complications

Kyphoscoliosis
Pressure effects of the neurofibromata on peripheral nerves and cranial nerves, especially:
 Acoustic neuroma (?Vth, VIth, VIIth, VIIIth nerve lesions, nystagmus and cerebellar signs; may be bilateral—p. 285)
 Vth nerve neuroma
Spinal nerve root involvement which may cause
 Cord compression
 Muscle wasting
 Sensory loss (Charcot's joints may occur)
Sarcomatous or other malignant change (5–16%)

For colour photograph see p. 379.

Lung cysts (honeycomb lung)
Pseudoarthrosis and other orthopaedic abnormalities
Plexiform neuroma†
Other intracranial tumours which can occur in this condition are:
 Gliomas (optic nerve and chiasma; cerebral)
 Meningiomas
 Medulloblastomas

Other features of neurofibromatosis

An association with phaeochromocytoma—5% of cases (?blood pressure)
Nodules of the iris
Hamartomas of the retina
Rib notching

---

*Neurofibromatosis should not be confused with lipomatosis with its characteristic soft subcutaneous lumps. In Dercum's disease (usually middle-aged females) subcutaneous lipomata may be painful and associated with marked obesity.

†An entire nerve trunk and all its branches are involved in diffuse neurofibromatosis with associated overgrowth of overlying tissues leading to gross deformities (temporal and frontal scalp are favourite sites but it may occur anywhere).

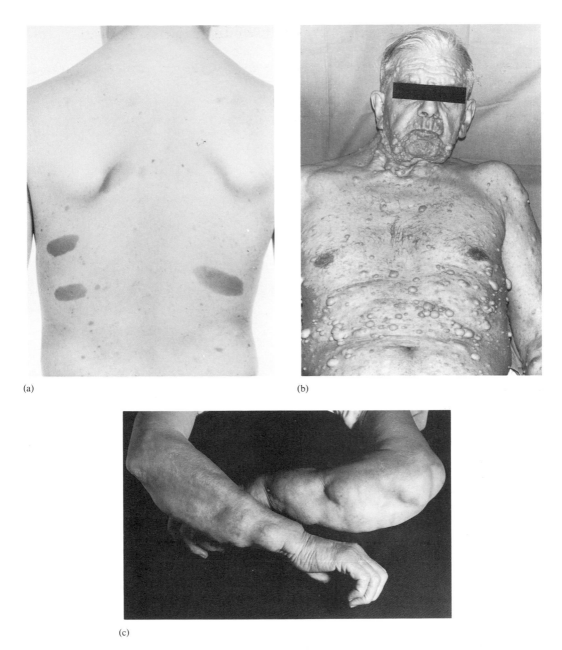

(a)

(b)

(c)

Fig. 3.50. (a) Café-au-lait spots. (b) Gross neurofibromatosis.
(c) Lipomatosis.

51 / Erythema nodosum

Frequency in survey: 3% of attempts at MRCP short cases.

Survey note: This usually occurs as a spot diagnosis followed by questions about the possible causes. Histology was asked for on one occasion.

Record

There are in this (usually) female patient *raised* (become flat with healing) *red* (pass through the changes of a *bruise* with healing), *tender* lesions 2–6 cm in diameter on the *shins* (and occasionally thighs and upper limbs).

The diagnosis is erythema nodosum (?fever, arthralgia).

Possible causes

1   Acute sarcoidosis (bilateral hilar lymphadenopathy; fever, arthralgia, palpable cervical and axillary lymph nodes, mild iridocyclitis).
2   Streptococcal infection (e.g. throat).
3   Rheumatic fever (tachycardia, murmur, nodules, etc.).
4   Primary tuberculosis (?ethnic origin, chest signs, etc.).
5   Drugs (sulphonamides, penicillin, oral contraceptives, codeine, salicylates, barbiturates).

Other causes

Pregnancy
Ulcerative colitis
Crohn's disease
Syphilis
Leprosy (important cause on a worldwide basis)
Tinea and other fungal infections
Coccidioidomycosis
Toxoplasmosis
Lymphogranuloma venereum
Behcet's disease (orogenital ulceration, iridocyclitis, etc.)
Idiopathic

For colour photograph see p. 379.

Histology

Perivascular mixed cell infiltrate followed by giant cell formation. There is oedema and a variable amount of extravascular blood. The inflammation spreads into the subcutaneous fat.

or

In a nutshell: subcutaneous inflammatory changes which are vasculitic in origin.

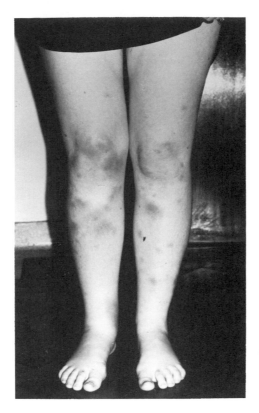

Fig. 3.51. Erythema nodosum.

52 / Horner's syndrome

Frequency in survey: Main focus of a short case in 3% of attempts at MRCP short cases. Additional feature in a further 1%.

Record

There is *miosis,** *enophthalmos* and slight *ptosis* on the R/L side (the other features are ipsilateral *anhydrosis* and vasodilatation of the head and neck).

This is a R/L sided Horner's syndrome (now examine the *neck* [scars, nodes, aneurysms], *hands* [wasting of the small muscles], and *chest* [ipsilateral apical signs]).

Causes of Horner's syndrome

1 Pancoast's syndrome (?wasting of ipsilateral small muscles of the hand, T1 and sometimes C7/C8 sensory loss and pain, clubbing, tracheal deviation, lymph nodes, ipsilateral apical signs).
2 Enlarged cervical lymph nodes especially malignant (?evidence of primary).
3 Neck surgery or trauma (?scars).
4 Brain-stem vascular disease (e.g. Wallenberg's syndrome†).
5 Brain-stem demyelination (?nystagmus, cerebellar signs, pyramidal signs, pale discs, etc.).
6 Carotid and aortic aneurysms.
7 Syringomyelia (?bilateral wasting of the small muscles of the hand, dissociated sensory loss, scarred hands, bulbar palsy, pyramidal signs, nystagmus—p. 268).

The syndrome can be caused by any other lesion in the sympathetic nervous system as it travels from the sympathetic nucleus, down through the brain-stem to the cord, out of the cord at C8/T1/T2, to the sympathetic chain, stellate ganglion and carotid sympathetic plexus (see Fig. 3.52b). Some cases of Horner's are idiopathic (usually females).

*NB Argyll Robertson pupils in neurosyphilis are usually bilateral, irregular and very small.
†Ipsilateral Vth, IXth, Xth, XIth nerve lesions, cerebellar ataxia and nystagmus. Contralateral pain and temperature loss—p. 320.

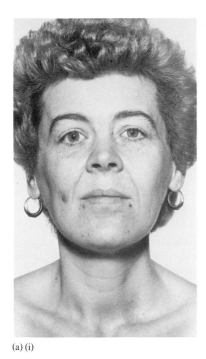

(a) (i)

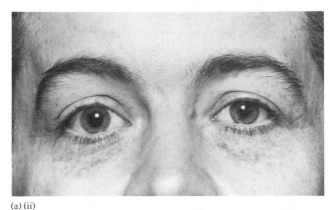

(a) (ii)

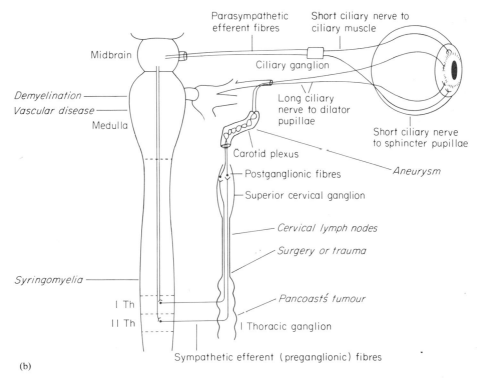

(b)

Fig. 3.52. (a): (i), (ii) left Horner's syndrome (note the scar over the left clavicle). (b) Sympathetic and parasympathetic nerve supply to dilator and sphincter pupillae. The diagram shows the sympathetic pathway and the sites where it may be interrupted to produce Horner's syndrome. (Pathways diagram adapted from *Gray's Anatomy of the Human Body* by kind permission of the publisher, Lea Febiger.)

53 / Old polio

Frequency in survey: Main focus of a short case in 3% of attempts at MRCP short cases. Additional feature in a further 1%.

Record

The R/L leg is *short, wasted, weak* and *flaccid* with *reduced (or absent) reflexes* and a normal plantar response. There is *no sensory defect*. The disparity in the length of the limbs suggests growth impairment in the affected limb since early childhood. The complete absence of sensory and pyramidal signs point to a condition affecting only lower motor neurones.*

The diagnosis is old polio affecting the R/L leg.

If you see one limb smaller than the other a possible differential diagnosis to consider is infantile hemiplegia. In this there is usually hemismallness of the whole of that side of the body and the neurological signs will reflect a contralateral hemisphere lesion (i.e. upper motor neurone).

---

*Fasciculation is only occasionally seen in old polio. Very rarely patients with old polio for many years develop a progressive wasting disease (with prominent fasciculation) which is indistinguishable from progressive muscular atrophy motor neurone disease or chronic asymmetrical spinal muscular atrophy (see p. 116).

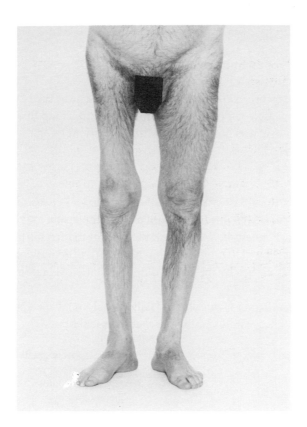

Fig. 3.53. Generalized wasting of the right lower limb due to old poliomyelitis.

54 / Ankylosing spondylitis

Frequency in survey: 3% of attempts at MRCP short cases.

Survey note: Candidates were asked to examine either the chest, the back, the neck, to watch the patient walk, or to watch the patient 'look at the ceiling'. One third of candidates made the point that the diagnosis was not apparent with the patient lying down.

Record

There is (in this male patient) *loss of lumbar lordosis* and *fixed kyphosis* which is compensated for by extension of the cervical spine (to attempt to keep the visual axis horizontal) producing a *stooped*, 'question mark' posture. When I ask the patient to turn his head to look to the side his whole body turns as a block (the spine being rigid with little movement). *Chest expansion* is *reduced*; the patient breathes by increased diaphragmatic excursion which is the cause of the *prominent abdomen*.

The diagnosis is ankylosing spondylitis. (If allowed, look at the *eyes*—iritis, listen to the *heart*—aortic incompetence, and examine the *chest*—apical fibrosis).

Males : Females = 8 : 1

Complications and extra-articular manifestations

Iritis—30% (acute, deep aching pain, redness, photophobia, miosis, sluggish pupillary reflex, circumcorneal conjunctival injection; may result in synechiae or cataracts)

Aortitis—4% (?collapsing pulse and early diastolic murmur of aortic incompetence; ascending aortic aneurysm)

Apical fibrosis—rare (?apical inspiratory crackles; probably secondary to diminished apical ventilation; there may be calcification and cavitation; may get secondary aspergillus infection)

Cardiac conduction defects—10% (usually AV block; other cardiac abnormalities may occur—pericarditis and cardiomyopathy)

Neurological (atlanto-axial dislocation or traumatic fracture of a rigid spine may injure the spinal cord—tetra/paraplegia; involvement of the sacral nerves at the sacroiliac joints may cause sciatica; rarely cauda equina involvement can cause urinary or rectal sphincter incompetence)

Secondary amyloidosis (kidneys, adrenals, liver—?hepatomegaly)

Other features

There is a strong (87%) association with HLA-B27. There is a familial tendency; 50% of relatives are HLA-B27 and 9% have sacroiliitis which may be symptomless. Ankylosing spondylitis usually starts before the age of 45.* It may present as an asymmetrical peripheral arthritis usually of large, weight-bearing joints; the small joints of the hands and feet are only rarely involved. It commonly presents with low back pain:

Ankylosing spondylitis—pain worse on waking, eases with exercise

Compared with

Mechanical back pain—no pain on waking; pain brought on by exercise

---

*In the early stages, loss of lateral flexion of lumbar spine is usually the first sign of spinal involvement, followed by loss of lumbar lordosis.

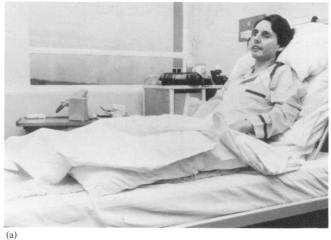

(a)

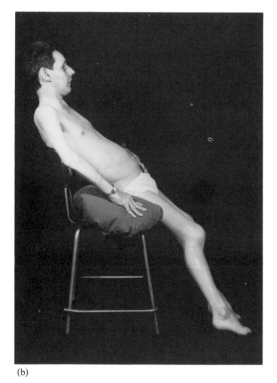

(b)

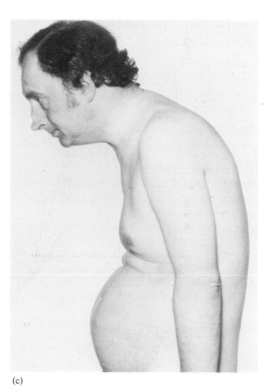

(c)

Fig. 3.54. (a) The ankylosing spondylitis is less obvious when reclining in bed. (b) In the same patient as Fig. 3.54a, a rigid and immobile spine was revealed by his attempt at sitting up (note the generalized involvement of the joints in this severe case). (c) Patient attempting to look straight ahead (note the kyphosis, loss of lumbar lordosis and protuberant abdomen).

Frequency in survey: Main focus of a short case in 3% of attempts at MRCP short cases. Additional feature in a further 3%.

Survey note: Relative frequencies in the survey: cerebellar ataxia 45%, spastic paraplegia 27%, sensory ataxia 9%, Parkinson's disease 9%, Charcot–Marie–Tooth (steppage) 9%. Neither hemiplegia, waddling gait nor gait apraxia occurred in our survey.

Record 1

The gait is *wide-based* and the arms are held wide (both upper and lower limbs tend to tremble and shake). The patient is *ataxic* and tends to fall to the R/L, especially during the *heel-to-toe* test which he is unable to perform. Romberg's test is negative.

This suggests *cerebellar disease* which is predominantly R/L sided. (Now, if allowed, examine for other cerebellar signs: finger–nose, rapid alternate motion, nystagmus, staccato dysarthria, etc.—p. 130).

Possible causes

1 Demyelinating disease (?pale discs, pyramidal signs, etc.—p. 316).
2 Tumour (primary or secondary—?evidence of primary—e.g. bronchus, breast, etc.).
3 Non-metastatic syndrome of malignancy (?evidence of primary especially bronchus—clubbing, cachexia, etc.).
4 Alcoholic cerebellar degeneration.
5 Familial degenerations (?pes cavus, kyphoscoliosis, absent ankle jerks and extensor plantars, etc. of Friedreich's ataxia).

Record 2

The patient has a *stiff*, awkward 'scissors' or 'wading through mud' gait.

This suggests *spastic paraplegia*. (Now, if allowed, examine tone, reflexes, plantars, sensation, etc.—p. 96.)

Possible causes

1 Demyelinating disease (?impaired rapid alternate motion in arms, pale discs, etc.—p. 316).
2 Cord compression (?sensory level with no signs above).
3 Hereditary spastic paraplegia (rare).
4 Cerebral diplegia (rare).

Record 3

The gait is ataxic and *stamping* (his feet tend to 'throw'; both the heels and the toes slap on the ground). The patient walks on a wide base, *watching his feet and the ground* (to some extent he can compensate for lack of sensory information from the muscles and joints by visual attention). He has difficulty walking heel-to-toe and the ataxia becomes much worse when he closes his eyes; *Romberg's* test is *positive*.

He has *sensory ataxia* (now look for Argyll Robertson pupils and for clinical anaemia).

Possible causes

1 Subacute combined degeneration of the cord (?pyramidal signs, absent ankle jerks plus peripheral neuropathy; anaemia, spleen, etc.; no Argyll Robertson pupils;—p. 273).
2 Tabes dorsalis (?facies, pupils, pyramidal signs if taboparesis, etc.—p. 310).
3 Cervical myelopathy (?midcervical reflex pattern in the arms; pyramidal signs in legs— p. 198).
4 Diabetic pseudotabes (?fundi).
5 Friedreich's ataxia (pes cavus, scoliosis, cerebellar signs, etc.—p. 220).
6 Demyelinating disease (ataxia in multiple sclerosis is usually mainly cerebellar).

Record 4

This (depressed, expressionless, unblinking and stiff) patient *stoops* and his gait, initially *hesitant*, is *shuffling* and has lost its spring. The *arms* are held flexed and *do not swing*. The hands show a *pill-rolling tremor*. His gait is *festinant* i.e. he appears to be continually about to fall forward as if chasing his own centre of gravity.

He has *Parkinson's disease*.* (Now examine the wrists for cog-wheel rigidity, elbows for lead-pipe rigidity, and for the glabellar tap sign, etc.—p. 134.)

Record 5

The patient has a *steppage* gait. He lifts his R/L foot high to avoid scraping the toe because he has a R/L *foot drop*. He is unable to walk on his R/L heel.

Possible causes

1 Lateral popliteal nerve palsy (?evidence of injury just below and lateral to the knee—p. 294).
2 Charcot–Marie–Tooth disease (?pes cavus, atrophy which stops abruptly part of the way up the leg, wasting of the small muscles of the hand, palpable lateral popliteal ± ulnar nerve—p. 230).
3 Old polio (?affected leg short as polio in childhood—p. 166).
4 Heavy metal poisoning such as lead (rare).

Record 6

The R/L leg is stiff and with each step he tilts the pelvis to the other side trying to keep the toe off the ground; the R/L leg describes a *semicircle* with the toe scraping the floor and the forefoot flops to the ground before the heel. The R/L arm is flexed and held tightly to his side and his fist is clenched.

The patient has a *hemiplegic gait*.

---

*In the mild case, tell-tale signs are (i) the lesser swing of one arm compared to the other; (ii) the tremor which is often unilateral.

Record 7

The patient has a lumbar lordosis and walks on a wide base with a *waddling gait*, his trunk moving from side to side and his pelvis dropping on each side as his leg leaves the ground. At each step his toes touch the gound before his heel. (This is a description of the typical gait of a patient with Duchenne muscular dystrophy—the commonest cause of a waddling gait. Other conditions causing wasting or weakness of the proximal lower limb and pelvic girdle muscles may also cause it—e.g. polymyositis.)

Record 8

The patient (an elderly person) walks with a broad-based gait, taking short steps and placing his feet flat on the ground like a person 'walking on ice'. (There is a tendency to retropulsion which increases the danger of falling.) The patient cannot hop on one foot.

This is *gait apraxia* (a common but little recognized disorder of the elderly; frontal lobe signs including dementia and grasp and suck reflexes will confirm the diagnosis). The commonest cause is a degenerative process similar to Alzheimer's disease. Other causes include subdural haematoma, tumour, normal pressure hydrocephalus, or a lacunar state. (Treatments include: small doses of L-dopa, mild stimulants, balancing exercises, use of a cane, daily walking.)

Frequency in survey: Main focus of a short case in 3% of attempts at MRCP short cases. Additional feature in at least a further 22%.

Survey note: Though an irregular pulse was usually encountered in the examination as a feature in the common valvular short cases, occasionally it was itself the main focus of a short case. This was often because the patient had a goitre.

Record

The pulse is . . . ./min and *irregularly irregular* in rate and volume suggesting controlled* (or uncontrolled if rate fast) atrial fibrillation. (Now look at the *neck* [goitre], *eyes* [exophthalmos], *face* [mitral facies, hypothyroidism,† or hemiplegia due to an embolus] and *chest* [thoracotomy scar]).‡

Differential diagnosis

The differentiation of an irregular pulse due to controlled atrial fibrillation from that of multiple extrasystoles, will depend upon the observation that only in atrial fibrillation do long pauses occur in groups of two or more (with ectopic beats the compensatory pause follows a short pause because the ectopic is premature). Furthermore exercise may abolish extrasystoles but worsen the irregularity of atrial fibrillation. Atrial fibrillation can be difficult to distinguish from atrial flutter with variable block, from multiple atrial ectopics due to a shifting pacemaker, and sometimes from paroxysmal atrial tachycardia with block. Only in atrial fibrillation is the rhythm truly *chaotic*.

Causes of atrial fibrillation

Ischaemic heart disease (especially myocardial infarction)
Rheumatic heart disease
Hypertensive heart disease
Thyrotoxicosis
Cardiomyopathy§
Acute infections (especially lung)
Constrictive pericarditis

---

*Though controlled atrial fibrillation may sometimes feel regular initially, if you concentrate there is a definite irregular variation in beat-to-beat time interval (NB experience 70, p. 340.)

†Previously treated Graves' disease now on inadequate thyroxine replacement—pulse rate slow, ankle jerk relaxation slow, etc.

‡If allowed follow up any positive findings from this *visual survey* by appropriate examination of the relevant system. If there is no visible abnormality proceed, if allowed, to examine the heart, the neck for a goitre, and thyroid status.

§Though in most patients with cardiomyopathy no cause can be found ('idiopathic'), sometimes the causal disorder can be identified. Some of the usual causes can be grouped as follows:
(a) Toxic (alcohol, adriamycin, cyclophosphamide, emetine, corticosteroids, lithium, phenothiazines, etc.).

(b) Metabolic (thiamine deficiency, kwashiorkor, pellagra, obesity, porphyria, uraemia, electrolyte imbalance).
(c) Endocrine (thyrotoxicosis, acromegaly, myxoedema, Cushing's, diabetes mellitus).
(d) Collagen diseases (SLE, polyarteritis nodosa, etc.).
(e) Infiltrative (amyloidosis, haemochromatosis, neoplastic, glycogen storage disease, sarcoidosis, mucopolysaccharidosis, Gaucher's disease, Whipple's disease).
(f) Infective (viral, rickettsial, mycobacterial).
(g) Genetic (hypertrophic obstructive cardiomyopathy, muscular dystrophies).
(h) Fibroplastic (endomyocardial fibrosis, Löffler's endocarditis, carcinoid).
(i) Miscellaneous (ischaemic heart disease, postpartum).

57 / Single palpable kidney

Frequency in survey: Main focus of a short case in 3% of attempts at MRCP short cases. Additional feature in a further 3%.

Record

There is a mass (describe consistency, edges, size, etc.) on the R/L side* of the abdomen in the mid-zone. It is *bimanually ballotable*, I can *get above it*, and the percussion note is *resonant* over it.

It is, therefore, likely to be renal in origin (check for the pale, brownish-yellow tinge of uraemia, dialysis fistula/shunt/scars, etc.).

Possible causes

1   Polycystic disease (p. 80) with only one kidney palpable.
2   Carcinoma (?weight loss, evidence of secondaries, anaemia, polycythaemia, pyrexia).
3   Hydronephrosis.
4   Hypertrophy of a single functioning kidney.

---

*NB A palpable right kidney may be normal in a thin person.

Frequency in survey: Main focus of a short case in 3% of attempts at MRCP short cases. Additional feature in a further 5%.

Survey note: Occurred in the examination (i) as part of cirrhosis; (ii) on its own without a clearly defined underlying cause, in which case it was the main focus and possible causes were often discussed; and (iii) in association with an obvious mass or the irregular liver of malignancy.

Record

There is *generalized swelling* of the abdomen and the umbilicus is *everted*. The flanks are *stony dull* to percussion but the centre is resonant (floating, gas-filled bowel). The dullness is *shifting* and a *fluid thrill* can be demonstrated (in tense, large ascites).

This is ascites.

Usual causes

1 Cirrhosis with portal hypertension (?hepatomegaly, icterus, spider naevi, leuconychia, etc.—p. 78).

2 Intra-abdominal malignancy (especially ovarian and gastrointestinal—?hard knobbly liver, mass, cachexia, nodes, e.g. Troisier's sign).

3 Congestive cardiac failure (?JVP↑, ankle and sacral oedema, hepatomegaly [pulsatile if tricuspid incompetence], large heart, tachycardia, S3 or signs of the cardiac lesion).

Other causes

Nephrotic syndrome (?young, underlying diabetes [fundi], evidence of chronic disease underlying amyloid, evidence of collagen disease, etc.—p. 275)

Other causes of hypoalbuminaemia (e.g. malabsorption)

Tuberculous peritonitis* (?ethnic origin, chest signs)

Constrictive pericarditis (JVP raised, abrupt x and y descent, loud early S3 ['pericardial knock'] though heart sounds often normal, slight 'paradoxical' pulse, *no signs in lung fields*; chest X-ray may show calcified pericardium; rare but important as response to treatment may be dramatic)

Budd–Chiari syndrome (ascites develops rapidly with pain, icterus but no signs of chronic liver disease, smoothly enlarged tender liver; causes include tumour infiltration, oral contraceptives, polycythaemia rubra vera, ulcerative colitis and severe dehydration)

Myxoedema (?facies, ankle jerks, etc.—very rare)

Meigs' syndrome (ovarian fibroma—important as easily correctable by surgery)

Pancreatic disease

Chylous ascites (due to lymphatic obstruction—milky fluid)

---

*NB Tuberculous peritonitis may attack debilitated alcoholics. Therefore it should always be considered when ascites is present in a cirrhotic. Fever or abdominal pain are suggestive but may not be present. Examination of the ascitic fluid may help—an exudative protein content (>25 g l⁻¹) with lymphocytes is also suggestive. Staining of the fluid for AFB is rarely positive and culture only positive in 20%. Diagnostic procedures include peritonoscopy (bowel adhesions may cause difficulty) and open peritoneal biopsy.

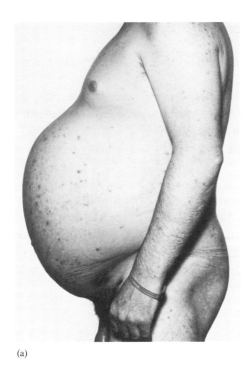

(a)

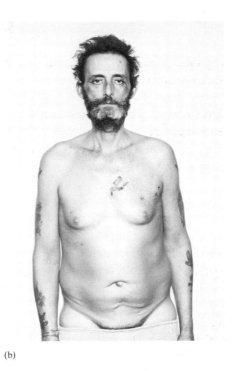

(b)

Fig. 3.58. (a) Gross ascites. (b) Residual ascites in another patient on treatment with diuretics (see also p. 79).

Frequency in survey: 3% of attempts at MRCP short cases.

Survey note: Patients with unilateral and bilateral lesions were seen. One case had buphthalmos. There was discussion on the skull X-ray appearance including the site of calcification and, on one occasion, on temporal lobe epilepsy.

Record

There is a *port-wine stain* (capillary haemangioma) involving the area supplied by the first (and/or second) division of the trigeminal nerve on the R/L side. There may be an associated ipsilateral intracranial capillary haemangioma* of the pia arachnoid with *tramline calcification* (which outlines the cortical mantle in an undulating manner) on skull X-ray and a history of *epilepsy*, in which case the diagnosis would be Sturge–Weber syndrome.

There may be a genetic predisposition.

Congenital abnormalities may be found in the eye on the affected side:
   Glaucoma (blindness frequent)
   Strabismus
   Buphthalmos or ox eye
   Angiomata of the choroid
   Optic atrophy

If the port-wine stain is in the area supplied by the first division of the trigeminal nerve the intracranial lesion is often in the occipital lobe. A facial naevus is more commonly associated with involvement of parietal and frontal lobes. The calcification seen on skull X-ray is in the cortical capillaries. The capillary haemangioma does not contain large vessels and does not fill on arteriography. The underlying brain damage is a rare cause of infantile hemiplegia (?hemismallness) and mental retardation as well as epilepsy.

For colour photograph see p. 375.

---

*Rare association with port-wine stain in real life but common in the examination!

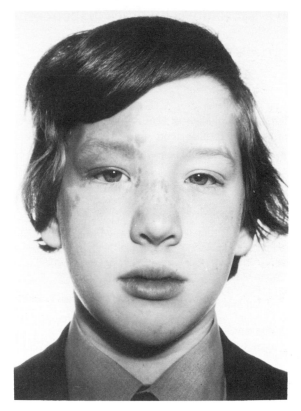

Fig. 3.59. Sturge–Weber syndrome (note strabismus).

60 / Necrobiosis lipoidica diabeticorum

Frequency in survey: 3% of attempts at MRCP short cases.

Record

There are *sharply demarcated*, coalescing *oval plaques* on the *shins* (occasionally arms and elsewhere) of this lady (usually a female aged < 40). The lesions have a *shiny atrophic surface*, with characteristic *waxy yellow* centres and *brownish-red edges*. There is (usually) telangiectasia over the surface.

The diagnosis is necrobiosis lipoidica diabeticorum.

It is rare, usually associated with diabetes, but can occur in the prediabetic and on its own. It may have to be differentiated from granuloma annulare, from nodular vasculitis when small, and from localized scleroderma or sarcoidosis when larger.

The lesions may ulcerate. Opinions vary as to whether good diabetic control can improve healing, but this should be tried. Gradual healing, with scarring, occurs over a period of years. Steroids (topical or local injection) administered cautiously (to avoid local atrophy) may help. Severe cases can be treated by excision and skin grafting. The histology varies, some containing large amounts of lipid, some not. There is necrosis of collagen, surrounded by pallisades of granulomatous epithelial cells, glycogen deposition is usual, and the aetiology is obscure.

Granuloma annulare (did not occur in survey): Pale or flesh coloured papules coalescing in rings of 1– 3 cm diameter on the backs of the hands and fingers. Blanching by pressure reveals a characteristic beaded ring of white dermal patches. It is sometimes associated with diabetes (latent or overt) especially when the lesions are extensive and atypical. The histology is almost identical to necrobiosis lipoidica diabeticorum. The lesions regress spontaneously.

Diabetic dermopathy (did not occur in survey): Atrophic pigmented patches (start as dull red oval papules; sometimes with a small blister) occurring mostly on the shins of diabetics. It has been suggested that they are precipitated by trauma in association with neuropathy.

Other skin lesions in diabetics

Infective (bacterial—boils, etc.; and fungal—candidiasis)

Foot/leg ulcers (ischaemic and neuropathic)

Vitiligo (?other associated organ-specific autoimmune disease—p. 254)

Fat atrophy (very rare with highly purified insulins)

Fat hypertrophy (recurrent injection of insulin into the same site)

Xanthomata (associated hyperlipidaemia—disappear with control of diabetes as this causes improvement in the hyperlipidaemia—p. 204)

Insulin allergy (immediate and delayed; though less likely this can even occur in patients on human insulin given subcutaneously)

Sulphonylurea allergy (erythema multiforme, phototoxic and other eruptions)

Chlorpropamide alcohol flush (a subtype of diabetes that may have a lower incidence of complications)

Pseudoxanthoma nigricans (like acanthosis nigricans but benign; occurs in obese diabetics and may improve with weight loss)

Peripheral anhydrosis (due to autonomic neuropathy)

For colour photograph see p. 380.

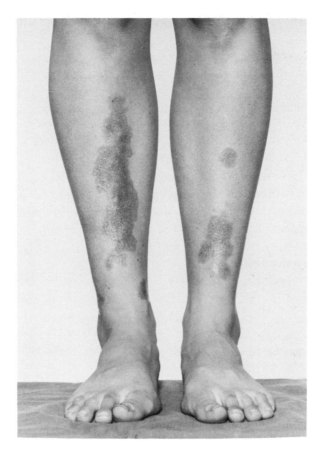

Fig. 3.60. Necrobiosis lipoidica diabeticorum.

61 / Ventricular septal defect

Frequency in survey: Main focus of a short case in 3% of attempts at MRCP short cases. Additional feature in a further 1%.

Survey note: Youthfulness of patient sometimes a clue to the diagnosis.

Record

The pulse is regular (give rate) and the venous pressure is not raised. The apex beat is (may be) palpable half-way between the midclavicular line and the anterior axillary line, and there is a *left parasternal heave* (there may be a systolic thrill). There is a *pansystolic murmur* at the lower left sternal edge which is also audible at the apex. (The pulmonary second sound may be loud due to pulmonary hypertension and there may be an early diastolic murmur of secondary pulmonary incompetence.)

The diagnosis is ventricular septal defect.

Other features of VSD

Maladie de Roger (small haemodynamically insignificant hole, loud murmur, normal heart size, etc.; tends to close spontaneously)

Development of Eisenmenger's complex (p. 192) if a significant defect is left untreated

Susceptibility to subacute bacterial endocarditis (defects of all sizes—NB chemoprophylaxis)

Association with aortic incompetence in 5% of cases (10% in Japan)

Possibility of a mitral mid-diastolic flow murmur if shunt is large

May occur following acute myocardial infarction with septal rupture

Sometimes associated with Down's syndrome and Turner's syndrome

62 / Lower motor neurone VIIth nerve palsy

Frequency in survey: 3% of attempts at MRCP short cases.

Record

On the R/L side there is *paralysis* of the *upper* and lower face*, so that the *eye cannot be closed* (or it can easily be opened by the examiner); the eyeball turns up on attempted closure (*Bell's phenomenon*) and the patient is unable to raise his R/L eyebrow. The corner of the *mouth droops*, the *nasolabial fold* is *smoothed* out, and the voluntary and involuntary (i.e. including emotional) movements of the mouth are paralysed on the R/L side (the lips may be drawn to the opposite side and the tongue may deviate as well—not necessarily hypoglossal involvement—see footnote, p. 56).

This is a R/L lower motor neurone VIIth nerve lesion (now check the ipsilateral ear for evidence of *herpes zoster*).

Causes of a lower motor neurone VIIth nerve lesion

1 Bell's palsy.†
2 Ramsay Hunt syndrome (herpes zoster on the external auditory meatus and the geniculate ganglion—taste to the anterior two-thirds of the tongue is lost; there may be lesions on the fauces and palate).

Other differential diagnoses

Cerebello-pontine angle compression (acoustic neuroma or meningioma; Vth, VIth, VIIth, VIIIth nerve palsy, cerebellar signs and loss of taste to the anterior two-thirds of the tongue—p. 285)
Parotid tumour (?palpable; taste not affected)
Trauma
A pontine lesion (e.g. multiple sclerosis, tumour or vascular lesion)
Middle ear disease (deafness)
The causes of mononeuritis multiplex (diabetes, polyarteritis nodosa and Churg–Strauss syndrome, rheumatoid, SLE, Wegener's, sarcoid, carcinoma, amyloid and leprosy)

Myasthenia gravis (?ptosis, variable strabismus, proximal muscle weakness, etc.—p. 246)
Congenital facial diplegia
Some forms of muscular dystrophy
Motor neurone disease (rarely)

The chorda tympani leaves the facial nerve in the middle ear to supply taste to the anterior two-thirds of the tongue. The superficial petrosal branch to supply the lachrymal glands, and the nerve to stapedius both leave higher in the facial canal than the chorda tympani. The level of the lesion in the facial canal can sometimes be assessed (very unlikely to be required in the examination) by assessing the relative involvement of these nerves.

Causes of bilateral lower motor neurone VIIth nerve paralysis‡

Guillain–Barré syndrome (occasionally only VIIth nerves affected)
Sarcoidosis (parotid gland enlargement not always present)
Bilateral Bell's palsy

Variation of the Ramsay Hunt syndrome Occasionally facial palsy is associated with trigeminal, occipital or cervical herpes with or without auditory involvement (see anecdote 24, p. 343). In some of these cases the geniculate ganglion may be spared—see p. 278.

---

*i.e. including frontalis ('raise eyebrows'), corrugator superficialis ('frown') and orbicularis oculi ('close your eyes tight').
†In the mild case of Bell's palsy taste over the anterior two-thirds of the tongue is usually preserved, because the lesion is due to swelling of the nerve in the confined lower facial canal.

In cases with more extensive involvement this taste is lost and the patient may also show increased susceptibility to high-pitched or loud sounds (hyperacusis due to stapedius paralysis).
‡Bilateral lower motor neurone VIIth nerve lesions are easily missed because there is no asymmetry.

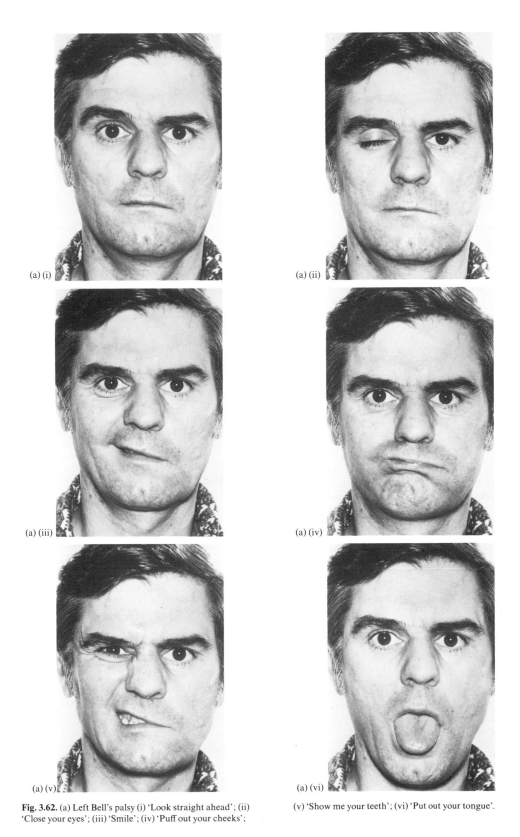

(a) (i)

(a) (ii)

(a) (iii)

(a) (iv)

(a) (v)

(a) (vi)

Fig. 3.62. (a) Left Bell's palsy (i) 'Look straight ahead'; (ii) 'Close your eyes'; (iii) 'Smile'; (iv) 'Puff out your cheeks'; (v) 'Show me your teeth'; (vi) 'Put out your tongue'.

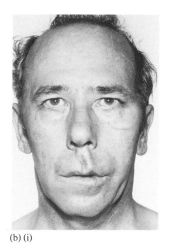

(b) (i)

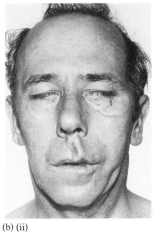

(b) (ii)

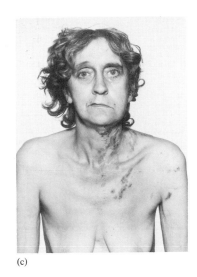

(c)

Fig. 3.62 (*continued*) (b)(i) Bilateral lower motor neurone seventh nerve palsy (Guillain–Barré syndrome), (ii) 'Close your eyes'. (c) Ramsay Hunt syndrome.

63 / Clubbing

Frequency in survey: Main focus of a short case in 2% of attempts at MRCP short cases. Additional feature in a further 13%.

Record

There is finger clubbing* (*thickening of the nail bed*† with *loss of the obtuse angle* between the nail and the dorsum of the finger—becomes > 180°; *increased curvature* of the nail bed—both side-to-side and lengthwise; increased *sponginess or fluctuation* of the nail bed; and sometimes, when there is marked swelling of the nail bed, the fingers may have a *drumstick appearance*).

Causes of clubbing

1 Carcinoma of the bronchus (the commonest cause—?nicotine staining, obvious weight loss with temporal dimples, lymph nodes, chest signs, evidence of secondaries, etc.—p. 132).
2 Fibrosing alveolitis (?basal crackles—p. 97).
3 Cyanotic congenital heart disease (?cyanosis, thoracotomy scars, Fallot's—p. 258, Eisenmenger's—p. 192).
4 Bronchiectasis (?productive cough, crepitations, etc.—p. 146).
5 Cirrhosis (?icterus, spider naevi, palmar erythema, Dupuytren's, xanthelasma—especially in primary biliary cirrhosis, hepatosplenomegaly, etc.—p. 78).

Other causes

Subacute bacterial endocarditis (heart murmur, fever, splenomegaly, petechiae, splinter haemorrhages, Osler's nodes, Janeway's lesions, Roth spots, etc.)
Empyema
Lung abscess
Crohn's disease
Ulcerative colitis
Asbestosis (especially with mesothelioma)
Thyroid acropachy (?exophthalmos, pretibial myxoedema, goitre, thyroid status, etc.—p. 108)
Hereditary (rare; dominant)

*Indisputable clubbing is one of the important fundamental clinical signs which, when present, have clear implications. Less clear-cut changes in the finger nails are susceptible to assessment which (even if dogmatic) may be very subjective. Such finger nails are best described as showing 'debatable clubbing' (in that physicians will disagree as to whether there are significant changes or not). Genuine 'debatable clubbing' occurring in the examination may cause trouble if you recognize it as such, but you are not sure what your examiners' opinion is. The safest course in a case of doubt is to use nail bed thickening as your guide and quote the nail angle rule in a way that cannot be argued with. For example: 'The appearance of the nails (e.g. increased curvature) is initially suggestive of clubbing, but the obtuse angle between the nail and the dorsum of the finger is preserved, and therefore by definition (loss of the angle being the "official" first sign) the diagnosis of definite clubbing cannot be accepted in this case'.
†Before palpating always inspect the fingers in profile for a slightly bulbous appearance due to thickening of the nail bed.

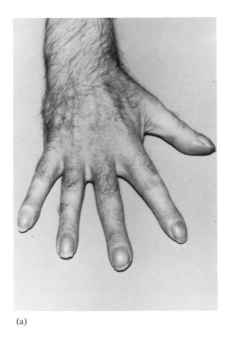

(a)

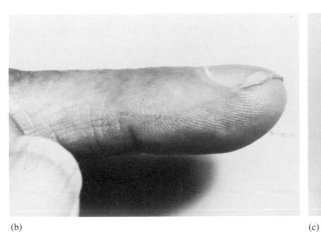

(b)

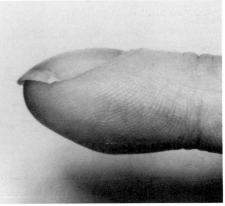

(c)

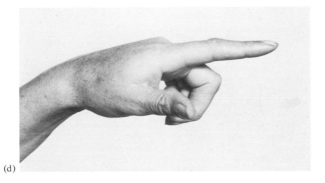

(d)

Fig. 3.63. (a) Clubbing (carcinoma of the bronchus). (b) Loss of the angle. (c) Thickening of the nail bed (early drumstick appearance—same patient as in (a)). (d) Clubbing and leuconychia (cirrhosis of the liver).

64 / Retinal vein thrombosis

Frequency in survey: 2% of attempts at MRCP short cases.

Record

The veins are *tortuous* and *engorged*. *Haemorrhages* are *scattered riotously* over the whole retina, irregular and superficial, like bundles of straw alongside the veins (*papilloedema* and *soft exudates* may also be seen).

The diagnosis is central retinal vein thrombosis. There may be an underlying *hyperviscosity syndrome,** especially *Waldenstrom's macroglobulinaemia* (?lymphadenopathy, hepatosplenomegaly, bruising and purpura), but also occasionally *myeloma* (?urinary Bence–Jones protein) and *connective tissue disorders*.

The condition is commoner in eyes prone to simple glaucoma (which should, therefore, be excluded in the other eye), in the elderly arteriosclerotic, and the hypertensive, but may also arise in young adults (especially women). It causes incomplete loss of vision and improvement may be scant. About three months after the acute event 20% of cases lose the remaining sight in the affected eye because of an acute secondary glaucoma. This is due to new vessels on the iris root developing as a result of retinal hypoxia.

In **thrombosis of a branch of the retinal vein** (also occurred in our survey) the occlusion usually occurs at an arteriovenous crossing with the changes confined to the sector beyond this (any loss of sight† recovers; no secondary glaucoma). In view of the association with hypertension, hypertensive changes may be visible in the rest of the fundus (thin arterioles, a-v nipping, etc.).

For colour photographs see pp. 372–3.

---

*The symptoms and signs of a hyperviscosity syndrome are principally neurological due to sluggish cerebral circulation. Cardiac failure may occur in the elderly. Waldenstrom's macroglobulinaemia is the cause in 90% of hyperviscosity syndromes.

†Think of this diagnosis if you find a quandrantic field defect in one eye only.

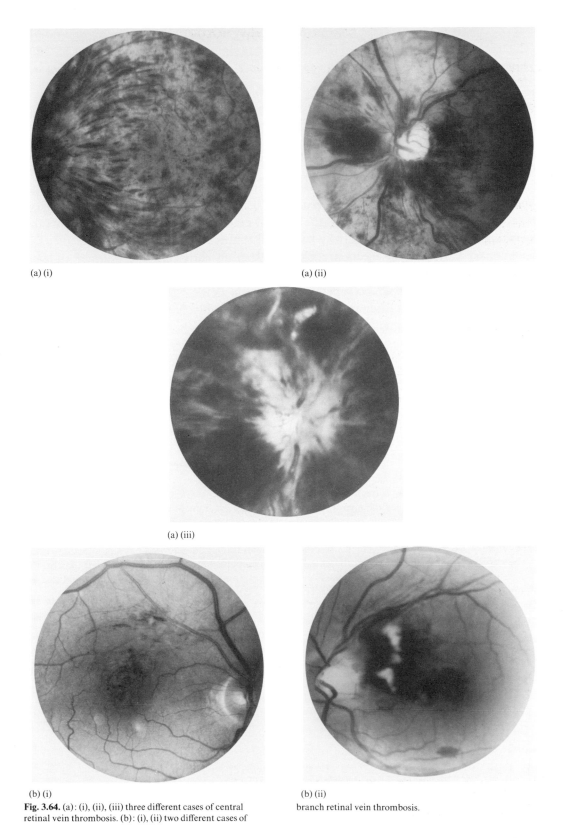

(a) (i)

(a) (ii)

(a) (iii)

(b) (i)

(b) (ii)

Fig. 3.64. (a): (i), (ii), (iii) three different cases of central retinal vein thrombosis. (b): (i), (ii) two different cases of branch retinal vein thrombosis.

65 / Eisenmenger's syndrome

Frequency in survey: Main focus of a short case in 2% of attempts at MRCP short cases. Additional feature in a further 1%.

Record

There is *central cyanosis* and *clubbing* of the fingers (may be only in the toes in patent ductus arteriosus). The pulse (give rate) is regular (and small in volume). A large *a* wave is (may be) seen in the venous pulse (due to forceful atrial contraction in the face of the right ventricular hypertrophy). There is a marked *left parasternal heave* and (often) a palpable (pulmonary) second heart sound. On auscultation (the signs of pulmonary hypertension are heard) the *second heart sound* is *loud*, there is (may be) a right ventricular fourth heart sound, (may be) a pulmonary early systolic ejection click, (may be) an early diastolic murmur (dilated pulmonary artery leads to secondary pulmonary incompetence), and (may be) a pansystolic murmur (secondary tricuspid incompetence—*v* wave in JVP).

These findings suggest Eisenmenger's syndrome with pulmonary hypertension leading to reversal of a left-to-right shunt.

Causes

1   Ventricular septal defect* (single or closely split second heart sound because the right and left venticular pressures are similar).
2   Atrial septal defect (fixed and wide splitting of the second sound).
3   Patent ductus arteriosus† (normal splitting of the second sound—*P2* follows *A2* and the split widens with inspiration; only the lower limbs are cyanosed—differential cyanosis).

Once Eisenmenger's syndrome has developed it is too late (high mortality) for corrective surgery. Death commonly occurs between the ages of twenty and forty years and is usually due to pulmonary infarction, right heart failure, dysrhythmias and, less often, infective endocarditis or cerebral abscess.

The absence of chest signs helps to differentiate Eisenmenger's syndrome from the cyanosis and pulmonary hypertension of cor pulmonale. The features which may be helpful in differentiating Eisenmenger's syndrome from Fallot's tetralogy (the commonest cause of central cyanosis in the adolescent or young adult) are shown in Table 3.65. Furthermore, the patient with Fallot's tetralogy in the examination may well have thoracotomy scars and a pulse which is weaker on the left than on the right, from a previous Blalock shunt operation (see p. 258).

---

*When due to a VSD it is termed Eisenmenger's complex. The classical pansystolic murmur of the VSD tends to disappear as the right and left ventricular pressures equalize. A pansystolic murmur in Eisenmenger's complex is more likely to be from tricuspid incompetence.

†Again the classical PDA murmur tends to shorten to a soft systolic murmur, and then disappear as the pressures in the pulmonary artery and descending aorta equalize.

Table 3.65 The features which may be helpful in differentiating Eisenmenger's syndrome from the tetralogy of Fallot

	Eisenmenger's syndrome	Fallot's tetralogy
Pulmonary systolic thrill	Absent	Present
Pulmonary systolic murmur	Absent	Intense (unless such severe stenosis that no flow)
Right ventricle	Very hypertrophied	Hypertrophied
Chest X-ray	Large pulmonary arteries	Small pulmonary arteries

66 / Crohn's disease

Frequency in survey: 2% of attempts at MRCP short cases.

Survey note: There were several different presentations: as a right iliac fossa mass, as multiple scars and sinuses on the abdomen, as perianal Crohn's disease and as Crohn's disease of the lips. In one-third of cases the clue was given that the patient had diarrhoea.

Record 1

The *multiple laparotomy scars* suggest a chronic, relapsing, abdominal condition which has led to crises requiring surgical intervention on several occasions. In view of the associated *fistula* formation, Crohn's disease is likely.

Record 2

The chronically *swollen lips* and history of chronic diarrhoea are suggestive of Crohn's disease (examine inside the *mouth for ulcers* which vary in size).

Record 3

There is a (characteristic) *dusky blue discolouration* of the perianal skin. There are *oedematous skin tags* (which look soft but are very firm), there is *fissuring, ulceration* and *fistula* formation.
   The diagnosis is perianal Crohn's disease (may antedate disease elsewhere in the bowel).

Record 4

Right iliac fossa mass—see p. 142.

Other physical signs in Crohn's disease

Fever
Anaemia (malabsorption, chronic disease and gastrointestinal blood loss)
Clubbing
Arthritis (including sacroiliitis)

For colour photograph see p. 382.

Erythema nodosum (p. 162)
Pyoderma gangrenosum (p. 314)
Iritis
Ankle oedema (hypoproteinaemia)

Other causes of anal fistulae (rare)

Simple fistula from an abscess of an anal gland
Tuberculosis
Ulcerative colitis
Carcinoma of the rectum

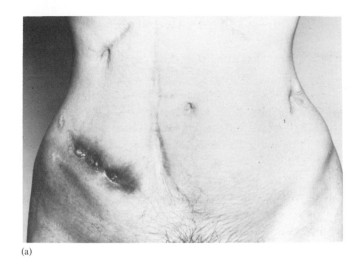

(a)

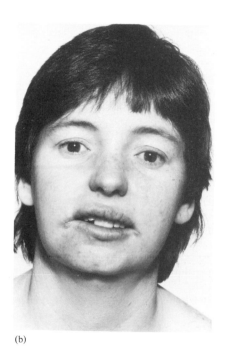

(b)

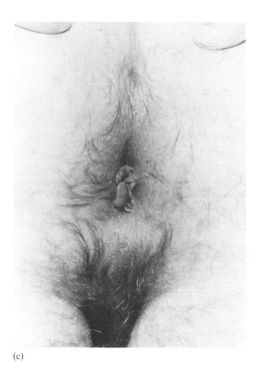

(c)

Fig. 3.66. (a) Multiple scars and fistulae. (b) Crohn's lips. (c) Perianal lesions.

67 / Mitral valve prolapse

Frequency in survey: 2% of attempts at MRCP short cases.

Record

The pulse (in this well-looking patient) is regular (give rate) and the venous pressure is not raised. The apex beat is palpable in the fifth intercostal space in the midclavicular line. There are no heaves or thrills. On auscultation the heart sounds are normal but there is a *midsystolic click** (which is usually but not always) followed by a late *systolic crescendo–decrescendo murmur* loudest at the left sternal edge (as the condition progresses the murmur develops the characteristics of mitral incompetence—p. 114).

These findings suggest mitral valve prolapse (floppy posterior mitral valve leaflet—echocardiography useful for confirmation).

The prolapse is increased by anything which decreases cardiac volume (standing position; Valsalva manoeuvre) and as a result the click and murmur occur earlier during systole and the murmur is prolonged. Increasing cardiac volume (squatting position, propranolol) has the reverse effect. Phonocardiography documents these effects well. Mitral valve prolapse (said to occur in 5–10% of the population†, more commonly in females) is usually asymptomatic but may be associated with atypical chest pain, palpitations, fatigue and dyspnoea. The symptoms may become worse once the patient knows there is a murmur. The prognosis is good† but complications can include infective endocarditis, atrial and ventricular dysrhythmias, worsening mitral incompetence, embolic phenomena (transient ischaemic attacks, amaurosis fugax, acute hemiplegia), rupture of the mitral valve (age-related degenerative changes) and sudden death. The condition may be familial and there may be a family history of sudden death. There is a serious risk of precipitating cardiac neurosis which may, at least in part, contribute to the association with atypical chest pain. There is often myxomatous degeneration of the mitral valve, deposition of acid mucopolysaccharide material and redundant valve tissue.

Causes and associations

Marfan's syndrome
Rheumatic heart disease
Coronary artery disease
Congenital heart disease
Congestive cardiomyopathy
Hypertrophic obstructive cardiomyopathy
Myocarditis
Mitral valve surgery
Left atrial myxoma
Ehlers–Danlos syndrome
Osteogenesis imperfecta
Systemic lupus erythematosus
Muscular dystrophy
Turner's syndrome
Athlete's heart
Primary mitral valve prolapse

Other causes of a short systolic murmur audible at the apex should always be thought of and excluded. These are:

Trivial mitral incompetence (the usual cause—the murmur may not be pansystolic but there is no click)
Aortic stenosis/sclerosis (p. 106)
Hypertrophic obstructive cardiomyopathy (p. 318).

---

*The click is characteristic but easily missed if you have not heard one before. This may be because of the distraction of the murmur. Concentrate on listening for other sounds at different frequencies from the murmur and you will hear it.
†It may be that the clinically silent, echocardiographic mitral valve prolapse which is common in thin, young women is a variant of normal, distinct from the floppy valve or complication of chordal lengthening or rupture needing mitral valve

replacement, which is commonest in elderly men. It seems likely that 'echo only' mitral valve prolapse carries a good prognosis whereas the complications are associated with the clinical variety. Since patients with auscultatory and echocardiographic evidence of mitral valve prolapse may be candidates for endocarditis, they should be recommended for antimicrobial prophylaxis before dental procedures, etc.

Frequency in survey: Main focus of a short case in 2% of attempts at MRCP short cases. Additional feature in a further 2%.

Survey note: Cervical collar may be a clue.

Record

The legs (of this middle-aged or elderly patient) show *spastic weakness,** the *tone* being *increased*, the *reflexes brisk* (?clonus) and the *plantar responses extensor. Vibration* sense is (may be) lost in the lower limbs (joint position and spinothalamic loss may also occur but are uncommon). In the upper limbs there is (often asymmetrical) *inversion*† of the biceps and supinator jerks.

These features suggest cervical myelopathy as the cause of the spastic paraparesis. *Cervical spondylosis* is the commonest cause though a *spinal cord tumour* cannot be excluded clinically.

In the upper limbs there may be segmental muscle wasting and weakness particularly if there is an associated radiculopathy. Gross wasting of the small muscles of the hand due to cervical spondylosis is uncommon because the latter usually affects C5/6 or C6/7 and the small muscles are supplied by C8/T1. Mild wasting of the small muscles does sometimes occur probably due to vascular changes in the cord below the lesion.

There is often no sensory loss in the hand. Sometimes in the elderly a complaint of numb, useless hands may be accompanied by constant unpleasant parasthesiae and writhing ('sensory wandering' or 'pseudo-athetosis') of the fingers when the eyes are closed. Position and vibration senses are lost in such hands.

Neck pain is surprisingly rare in cervical spondylosis causing cervical myelopathy, and sphincter function is seldom disturbed. Among patients with cervical spondylosis (which is very common) those with a narrow cervical canal are most likely to develop cervical myelopathy. Lhermitte's phenomenon may occur (see p. 273).

---

*In this condition signs often exceed symptoms and spasticity often exceeds weakness.

†When attempts are made to elicit the normal biceps and supinator tendon reflexes, there is a brisk finger flexion despite little or no response of the biceps and supinator jerks themselves. This is because the lower motor neurones and pyramidal tracts are damaged at the C5/6 level producing lower motor neurone signs at that level and upper motor neurone signs below. The combination of inverted biceps and supinator jerks (the C5/6 jerks) and a brisk triceps jerk (C7/8) is termed the 'midcervical reflex pattern'.

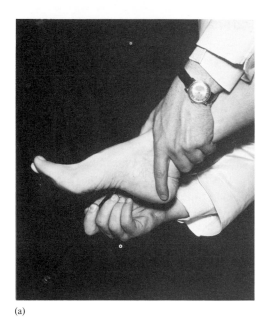

(a)

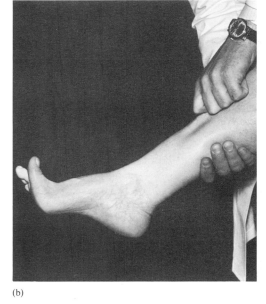

(b)

Fig. 3.68. (a) Babinski's sign. (b) Oppenheim's sign (see p. 27).

Frequency in survey: 2% of attempts at MRCP short cases.

Record

The *pulse* is *collapsing* (may be normal if the duct is narrow and the 'run-off' from the aorta to the left pulmonary artery is small) in character, regular (give rate) and the venous pressure is not raised. The apex is *thrusting* in the anterior axillary line (may be normal if the ductus is small), and there is a *left parasternal heave*. On auscultation there is a continuous *'machinery' murmur** with systolic *accentuation* heard in the second left intercostal space near the sternal edge (but maximal 5 to 7.5 cm above or to the left of this, *beneath the clavicle*, and also *heard posteriorly*).

    The diagnosis is patent ductus arteriosus.

Males : Females = 1 : 3.
The incidence is higher in patients born at a high altitude. Spontaneous closure is rare except in premature infants.

Other causes of a continuous murmur†

(a) With collapsing pulse
    Mitral incompetence and aortic incompetence
    Ventricular septal defect and aortic incompetence
(b) Without collapsing pulse
    Venous hum (common in normal children— maximal to the right of the sternum— diminishes or disappears when the child lies flat or when the right JVP is compressed)
Pulmonary arteriovenous fistula

Complications of patent ductus arteriosus

Infective endocarditis (infection of the ductus— even small ones; therefore closure is always recommended unless Eisenmenger's is already present)
Heart failure
Eisenmenger's syndrome (p. 192)

---

*The murmur seldom lasts for the whole of systole and diastole. It may occupy only the latter part of systole and the early part of diastole. Occasionally, particularly in young children, it may occur as a crescendo in late systole only.

†NB The murmur of patent ductus distinguishes itself by being loudest below the left clavicle. There should not usually be any diagnostic difficulty.

Frequency in survey: Main focus of a short case in 2% of attempts at MRCP short cases. Additional feature in a further 2%.

Record

The JVP is elevated (say height*) and shows *giant v waves*† which oscillate the earlobe (if the venous pressure is high enough) and which are diagnostic of tricuspid incompetence. (Now, if allowed, examine the heart, respiratory system and abdomen.‡)

The commonest cause of tricuspid incompetence is *not* organic, but dilatation of the right ventricle and of the tricuspid valve ring due to right ventricular failure in conditions such as:
   Mitral valve disease
   Cor pulmonale
   Eisenmenger's syndrome
   Atrial septal defect
   Right ventricular infarction
   Primary pulmonary hypertension
   Thyrotoxicosis

Causes of primary tricuspid incompetence

Rheumatic heart disease (usually associated with tricuspid stenosis; almost invariably associated with other valvular disease—if there is pulmonary hypertension it may not be possible to differentiate organic from functional tricuspid incompetence on clinical grounds alone)
Infective endocarditis (especially 'main-lining' drug addicts—recurrent septicaemia with pulmonary infiltrates should raise suspicion)
Congenital heart disease (e.g. Ebstein's anomaly)
Carcinoid syndrome (flushing, diarrhoea, hepatomegaly, sometimes asthma; fibrous plaques on the endothelial surface of the heart are associated with tricuspid incompetence and pulmonary stenosis)
Myxomatous change (may be associated with mitral valve prolapse or ASD)
Trauma

---

*In centimetres vertically above the sternal angle, not the suprasternal notch or supraclavicular fossa. In tricuspid incompetence which is secondary to right ventricular dilatation, the venous pressure is usually of the order of 8–10 cm or more.
†These *v* waves are in fact *cv* waves because systole spans the time between *c* and *v* waves of the normal jugular pulse.
‡In the *heart* you would expect to find the systolic murmur of tricuspid incompetence which may be louder on inspiration (Carvallo's sign) and augmented by the Müller manoeuvre (attempted inspiration against a closed glottis). There may be murmurs of associated or underlying disease of the heart valves, especially mitral. There may be a tricuspid diastolic murmur louder on inspiration and augmented by the Müller manoeuvre. This could be due to increased flow across the tricuspid valve or to concomitant tricuspid stenosis. In the *respiratory system* you would be looking for underlying cor pulmonale. In the *abdomen* you may find forceful epigastric pulsations and hepatomegaly which is tender and pulsatile. In severe, long-standing tricuspid incompetence, ascites and signs of chronic liver disease (p. 78) can occur.

71 / Purpura

Frequency in survey: Main focus of a short case in 2% of attempts at MRCP short cases. Additional feature in a further 3%.

Record

There is purpura.* (Now look at the patient and note:
  ?*Age* ['senile purpura']
  ?*Cushingoid features* with thin skin [if present observe for features of underlying steroid treated disease, e.g. asthma, rheumatoid arthritis, cryptogenic fibrosing alveolitis]
  ?*Rheumatoid arthritis* [phenylbutazone and gold as well as steroids]
  ?*Anaemia* [leukaemia, bone marrow aplasia or infiltration]
—as well as the distribution and type of purpura).

Causes of purpura can be divided into
Thrombocytopenic purpura such as:
  Idiopathic thrombocytopenic purpura (purpuric rash in a young female, ?spleen—may respond to steroids and/or splenectomy).
  Marrow replacement by leukaemia (acute and chronic; ?spleen, nodes, liver, anaemia, oral and pharyngeal infection).
  Marrow replacement by secondary malignancy (?cachexia, evidence of primary).
Capillary defect (vascular) such as:
  Senile and steroid-induced purpura (purpura over loose skin areas).
  Henoch–Schönlein purpura (children > adults; purpuric rash over the extensor surfaces of the limbs particularly at the ankles and on the buttocks; associated with arthritis of medium-sized joints, colicky abdominal pains, occasionally GI bleeding and acute nephritis).
Coagulation deficiency such as:
  Haemophilia.
  Christmas disease.
  Anticoagulant therapy.

Other causes of purpura

Other drugs (e.g. sulphonamides, chloramphenicol, thiazides)
Hypersplenism (large spleen)
Von Willebrand's disease
Infective endocarditis (?heart murmur, splenomegaly, splinters, clubbing, Osler's nodes, etc.)
Systemic lupus erythematosus (?typical rash)
Polyarteritis nodosa (?arteritic lesions)
Osler–Weber–Rendu syndrome (p. 141)
Venous stasis (ankle and lower legs; obesity or varicose veins; accompanied by progressive pigmentation due to deposition of haemosiderin)

Scurvy (NB the neglected elderly patient with ecchymoses on the legs)
Paroxysmal nocturnal haemoglobinuria
Amyloidosis (periorbital purpura)
Uraemia (pale, brownish-yellow tinge to skin)
Disseminated intravascular coagulation
Thrombotic thrombocytopenic purpura
Haemolytic-uraemic syndrome
Paraproteinaemia
Fat embolism
Meningitis (especially meningococcal)
Septicaemia (especially meningococcal)

*Purpura refers to a spontaneous extravasation of blood from the capillaries into the skin; petechiae = pin-head size, ecchy- ecchymoses = larger lesions.

Scarlet fever   Glandular fever
Measles   Typhoid
Rubella   Cyanotic congenital heart disease

For colour photograph see p. 379.

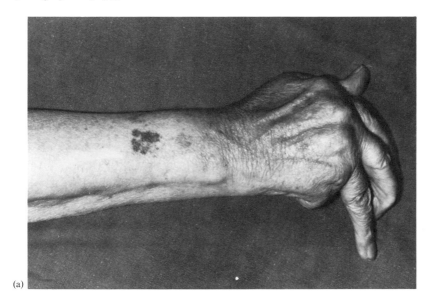
(a)

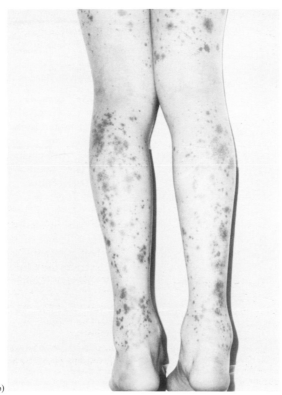
(b)

Fig. 3.71. (a) Purpura on forearm (note rheumatoid arthritis).
(b) Henoch–Schönlein purpura.

72 / Xanthomata

Frequency in survey: Main focus of a short case in 2% of attempts at MRCP short cases. Additional feature in a further 2%.

Record 1

There are *tendon xanthomata* (?corneal arcus, xanthelasma) in the *extensor tendons* on the back of the *hand*, and on the *Achilles* and *patella* tendons.

They suggest *familial hypercholesterolaemia*. (In this condition raised and nodular *tuberous xanthomata* may also occur, usually symmetrically, over the *extensor aspects of the joints* and on the *buttocks*. They may be several millimetres to several centimetres in size.)

Record 2

There are (orange or) *yellow papules* (up to 5 mm in diameter) on the *extensor surfaces* particularly over the *joints*, on the *limbs* and on the *buttocks* and *back*. They are (sometimes) surrounded by a rim of erythema (and may be tender).

This is *eruptive xanthomatosis* (?lipaemia retinalis on fundoscopy. There is often abdominal pain and there is a risk of acute pancreatitis. It suggests severe *hypertriglyceridaemia*—plasma triglycerides of the order of 20–25 mmol l^{-1}—'milky plasma' syndrome).*

Familial hypercholesterolaemia is associated with premature development of vascular disease. Familial hypertriglyceridaemia does not appear to be an important risk factor for atherosclerosis but equivalent hypertriglyceridaemia due to familial combined hyperlipidaemia† is associated with an increased risk.

Order of priorities in treating hyperlipidaemia‡

(i) Identify and treat any causes of secondary hyperlipidaemia such as:
    Diabetes mellitus (?fundi)
    Alcoholism (may be the occult underlying cause of treatment failure)
    Nephrotic syndrome (?generalized oedema)
    Myxoedema (?facies, pulse, ankle jerks)
    Cholestasis (?icterus)
    Myelomatosis
    Oral contraceptives (exogenous oestrogens)
(ii) Dietary treatment for obesity. If that fails:

For colour photographs see p. 377.

(iii) Dietary treatment for hyperlipidaemia, and only if that fails:
(iv) Lipid lowering drugs

Types of hyperlipidaemia simplified

Comparatively common
Type IIa (e.g. familial hypercholesterolaemia)—raised cholesterol only
Type IIb (e.g. familial combined hypercholesterolaemia)—raised cholesterol and triglycerides
Type IV (e.g. familial hypertriglyceridaemia)—raised triglycerides

Rare
Type I—raised chylomicrons
Type III—a defect in a particular step in lipid catabolism resulting in a rise in cholesterol and triglycerides to an equal extent
Type V—raised chylomicrons and triglycerides

---

*This level of hypertriglyceridaemia is usually due to combined primary and secondary hypertriglyceridaemia; i.e. over-production of triglycerides occurring at the same time as hinderance of removal. For example, the coexistence of familial hypertriglyceridaemia (type IV), diabetes, and/or alcohol consumption. Treatment of the secondary cause usually leads to a dramatic reduction in triglyceride levels and greatly reduces the risk of acute pancreatitis which is the main threat of this condition.

†Affected family members show either a combined rise in plasma cholesterol and triglycerides, or hypercholesterolaemia alone, or hypertriglyceridaemia alone.

‡NB the screening and treatment of families with hypercholesterolaemia.

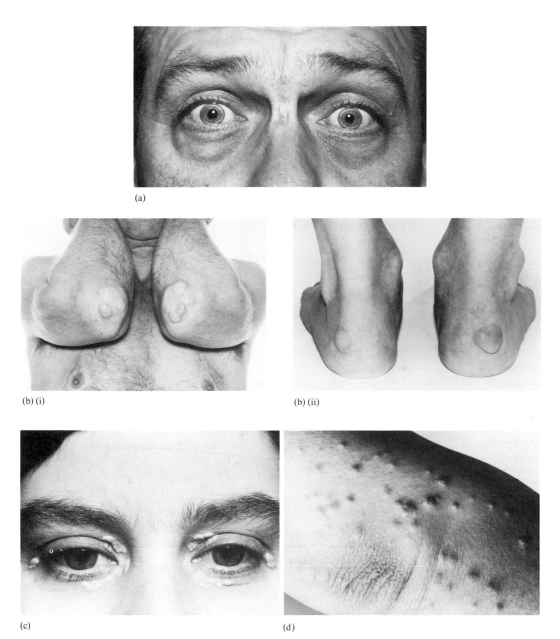

(a)

(b) (i)

(b) (ii)

(c)

(d)

Fig. 3.72. (a) Arcus senilis. (b): (i), (ii) elbows and Achilles of the same patient. (c) Xanthelasma. (d) Eruptive xanthomata.

73 / Drug-induced extrapyramidal syndrome

Frequency in survey: 2% of attempts at MRCP short cases.

Record

There are (in this ?elderly, chronic schizophrenic) stereotyped tic-like *orofacial dyskinesias* (involuntary movements) including *lip-smacking, chewing, pouting* and *grimacing*. There is (may be) *choreoathetosis* of the limbs and trunk.

The diagnosis is tardive dyskinesia. (It is likely that the patient has been on sustained phenothiazine treatment for at least six months. The condition often persists when the drug is withdrawn, in which case tetrabenazine may help.)

Neuroleptics which may cause abnormal involuntary movements (by inhibiting dopamine function):
Phenothiazines (e.g. chlorpromazine)
Butyrophenones (e.g. haloperidol)
Substituted benzamides (e.g. metoclopramide)
Reserpine
Tetrabenazine

The other neuroleptic-induced extrapyramidal adverse reactions (apart from tardive dyskinesia):
Acute dystonias (soon after starting the drug; e.g. oculogyric crises)
Akathisia (uncontrollable restlessness with an inner feeling of unease)
Parkinson's syndrome (indistinguishable from Parkinson's disease though tremor less common; tends to respond to anticholinergics rather than L-dopa)

Frequency in survey: 2% of attempts at MRCP short cases.

Survey note: All patients with sicca symptoms (dry eyes and dry mouth) in our survey had parotid enlargement.

Record

There is *bilateral parotid enlargement*. The conjunctivae are injected (the patient complains of *gritty eyes*—the dry eyes of keratoconjunctivitis sicca) and the tongue (touch it) is dry (or the patient complains of a *dry mouth*).

This is Mikulicz's syndrome (diffuse swelling of lachrymal and salivary glands) which is most likely to be produced by:

1   Sarcoidosis (?lupus pernio, chest signs) but may also be caused by
2   Lymphoma (?lymph nodes, hepatosplenomegaly—both signs, of course, may also occur in sarcoid)
3   Leukaemia (?pallor, hepatosplenomegaly)

Reduction in tear secretion can be demonstrated with *Schirmer's test* in which a 5 mm wide strip of filter paper is folded 3 mm from one end and hooked into the lower conjunctival sac. Normal tear secretion moistens more than 15 mm of strip within five minutes.

Sjögren's syndrome (*Mikulicz's disease*) is the triad of dry mouth (xerostomia), keratoconjunctivitis sicca and a connective tissue disease—most commonly rheumatoid arthritis (50%) but also including autoimmune liver disease and fibrosing alveolitis. Bronchial, pancreatic and vaginal secretions may also be diminished. The lachrymal and salivary glands are not swollen as in *Mikulicz's syndrome* (the issue is complicated, though, by the fact that there is a high incidence of lymphoma in Sjögren's syndrome!). Sjögren's syndrome without associated connective tissue disease (30%) is referred to as the *sicca syndrome*.

75 / Primary biliary cirrhosis

Frequency in survey: 2% of attempts at MRCP short cases.

Record

This middle-aged lady is *icteric* (may not be) with *pigmentation* of the skin. There are *excoriations* (due to scratching) and she has *xanthelasma* (other xanthomas frequently occur over joints, skin folds and at sites of trauma). The liver is enlarged . . . cm (may be very large; there may be splenomegaly).

The clinical diagnosis is primary biliary cirrhosis (there may be *clubbing*). The scratch marks are due to *pruritus* (the predominant presenting symptom).

Serum antimitochondrial antibody positive in 95–99%
Smooth muscle antibody positive in 50%
Antinuclear factor positive in 20%

Impaired biliary excretion of copper occurs with excessive copper deposition in the liver. This may not be an important factor in the pathogenesis of the progressive liver disease, but it can be helpful in the diagnosis—sometimes differentiation from chronic active hepatitis (25% have antimitochondrial antibody) can be difficult (clinically and histologically) and the issue can be resolved by staining the biopsy specimen for copper. Kayser–Fleischer rings occasionally occur. Penicillamine (immunological, antifibrotic, as well as chelating effects) may improve survival in advanced disease but should not be given in the early stages when the prognosis is excellent. Azathioprine has not proved effective, corticosteroids are contraindicated (bone disease) but initial results with cyclosporin A are encouraging. Supplements of fat-soluble vitamins, calcium and phosphate are given in view of malabsorption. The pruritus often responds to cholestyramine (taken before and after meals) though antihistamines and phenobarbitone may also help. Resistant pruritus responds to norethandrolone but this deepens jaundice.

The patient is at risk of
Bleeding oesophageal varices
Steatorrhoea and malabsorption, leading to
Osteomalacia

Associated conditions*
Sjögren's syndrome
Systemic sclerosis
CRST syndrome
Rheumatoid arthritis
Hashimoto's thyroiditis
Renal tubular acidosis
Coeliac disease
Dermatomyositis

*The incidental finding of a raised alkaline phosphatase in patients with the conditions on this list should raise the suspicion of an associated primary biliary cirrhosis.

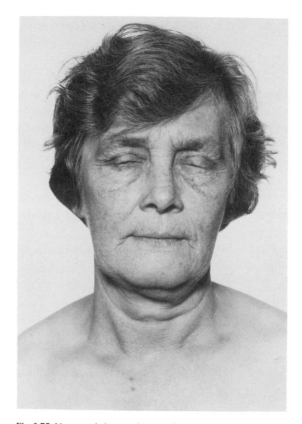

Fig. 3.75. Note xanthelasma, pigmentation and spider naevi.

76 / Lupus pernio

Frequency in survey: 2% of attempts at MRCP short cases.

Survey note: Candidates often gave differential diagnoses such as SLE and rosacea before being led to the correct diagnosis. We suggest that candidates try to see real-life cases of all three conditions affecting the face before the examination so that they may recognize the differences.

Record

There is (in this female patient) a *diffuse*, livid, *purple-red infiltration* of the *nose* (and/or cheeks, ears, hands and feet).

The diagnosis is lupus pernio (usually associated with *chronic pulmonary sarcoidosis* which progresses to *fibrosis*; *chronic uveitis* and *bone cysts* in the phalanges are often present).

Other complications which may occur in chronic sarcoidosis

Facial palsy (may be bilateral; parotid enlargement not always present)
Peripheral neuropathy
Meningeal infiltrations and tumour-like deposits
Hypopituitarism and diabetes insipidus (granulomas extending from the meninges into the hypothalmus)
Hypercalcaemia and its nephropathy (probably hypersensitivity to vitamin D)
Mikulicz's syndrome (diffuse swelling of lachrymal and salivary glands by conditions such as sarcoidosis, lymphoma or leukaemia—p. 207)
Cardiomyopathy (clinical evidence rare; cor pulmonale is more likely to be the cardiac lesion)
Chronic arthritis
Hypersplenism if sufficient splenomegaly
Infiltration of old scars by sarcoid tissue
Polymyositis (progressive muscle wasting)

Hepatic granulomas can be found in two-thirds of patients with sarcoidosis (symptoms rare). Sarcoidosis may affect most tissues.

For colour photograph see p. 374.

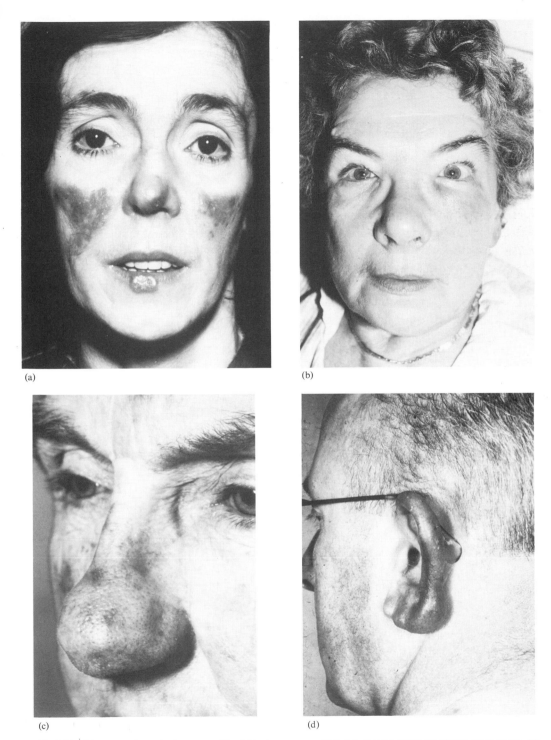

(a)

(b)

(c)

(d)

Fig. 3.76. (a) Lupus pernio on cheeks, nose and lip. (b) Lesions under the eyes especially on the left. (c) A close-up of lupus pernio on the nose. The treated case may just show a faint purplish discoloration on the end of the nose or cheeks. (d) Lupus pernio of the ear.

77 / Muscular dystrophy

Frequency in survey: 2% of attempts at MRCP short cases.

Survey note: All cases were of facio-scapulo-humeral except one possible case of limb-girdle type.

Record 1

The patient has a dull, unlined, expressionless face (*myopathic facies*) with lips that are (usually) open and slack. There is *wasting* of the *facial* and *limb-girdle muscles*,* and the superior margins of the scapulae (viewed from the front) are (may be) visible above the clavicles. The movements of smiling, whistling and closing the eyes are impaired. There is *winging of the scapulae* (when the patient leans against a wall with arms extended). There is (may be) involvement of the trunk and legs (anterior tibials may cause bilateral foot drop) now or in the future.

The diagnosis is *facio-scapulo-humeral* (Landouzy–Déjérine) muscular dystrophy (autosomal dominant, course variable but usually relatively benign).

Record 2

There is *limb-girdle wasting* and *weakness* which affects some groups of muscles more than others (e.g. deltoid and spinati usually spared), and the *face* is *spared*. There is (not uncommonly) enlargement of the calf muscles.

These features suggest *limb-girdle* (Erb) muscular dystrophy (autosomal recessive, both sexes affected equally, more benign if the upper limb is involved first, usually begins in the 2nd or 3rd decade, sometimes arrests but usually patients are severely disabled within twenty years of onset).

Other muscular dystrophies

Duchenne or pseudohypertrophic (X-linked, severe, onset age three to four years, initially enlargement of calves, buttocks and infraspinati [this disappears later] while other muscles [especially the proximal lower limb] waste; waddling lordotic gait; usually confined to wheelchair by age of ten years; cardiac muscle involved; face spared; death from respiratory infection and/or cardiac failure commonly at about age of twenty)

Benign X-linked (Becker) muscular dystrophy (similar to Duchenne but much less severe—onset five to twenty-five years; confined to wheelchair twenty-five years later)

Distal muscular dystrophy (dominant; most cases occur in Sweden—eventually spreads to proximal muscles unlike peroneal muscular atrophy [p. 229] with which it is most often confused)

Ocular myopathy (sporadic or dominant—first ptosis, then ophthalmoplegia, face and neck muscles often mildly involved—see footnote p. 133)

Oculopharyngeal muscular dystrophy (similar to ocular myopathy but late onset and dysphagia prominent—often French-Canadian ancestry)

Childhood muscular dystrophy with autosomal recessive inheritance (rare, similar to Duchenne but more benign and girls may be affected)

Congenital muscular dystrophy (rare, hypotonia from birth, prognosis unfavourable)

---

*The sternal head of sternomastoid (which forms the anterior axillary fold) is affected earlier than the clavicular head, leading to a peculiar appearance of the axillary folds.

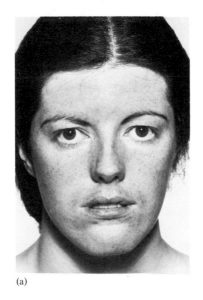

(a)

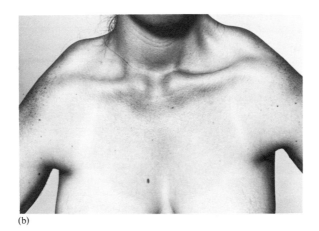

(b)

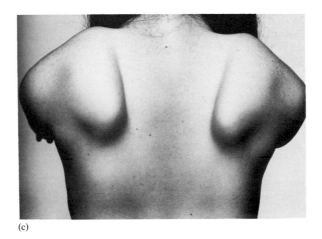

(c)

Fig. 3.77. (a) Myopathic facies (facio-scapulo-humeral muscular dystrophy). (b) The superior margins of the scapulae are visible from the front (same patient as Fig. 3.77a). (c) Winging of the scapulae (same patient).

Frequency in survey: Main focus of a short case in 2% of attempts at MRCP short cases. Additional feature in a further 1%.

Survey note: Both mitral and aortic prostheses occurred. Often leaking. There may also be murmurs from the unreplaced valve.

Record 1

There is a *midsternal, vertical thoracotomy scar*. There is a *click at the first heart sound* (closing of the mitral prosthesis) and an *opening click* in diastole (this may occasionally be followed by a mid-diastolic flow murmur).

These clicks represent the opening and closing of a *mitral valve prosthesis*. (The panystolic murmur ± signs of heart failure suggest it is leaking.)

Record 2

There is a *midsternal, vertical thoracotomy scar*. The first heart sound is normal (unless there is accompanying mitral stenosis), and is followed by an *ejection click* (opening of the prosthesis), an *ejection systolic murmur* and a *click at* (as part of) *the second sound* (closing of the prosthesis).

These clicks suggest an *aortic valve prosthesis*. (The early diastolic murmur and collapsing pulse [?wide pulse pressure] suggest it is leaking.)

Complications of prosthetic valves

Thromboembolic disease (anticoagulants or antiplatelet agents reduce but do not abolish)

Infective endocarditis (always consider when leakage develops)

Leakage due to wear of the valve

Leakage due to inadequacy or infection (SBE) of valve siting

Near total or even total dehiscence of the valve from its siting (the valve will be seen to rock on X-ray screening when there is serious leakage)

Ball embolus (the ball of the Starr–Edwards valve)

Valve obstruction from thrombosis/fibrosis clogging up the valve mechanics

Haemolysis (aortic valve)

NB Porcine heterografts and cadavaric homografts do not cause clicks, do not require long-term anticoagulants but may develop degenerative changes with calcium deposition.

Frequency in survey: 2% of attempts at MRCP short cases.

Survey note: Often the differential diagnosis of Addison's/Nelson's was given and further differentiation was not required.

Record

There is *generalized pigmentation* (due to the direct action of ACTH causing increased melanin in the skin), which is more marked in the *skin creases* (e.g. palmar), in *scars* (especially more recent ones), in the *buccal mucosa* (look in the mouth), in the *nipples* and at *pressure points*.

This suggests Addison's disease or Nelson's syndrome (?temporal field defect, ?abdominal scar of bilateral adrenalectomy).

Patchy, almost symmetrical, areas of skin depigmentation surrounded by areas of increased pigmentation may occur due to vitiligo (15% of patients with idiopathic Addison's) which is one of the associated organ-specific autoimmune diseases. (For the others, which include Hashimoto's thyroiditis, myxoedema, diabetes mellitus, pernicious anaemia and hypoparathyroidism, see p. 254. Premature ovarian failure is particularly associated with Addison's disease.)

The common causes of primary hypoadrenalism

Autoimmune adrenalitis
Tuberculosis (?lung signs)
Bilateral adrenalectomy (malignant disease, e.g. breast cancer; Cushing's syndrome)

Other causes of primary hypoadrenalism

Secondary deposits
Amyloidosis (hypoadrenalism preceded by nephrotic syndrome—see footnote, p. 65)
Haemochromatosis
Granulomatous disease (rarely sarcoidosis)
Fungal diseases (e.g. histoplasmosis)
Congenital adrenal hypoplasia
Meningococcal septicaemia
Adrenal haemorrhage (newborn especially breech delivery; patients on anticoagulants)
Adrenal vein thrombosis after trauma or adrenal venography

Skin pigmentation is usually racial (including buccal pigmentation) or due to sun-tanning. Other causes of abnormal generalized pigmentation include:

Endocrine
ACTH therapy (e.g. asthma)
Cushing's disease (?facies, truncal obesity, striae, etc.—p. 218)
Thyrotoxicosis (?exophthalmos, goitre, etc.—p. 108)
Ectopic ACTH (especially oat-cell carcinoma)

Chronic debilitating disorders (also, like Addison's, associated with lassitude and weight loss)
Malignancy (including reticuloses and leukaemias)
Malabsorption syndromes
Chronic infections (especially tuberculosis)
Cirrhosis (?icterus, spider naevi, etc.—pp. 78 and 208)
Uraemia (pale, brownish yellow tinge to skin)

Pigments other than melanin such as:
Haemochromatosis (slate-grey pigmentation, hepatosplenomegaly, etc.—p. 233)
Argyria
Chronic arsenic poisoning

For colour photographs see pp. 376–7.

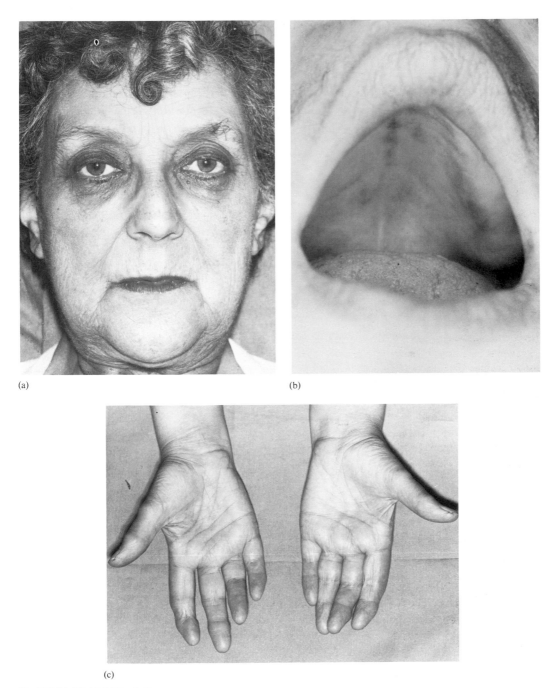

(a)

(b)

(c)

Fig. 3.79. (a), (b), (c) Addison's disease.

Frequency in survey: Main focus of a short case in 2% of attempts at MRCP short cases. Additional feature in a further 3%.

Survey note: Almost all cases were secondary to therapeutic steroids—especially for asthma and rheumatoid arthritis, but also for cryptogenic fibrosing alveolitis and chronic active hepatitis, amongst others.

Record

The patient has a *moon face* with *acne* and *truncal obesity* with a *buffalo hump*. The skin is thin and shows excessive bruising (*purpuric patches*) and there are purple *striae* on the abdomen (must be differentiated from the pale pink striae of obese adolescents and the stretch marks of pregnancy and simple obesity). He has *gynaecomastia* (and she is *hirsute* with a *deep voice*). There is *proximal muscle weakness* (few patients with Cushing's syndrome can rise normally from the squatting position).

The diagnosis is Cushing's syndrome (?evidence of underlying steroid responsive inflammatory or immunological disorder).

Other features of Cushing's syndrome

Hypertension and peripheral oedema (salt retention)
Irregular menstruation
Impotence
Back pain (osteoporosis and vertebral collapse leading to kyphosis and loss of height)
Diabetes mellitus
Pigmentation (especially ectopic or exogenous ACTH)
Psychiatric disorder (commonly depressive illness)

Causes of Cushing's syndrome*

Therapeutic corticosteroids
Therapeutic ACTH
Cushing's disease (pituitary [basophilic or chromo-phobe pituitary adenoma] or hypothalamic lesion leading to excessive ACTH)
Adrenocortical adenoma (occasionally part of *multiple endocrine adenopathy type I* with one or more of: primary hyperparathyroidism, islet-cell tumour, pituitary tumour—see also p. 104†)
Adrenocortical carcinoma
Ectopic ACTH secreting non-endocrine tumours:
Oat-cell carcinoma of bronchus (weight loss, pigmentation, hypokalaemic alkalosis and oedema)
Bronchial adenoma
Carcinoid tumour (usually bronchial)
Carcinoma of pancreas
Non-teratomatous ovarian tumour

---

* When the syndrome is not iatrogenic, then in about 80% of affected adults the cause is Cushing's disease; whereas adrenal adenoma, carcinoma and ectopic ACTH syndrome contribute equally to the remaining 20%.
† The islet-cell tumour may secrete gastrin (Zollinger–Ellison syndrome) or insulin (insulinoma). The pituitary tumour may be eosinophilic (acromegaly) or a chromophobe adenoma which is non-secreting (bitemporal hemianopia, headaches, blindness, hypopituitarism and other pressure symptoms—tumour may become very large). Pituitary tumours may also secrete prolactin (impotence, amenorrhoea, galactorrhoea) or ACTH (Cushing's disease).

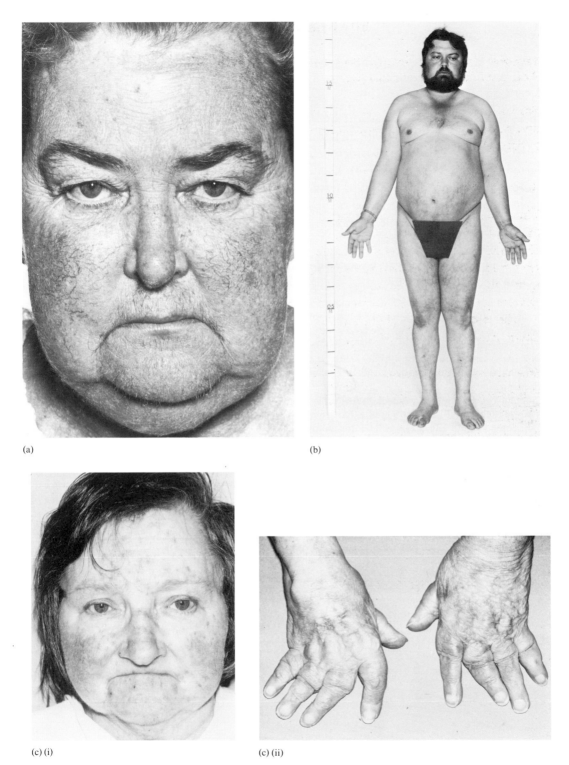

(a)

(b)

(c) (i)

(c) (ii)

Fig. 3.80. (a) Cushingoid facies (steroid therapy for cerebral lupus erythematosus). (b) Truncal obesity (Cushing's disease).

(c): (i), (ii) Corticosteroid therapy in a patient with rheumatoid arthritis.

81 / Friedreich's ataxia

Frequency in survey: 2% of attempts at MRCP short cases.

Record

There is *pes cavus*, (*kypho*) *scoliosis* and (may be) a deformed and high-arched palate. The patient is *ataxic* and clumsy with an *intention tremor* and his *head shakes*. There is *nystagmus* (often slow and coarse and observed before formal examination) and *dysarthria* (slow and slurred or scanning and explosive). There is (?gross) bilateral impairment of rapid alternate motion, finger–nose and heel–shin tests. Knee and *ankle jerks* are *absent* and the *plantar responses are extensor. Position and vibration* sense are diminished in the feet.

    The diagnosis is Friedreich's ataxia.

Other features (if asked)

1 Cardiomyopathy (may cause sudden death).

2 Optic and retinal atrophy.

3 Diabetes mellitus.

4 Mild dementia.

The condition is one of the hereditary spinocerebellar degenerations. It is usually recessive but in some families it is dominant. The fully-fledged syndrome is rare among affected family members who more commonly show slight signs of abnormality in the lower limbs, chiefly pes cavus and absent reflexes (*formes fruste*).

The major ataxic conditions which may need to be differentiated from Friedreich's ataxia, particularly if the latter is mild and presents late, are multiple sclerosis and tabes dorsalis. Typical features which may help to differentiate these conditions are shown in Table 3.81.

Other conditions which may have features of Friedreich's ataxia (all are recessive):

Bassen–Kornzweig syndrome (abetalipoproteinaemia*)—steatorrhoea, acanthosis, pigmentary retinal degeneration and a spinocerebellar degeneration which resembles Friedreich's ataxia

Refsum's disease (elevated serum phytanic acid due to defective lipid alpha-oxidase)—pupillary abnormalities, optic atrophy, deafness, pigmentary retinal degeneration, cardiomyopathy, icthyosis and a Friedreich-like ataxia

Roussy–Lévy syndrome (may be an intermediate between Charcot–Marie–Tooth disease and Friedreich's ataxia)—ataxia, areflexia, pes cavus and kyphoscoliosis but absence of nystagmus, dysarthria, extensor plantar responses and posterior column signs

Table 3.81 Features which may help to differentiate the major ataxic conditions

	Friedreich's ataxia	Multiple sclerosis	Tabes dorsalis
Family history	Major	Minor	None
Onset before age 15	Usual	Rare	Rare
Knee and ankle jerks	Absent	Usually exaggerated	Absent
Spine	(kypho-)scoliosis	Normal	Normal
Feet shape	Pes cavus	Normal	Normal
Pupils	Normal	Normal	Argyll Robertson
Plantars	↑	↑	↓ or → (unless taboparesis)
Pain and deep pressure	Normal	Normal	Absent
Rombergism	+/−	−	+

* LDL, VLDL and chylomicra are absent from the serum, cholesterol is very low and triglycerides are barely detectable.

82 / Peutz–Jeghers syndrome

Frequency in survey: 2% of attempts at MRCP short cases.

Record

There are (sparse or profuse) small brownish-black *pigmented macules* (2–5 mm) on the lips, around the *mouth* (and/or eyes or nose) and *buccal mucosa* (but never on the tongue). They are also (may be) seen on the hands and fingers.

This pigmentation (which tends to disappear in adult life) may be associated with *intestinal polyposis* (single or multiple polyps, which are *hamartomas*, may occur in small and large bowel) in which case the diagnosis would be Peutz–Jeghers syndrome.

Autosomal dominant

Complications

Recurrent colicky abdominal pain
Intestinal obstruction or intussusception

For colour photographs see p. 376.

Iron deficiency anaemia
Frank gastrointestinal haemorrhage
Malignant transformation (rare*)

Multiple polypectomy may be required for disabling symptoms but excision of bowel is to be avoided, if possible, as polyps may recur.

* cf. familial polyposis coli—adenomatous tumours in which malignant transformation is inevitable and for which premalignant treatment is colectomy, ileorectal anastomosis and fulgarization of remaining rectal polyps. This is followed by careful life-long six-monthly follow-up with sigmoidoscopy and polyp fulgarization.

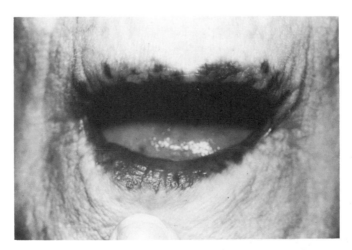

Fig. 3.82. Peutz–Jeghers syndrome.

83 / Systemic lupus erythematosus

Frequency in survey: 2% of attempts at MRCP short cases.

Record

There is (in this *young female* patient) a *red, papular butterfly rash* on the face (and elsewhere—especially light exposed areas) with *scaling, follicular plugging* * and *scarring*.

These features suggest lupus erythematosus (chronic discoid lupus erythematosus if only the skin is affected; SLE if there is evidence of multisystem involvement).

Discoid LE—Males:Females = 1 :2
SLE—Males:Females = 1 :9

Look for other features

Buccal mucosa (sharply defined whitish patches with red borders)

Scalp (scarring alopecia)

Hands and joints (arthritis; deformity may occur but usually mild; Raynaud's in 20%)

Skin (vasculitis—see below)

Lungs† (pleural effusions, or rarely crepitations from interstitial involvement)

Ankles (oedema—SLE is an important cause of nephrotic syndrome)

Heart (for pericardial friction rub, rarely pericardial effusion; cardiac enlargement or failure—myocarditis; or murmurs—Libman–Sachs endocarditis)

Proximal muscles (myalgia is common; polymyositis may occur)

Eyes (Sjögren's syndrome; fundal haemorrhages or white exudates called cytoid bodies; papilloedema)

Reticuloendothelial system (lymph nodes; splenomegaly)

Mucous membranes for pallor (anaemia is normochromic normocytic and/or haemolytic [Coomb's +ve or −ve]; thrombocytopenia often occurs; haematological changes may antedate the other features of the disease by years)

Hepatomegaly (chronic passive congestion—usually transient‡)

Urine (proteinuria and haematuria)

NB In SLE vasculitic rashes occur more commonly than the classic butterfly rash. They characteristically affect the elbows, knees, hands and feet. The rash may be a punctate erythematous rash, palmar erythema, periungual erythema, or livedo reticularis (see Fig. 3.98b, p. 243). Subcutaneous nodules may occur (5%) somewhat resembling those encountered in rheumatoid arthritis.

For colour photograph see p. 374.

---

* Very close examination of the butterfly rash reveals that the scales in many areas appear as dots. These dots indicate where the follicle has been plugged by a scale. When the scales are removed (very unlikely to be required in the examination) and the undersurface is inspected, they clearly appear as tiny spicules projecting from the scaly mass. No other scaly condition produces this phenomenon. Healing of the discoid lesions occurs with atrophy, scarring (telangiectasia), hyperpigmentation or hypopigmentation (vitiligo).

† Drug-induced SLE involves the lungs more commonly and kidneys less commonly than classical SLE. The commonest (90%) drugs are hydralazine (slow acetylators), isoniazid, phenytoin and procainamide (rapid acetylators). Other drugs include hydrochlorothiazide, oral contraceptives, penicillin, practotol, reserpine, streptomycin, sulphonamides, tetracycline.

‡ Liver biopsy may be normal or show fatty infiltration and/or fibrosis. These manifestations in SLE should not be confused with the form of chronic active hepatitis, which often has a positive antinuclear factor, called 'lupoid hepatitis'. The liver biopsy in the latter shows an inflammatory infiltrate extending into the liver lobule, causing erosion of the limiting plate and piecemeal necrosis. Fibrous septa isolate rosettes of cells. Cirrhosis is usually present and eventually hepatic failure may develop.

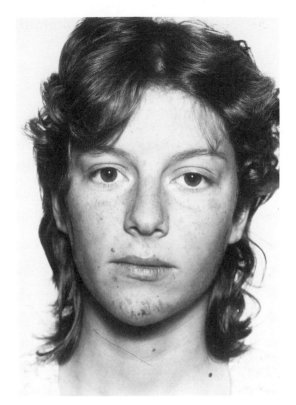

Fig. 3.83. Butterfly rash (see also p. 374).

84 / Superior vena cava obstruction

Frequency in survey: 2% of attempts at MRCP short cases.

Record

There is stridor. The face and upper extremities are *oedematous* (puffy) and *cyanosed*, and the eyes are *suffused*. The *superficial veins* over these areas are *dilated* and there is *fixed engorgement* of the *neck veins*. There is a radiation burn on the chest wall.

The diagnosis is superior vena cava obstruction, most likely due to carcinoma* of the bronchus (?lymph nodes, chest signs, clubbing, etc.—p. 132). It has been treated by radiotherapy (this treatment, or chemotherapy, is required urgently in this condition).

The patient may complain of headaches (may be severe on coughing), difficulty in breathing, dysphagia, dizziness or blackouts. Physical signs are frequently absent or minimal.

Other causes of SVC obstruction

Lymphoma
Aortic aneurysm
Mediastinal fibrosis
Mediastinal goitre

---

* The compression may either be by the tumour or by involved lymph nodes.

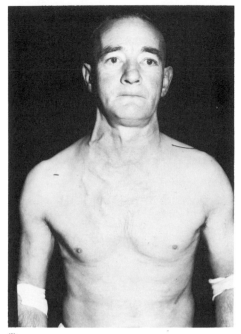

(i)

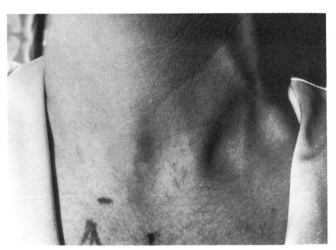

(ii)

Fig. 3.84 (i), (ii) Superior vena cava obstruction. Note the
radiotherapy ink marks in (ii).

85 / Vasculitis

Frequency in survey: Main focus of a short case in 2% of attempts at MRCP short cases. Additional feature in a further 2%.

Record

There are (may be) small *nail fold* and nail edge *infarcts* (due to small vessel vasculitis affecting the terminal digital arteries—in severe cases there may be *digital gangrene*). There is (may be) a purpuric rash (macules, papules or nodules). There are (may be) chronic leg ulcers. There is (may be) a peripheral neuropathy (due to involvement of the vasa nervorum). This patient has vasculitis (look for obvious signs of a cause, e.g. rheumatoid arthritis or SLE).

The term vasculitis refers to disorders involving the small vessels and larger arteries of the skin, either alone or in association with other organs (there is chronic inflammation in and around the vessel wall). This is usually caused by deposition of immunoglobulin and sustained by complement activation.

Other manifestations of vasculitis include nodular vasculitic lesions (e.g. erythema nodosum—p. 162), urticaria, erythema multiforme, and livedo reticularis (see p. 242).

Conditions associated with vasculitis

Rheumatoid arthritis (?hands, nodules, etc.—p. 68)
Systemic lupus erythematosus (?rash, etc.—p. 222)
Polyarteritis nodosa (medium and small arteries and adjacent veins—fever, hypertension, abdominal pain, mononeuritis multiplex, peripheral neuropathy, proteinuria, haematuria, renal failure, myocardial infarction)
Churg–Strauss syndrome (eosinophilic granulomatous vasculitis—similar to polyarteritis nodosa but asthma, eosinophilia, IgE elevation and pulmonary infiltrates are prominent; it may present as asthma)
Australia-antigenaemia and vasculitis (a variant of polyarteritis nodosa)
Wegener's granulomatosis (granulomatous ulceration of the upper and lower respiratory tract associated with generalized arteritis and glomerulitis)
Other connective tissue diseases (systemic sclerosis, etc.)
Drug reactions
Infective endocarditis
Mixed cryoglobulinaemia
Hypergammaglobulinaemia
Lymphoproliferative disorders
Henoch–Schönlein syndrome (children > adults; purpuric rash over the extensor surface of the limbs, particularly at the ankles and often on the buttocks; associated with arthritis of medium-sized joints, colicky abdominal pains, occasionally GI bleeding and acute nephritis)
Persistent urticaria
Giant-cell arteritis (large and medium-sized vessels; elderly patients—headache, temporal artery tenderness, polymyalgia rheumatica—danger of blindness)

Rheumatoid patients with vasculitis often have

Nodules
Circulating immune complexes
Cryoglobulins
Low complement levels
Rheumatoid factor
Antinuclear factor
Immunoglobulins and complement in the cutaneous lesions

For colour photograph see p. 378.

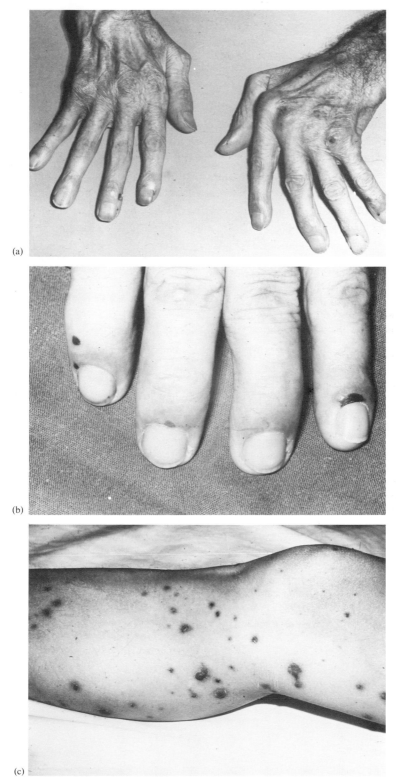

(a)

(b)

(c)

Fig. 3.85. (a) Rheumatoid arthritis. (b) Nail fold infarcts (rheumatoid arthritis). (c) Vasculitis on the lower limb.

86 / Cor pulmonale

Frequency in survey: 1% of attempts at MRCP short cases.

Record

The patient's fingers are *nicotine-stained* and there is *central cyanosis*. The pulse is regular, the *venous pressure* is *raised* (give height) with prominent small *a* waves and giant *v* waves (if there is secondary tricuspid incompetence), and there is *ankle* and *sacral oedema*. *Expiration is prolonged and noisy*. The *accessory muscles* of respiration are in use at rest, and there is a *tracheal tug*. The trachea is central, expansion is equal, the percussion note is resonant, and tactile fremitus and vocal resonance are normal. There is a *left parasternal heave* and a palpable second heart sound* (?pansystolic murmur of tricuspid incompetence). There are widespread *expiratory rhonchi* and the forced expiratory time (see p. 32) is 8 seconds. (There is no *flapping tremor* of the hands—if there were you would want to examine the fundi for papilloedema.)

These findings suggest cor pulmonale due to chronic bronchitis and emphysema. (Right heart failure is often precipitated by acute infection.)

The auscultatory cardiac signs of pulmonary hypertension, some of which may be audible,* are:

Loud pulmonary second sound
Pulmonary early systolic ejection click
Right ventricular fourth heart sound
Pansystolic murmur of functional tricuspid incompetence (giant *v* waves)
Early diastolic murmur of functional pulmonary incompetence (Graham–Steell murmur)

Causes of pulmonary heart disease

Chronic bronchitis (with or without emphysema; by far the commonest cause—p. 136)
Recurrent pulmonary emboli (signs of pulmonary hypertension without clinical evidence of other lung disease; ?DVT)
Primary pulmonary hypertension (signs of pulmonary hypertension without clinical evidence of other lung disease)
Non-pulmonary causes of alveolar hypoventilation (kyphoscoliosis, obesity, neuromuscular weakness)

Lung diseases which only rarely result in cor pulmonale including:

Emphysema (a much less common cause than chronic bronchitis—p. 136)
Progressive massive fibrosis (?coal dust tattoos on the skin; chronic bronchitis is the commonest cause of cor pulmonale in miners)
Bronchiectasis (especially cystic fibrosis; ?clubbing, cyanosis, full sputum pot, productive cough, crepitations—p. 146)
Cryptogenic fibrosing alveolitis (?clubbing, cyanosis, basal crackles—p. 97)
Systemic sclerosis (hands, facies—p. 90)
Sarcoidosis (?lupus pernio—p. 210)
Asthma (severe and chronic; may be missed if the reversibility is not checked in chronic small airways obstruction)

* These findings, which may be prominent in cor pulmonale due to other causes, may be difficult to elicit in cor pulmonale where a barrel-shaped chest and hyperinflation are present, and the heart is enfolded by over-inflated lungs.

87 / Myelinated nerve fibres

Frequency in survey: 1% of attempts at MRCP short cases.

Record

There are *bright white*, streaky, irregular patches with frayed margins at the edge of the disc. These are due to myelinated nerve fibres. They do not affect vision.

Normally the fibres of the optic nerve lose their myelin sheath as they enter the eye. Occasionally the sheath persists for some distance after the fibres leave the optic disc. If this phenomenon is extensive the disc and emerging vessels can be obscured.

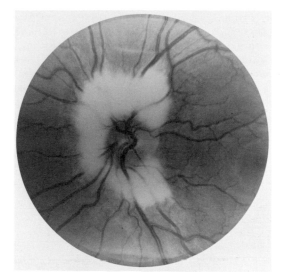

Fig. 3.87. Myelinated nerve fibres.

For colour photograph see p. 373.

Frequency in survey: 1% of attempts at MRCP short cases.

Record

There is *distal wasting* of the *lower limb muscles* which *stops abruptly* part of the way up the legs (say where).* The feet show *pes cavus* and clawing of the toes, and there is weakness of the extensors of the toes and feet. The *ankle jerks* are *absent* and the plantar reflexes show no response. There is only slight *distal involvement* of *superficial* modalities of *sensation* (though occasionally marked sensory loss may lead to digital trophic ulceration). The lateral popliteal (?and ulnar) nerves are palpable (in some families only). The patient has a *steppage gait* (bilateral foot drop). There is (may be) *wasting of the small muscles of the hand*.

   The diagnosis is peroneal muscular atrophy.

Patterns of inheritance are variable.

   The degree of disability in this condition is commonly surprisingly slight in spite of the remarkable deformities. Toe retraction and talipes equinovarus may occur and fasciculation (much less apparent than in motor neurone disease) is sometimes seen.

   The degeneration is mainly in the motor nerves.

It is sometimes also found in the dorsal roots and dorsal columns, and slight pyramidal tract degeneration is often seen (however in classical cases extensor plantars are not found). The condition usually becomes arrested in middle-life. Other members of the patient's family may have a *formes fruste* and show just minor signs such as pes cavus and absent ankle jerks only.

* As the disease progresses, the wasting creeps very slowly up the limb, inch by inch, involving all muscles. According to the stage of the disease, the characteristic appearances have been described as 'stork' or 'spindle' legs, 'fat bottle' calves, and 'inverted champagne bottles'. The same process may occur in the arms; wasting of the small muscles of the hands is common with a tendency for the fingers to curl and the patient to have difficulty in straightening and abducting them.

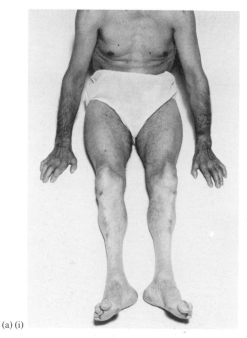

(a) (i)

Fig. 3.88. (a): (i), (ii), (iii) note that the muscle wasting stops in the thighs, foot-drop, pes cavus, and wasting of the small muscles of the hand all in the same patient. (b) Distal wasting in the upper limbs.

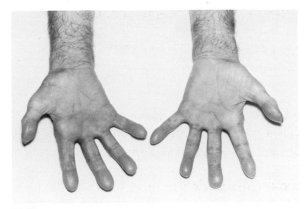

(a) (ii)

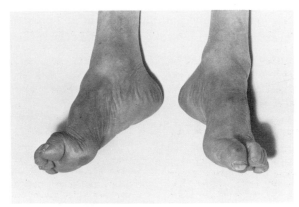

(a) (iii)

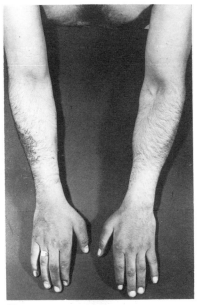

(b)

89 / Cataracts

Frequency in survey: Main focus of a short case in 1% of attempts at MRCP short cases. Additional feature in a further 4%.

Record

There are partial cataracts in both eyes (may be localized to the lens nucleus, or seen as flakes, dots or sector-shaped opacities within the lens periphery).

The commonest causes of cataracts are

1 Old age (usually nuclear, with a brownish discolouration, or of the cortical spoke variety).
2 Diabetic patients develop senile cataracts at younger ages than non-diabetics and this is the commonest type of cataract in diabetes. Rarely a 'snowflake' (dot cortical opacities) cataract can develop in a young, poorly controlled diabetic, and progress rapidly to a mature cataract in months or even days (good control may halt and even reverse development).

Other causes of cataract in adults

Trauma
Chronic anterior uveitis
Hypoparathyroidism (Chvostek's and Trousseau's signs, tetany, paraesthesiae and cramps, ectodermal changes, moniliasis, mental retardation and psychiatric disturbances, papilloedema, epilepsy, bradykinetic-rigid syndrome)
Radiation (infra-red, ultra-violet, X-rays and possibly microwaves)
Dystrophia myotonica (?frontal balding, ptosis, sternomastoid wasting, myopathic facies, myotonia, etc.—p. 144)
Retinitis pigmentosa (including Refsums, Laurence–Moon–Biedl—p. 131)
Steroid therapy (10 mg prednisolone daily for more than one year)
Chlorpromazine (500 mg daily for three years or more)
Chloroquine

Causes of cataracts in children include: perinatal hypoglycaemia, perinatal hypocalcaemia, maternal rubella, galactosaemia, galactokinase deficiency, genetically inherited, Down's syndrome (trisomy 21), Patau's syndrome (trisomy 13), Edward's syndrome (trisomy 18), Alport's syndrome, Lowe's syndrome.

90 / Idiopathic haemochromatosis

Frequency in survey: 1% of attempts at MRCP short cases.

Record

There is (in this thin patient) *slate-grey pigmentation,** *decreased body hair* and *gynaecomastia* (and *testicular atrophy**—iron deposition affecting hypothalamic pituitary function). The *liver** is *enlarged* at ... cm (in 95% of symptomatic patients; spleen is present in 50%).

The diagnosis is haemochromatosis.

Males > females.

In males it may present at any time in adult life. In females it usually presents after the menopause (physiological iron loss protects).

Autosomal recessive—association with HLA-A3.

Other features which may be present

Spider naevi

Palmar erythema

Ascites

Jaundice

Diabetes mellitus* (not entirely due to iron deposition in the pancreas because insulin levels may be normal and there is a higher incidence of diabetes in relatives without iron overload; high incidence of insulin resistance and fat atrophy)

Arthropathy* (pseudogout—especially the second and third metacarpophalangeal joints, wrists, hips, and knees)

Cardiac involvement* (large heart, dysrhythmias, congestive cardiac failure; it is the presenting manifestation in 15%—sometimes young adults; it may be *misdiagnosed* as idiopathic cardiomyopathy)

Hepatocellular carcinoma (develops in 33% of cirrhotic patients; it does not appear to occur if the disease is treated in the precirrhotic stage;

hence the importance of *family screening*)

Addison's disease, hypothyroidism and hypoparathyroidism are exceedingly rare

Treatment

Weekly *phlebotomy* (500 ml) until the haemoglobin concentration falls below 11 g dl^{-1} and the patient is marginally iron deficient (serum ferritin < 10 ug l^{-1}—this usually takes two to three years), then maintenance phlebotomy to keep the serum iron and ferritin in the low normal range (about once every three months). If anaemia and hypoproteinaemia preclude phlebotomy, *desferrioxamine* may be indicated. This is most practically administered by high dose subcutaneous infusion using a portable pump. *Ascorbic acid* given concurrently improves iron excretion.

NB Patients with alcoholic liver disease often have increased stainable iron on liver biopsy. These can be divided into two groups: (i) mild to moderate increase in stainable iron but relatively normal body iron stores (< 3 g); (ii) gross iron deposition and increased body iron stores. Phlebotomy may prolong survival in the latter (the majority of whom have idiopathic haemochromatosis) but not the former group.

---

* The association of hepatomegaly, skin pigmentation, diabetes mellitus, heart disease, arthritis and evidence of hypogonadism should always suggest haemochromatosis. These days the precirrhotic condition is often diagnosed in young relatives by family screening. The diagnosis should be considered in any patient with unexplained hepatomegaly, idiopathic cardiomyopathy, abnormal pigmentation or loss of libido (may antedate the other clinical manifestations of the disease). Ninety per cent of patients show bronzing of the skin due to excess melanin. In half, haemosiderin is also present, giving the skin the classic slate-grey appearance.

91 / Chest infection/consolidation/pneumonia

Frequency in survey: Main focus of a short case in 1% of attempts at MRCP short cases. Additional feature in many others (Ca bronchus and old TB—pp. 132 and 102).

Record

There is reduced movement of the R/L side of the chest. There is *dullness* to percussion over . . . (describe where) with *bronchial breathing, coarse crepitations, whispering pectoriloquy* and a *pleural friction rub*.

These features suggest consolidation (say where).

The commonest causes of consolidation

Bacterial pneumonia (pyrexia, purulent sputum, haemoptysis, breathlessness)

Carcinoma (with infection behind the tumour; ?clubbing, wasting, etc.—p. 132)

Pulmonary infarction (fever less prominent, sputum mucoid, occasionally haemoptysis and blood-stained pleural effusion)

92 / Coarctation of the aorta

Frequency in survey: Main focus of a short case in 1% of attempts at MRCP short cases. Additional feature in a further 1%.

Record

The radial pulses (in this young adult with a well-developed upper torso) are regular, equal,* and of large volume (give rate). The *carotid pulsations* are *vigorous,*† and the JVP is not elevated (unless there is heart failure). The *femorals* are *delayed* and of *poor volume* (palpate the radial and femoral simultaneously). The *blood pressure* in the right arm is elevated at 190/110 mmHg (it will be *low in the legs*). There are *visible arterial pulsations*‡ and *bruits* can be heard over and around the *scapulae, anterior axilla* and over the *left sternal border* (internal mammary artery). The cardiac impulse is heaving but not displaced (unless in failure). Systolic *thrills* are palpable over the collaterals and suprasternally. There is a *systolic murmur* which is loudest at the level of the *fourth intercostal space posteriorly* (the level of the coarctation), but is also audible in the *second intercostal spaces* close to the sternum (the murmur—if present—of the associated bicuspid aortic valve is often obscured by that from the coarctation).

These findings suggest a diagnosis of coarctation of the aorta.

Males:Females = 2:1

Other features and associations of coarctation of the aorta

Rib notching* and poststenotic dilatation on chest X-ray

Bicuspid aortic valve in 25% (site of infective endocarditis and may lead to coexisting aortic incompetence; diagnosis can be made by echocardiography)

Berry aneurysms of the circle of Willis (may cause death even in corrected cases)

Ventricular septal defect (?pansystolic murmur, etc.—p. 182)

Patent ductus arteriosus (?machinery murmur, etc.—p. 200)

Turner's syndrome (check for features of Turner's if your patient is female—webbed neck, increased carrying angle, short stature, etc.—p. 302)

Marfan's syndrome (?tall, arachnodactyly, high arched palate, lens dislocation, etc.—p. 244)

High mortality after the age of forty. Hypertension may not be cured even in corrected cases (low perfusion of kidneys may involve the renin-angiotensin system)

Other causes of rib notching

Neurofibromatosis (multiple neuromas on the intercostal nerves)

Enlargement of nerves (amyloidosis, congenital hypertrophic polyneuropathy)

Inferior vena cava obstruction

Blalock shunt operation (left-sided unilateral rib notching)

Congenital

---

* Rarely (2%) the coarctation is proximal to the origin of the left subclavian artery and the left arm pulses will be weaker than the right; rib notching will be unilateral and right sided.
† If you see vigorous carotid pulsations the likeliest cause is aortic incompetence (?collapsing pulse). The occasional patient, however, will have coarctation.
‡ Collaterals are best observed with the patient sitting up and leaning forward with the arms hanging by the side.

93 / Bulbar palsy

Frequency in survey: 1% of attempts at MRCP short cases.

Record

The *tongue* is *flaccid* and *fasciculating* (it is wasted, wrinkled, thrown into folds and increasingly motionless). The *speech* is *indistinct*, lacks modulations and has a *nasal twang*, and *palatal movement* is *absent*. There is (may be) saliva at the corners of the mouth (and while the patient talks he may be seen to pause periodically to gulp the secretions that have accumulated meanwhile in the pharynx; there may be dysphagia and nasal regurgitation).

This is bulbar palsy.

Possible causes
1   Motor neurone disease (?muscle fasciculation, absence of sensory signs, etc.—p. 116).
2   Syringobulbia (?nystagmus, Horner's, dissociated sensory loss, etc.—p. 268).
3   Guillain–Barré syndrome (?generalized including facial flaccid paralysis, absent reflexes, peripheral neuropathy or widespread sensory defect; monitor peak flow rate).
4   Poliomyelitis.
5   Neurosyphilis.

94 / Choreoathetosis

Frequency in survey: Main focus of a short case in 1% of attempts at MRCP short cases. Additional feature in a further 2%.

Survey note: Often hemichorea associated with a hemiplegia.

Record

There are *brief, jerky, abrupt, irregular, quasi-purposeful, involuntary movements* (which never integrate into a coordinated act but may match it in complexity). The movements *flit* from one part of the body to another in a random sequence; they are *present at rest* and *accentuated by activity* (at rest the movements prevent the patient's relaxation and they interrupt and distort voluntary movement). The patient has a general air of restlessness. He is *unable* to keep his *tongue protruded* (it darts in and out). There is *abnormal posturing* of the *hands* in which the wrist is flexed and the fingers are hyperextended at the metacarpophalangeal joints. When the upper limbs are raised and extended there is *pronation of the forearm*.
This is chorea.*

Causes of chorea

Sydenham's chorea (usually between age 5 and 15; ?heart murmur; one third have a history of rheumatic fever; it may recur during pregnancy and when on the oral contraceptive pill)
Huntington's chorea (affects the lower limbs more often than the upper, producing a dancing sort of gait; chorea may precede dementia; onset age 35–50; family history)
Drug-induced chorea (e.g. neuroleptics, L-dopa)
Senile chorea (idiopathic orofacial dyskinesia; no dementia)
Other causes of chorea include epidemic encephalitis, the encephalopathies occurring with exanthema, idiopathic hypocalcaemia, thyrotoxicosis, SLE, carbon monoxide poisoning, polycythaemia rubra vera, acanthosis, and hereditary.

Causes of hemichorea/hemiballism†

Cerebrovascular accident† (?hemiplegia, homonymous hemianopia)
Intracerebral tumour (?pyramidal signs on the side of the chorea, papilloedema)
Trauma
Post-thalamotomy

Other types of involuntary movement (dyskinesias)

Athetosis‡ (slow, coarse, irregular, writhing muscular distortion most commonly of the hands, feet and digits, though the face and tongue may be affected—many choreic and dystonic movements are indistinguishable from athetosis)
Dystonia‡ (sustained spasm of some portion of the body; the movements are powerful and deforming, torticollis is a common example of torsion dystonia; lordosis and scoliosis may also be caused)
Myoclonus (rapid shock-like muscular jerks often repetitious and sometimes rhythmic—most common causes include epilepsy, essential [familial], physiological [sleep, exercise, anxiety], metabolic disorders [renal, respiratory or hepatic failure], subacute encephalitis)
Tremors (e.g. Parkinson's, anxiety, thyrotoxicosis, drugs [e.g. alcohol, caffeine, salbutamol], multiple sclerosis, spinocerebellar degeneration, CVA, essential/familial)
Tics

* In choreoathetosis (cerebral palsy, tumours involving the pallidum, vascular insufficiency, Wilson's disease, carbon monoxide poisoning, etc.) the movements mainly involve the upper limbs and cranial nerves (grimacing, writhing movements of the tongue, etc.). The hands are repeatedly brought in front of the chest shaped like cups with flexion at the metacarpophalangeal joints and extension at the interphalangeal joints.
† Hemiballism is wild irregular flinging or throwing movements of whole limbs on one side. Vascular lesions are the commonest cause. The lesion is in the contralateral subthalamic nucleus. The ballistic movements often begin as the other neurological signs of the CVA start to clear (i.e. after an interval). They disappear during sleep. Though initially they may exhaust the patient, they usually die out gradually over 6–8 weeks.
‡ The common causes of the two closely linked dyskinesias, dystonia and athetosis, are drugs (neuroleptics, L-dopa) and post-hypoxia. There are many rare causes.

95 / Dysarthria

Frequency in survey: Main focus of a short case in 1% of attempts at MRCP short cases. Additional feature in at least a further 1%.

Survey note: The only dysarthria used as a short case in our survey was cerebellar (ataxic) dysarthria.

Record

There is dysarthria with *slurred, jerky* and *explosive* (slow, lalling, staccato, scanning) speech. (There may be inspiratory whoops indicating the lack of coordination between respiration and phonation).

This suggests cerebellar disease (?nystagmus, dysdiadochokinesis, finger–nose test, etc.— p. 130).

Other varieties of dysarthria

Spastic dysarthria (Conditions in which all or some of the articulatory parts are rigid or spastic)
Pseudobulbar palsy (indistinct, suppressed, without modulations, high-pitched, 'hot potato', 'Donald Duck' speech due to a tight, immobile tongue— ?bilateral spasticity with extensor plantars—p. 265)
Parkinson's disease (monotonous without accents or emphasis, somewhat slurred speech—?expressionless unblinking face, glabellar tap sign, tremor, etc.—p. 134)
Dystrophia myotonica (slurred and suppressed speech—?ptosis, frontal balding, etc.—p. 144)
Huntington's chorea (slurred and monotonous— ?chorea, dementia)
General paresis of the insane—very rare (slurred, hesitant or feeble voice—?dementia, vacant expression, trombone tremor of tongue, brisk reflexes, extensor plantars, etc.—p. 310)

Paralytic dysarthria
Bulbar palsy (nasal, decreased modulation, slurring of labial and lingual consonants—?lingual atrophy, fasciculations, etc.—p. 146)
Paralysis of the VIIth, IXth, Xth or XIIth nerves (CVA)

Myopathic dysarthria
Myasthenia gravis (weak hoarse voice with a nasal quality, pitch unsustained, soft accents—?ptosis, variable strabismus, facial and proximal muscle weakness all of which worsen with repetition, etc.—p. 246).

Variegated dysarthria
Hypothyroidism (low-pitched, catarrhal, hoarse, croaking, gutteral voice as if the tongue is too large for the mouth—?facies, pulse, ankle jerks, etc.—p. 138)
Amyloidosis—large tongue (rolling and hollow, hardly modulated)
Multiple ulcers or thrush in the mouth (some parts of the speech indistinct)
Parotitis or temporomandibular arthritis (monotonous, suppressed, badly modulated)

96 / Dysphasia

Frequency in survey: Main focus of a short case in 1% of attempts at MRCP short cases. Additional feature in a further 1%.

Survey note: Where the type of dysphasia was reported by the candidate, it was always expressive.

Record 1

The patient's speech *lacks fluency*. He has *difficulty finding certain words* and sometimes produces the *wrong word*. *Comprehension* however is *well-preserved* (as are the higher cerebral functions and general intellect—the prognosis for eventual adaptation of the patient to his disability is good) and his ability to repeat is better than his spontaneous speech.

The patient has Broca's (*expressive*, non-fluent) *dysphasia* (?associated *right hemiplegia*). The brain damage causing this condition is believed to involve the dominant* inferior frontal gyrus (Broca's area).

Record 2

Though the patient *speaks fluently* (often rapidly) with normal intonation, his speech is completely *unintelligible*. He puts words together in the wrong order and mixes them with non-existent words† and phrases (*jargon dysphasia*). Attempts to repeat result in paraphasic† distortions and irrelevant insertions. *Comprehension* is severely *impaired* (and the patient may seem unaware of his dysphasia).

The patient has Wernicke's (*receptive*, fluent) *dysphasia* (?associated *homonymous visual field defect* and/or *sensory diminution* down the right side of the body). The brain damage causing this condition is believed to involve the posterior part of the dominant* superior temporal gyrus (Wernicke's area).

Record 3

The patient shows combined expressive and receptive dysphasia. There is marked disturbance in comprehension (and inability to read or write).

The patient has *global dysphasia* (?dense right hemiplegia with sensory loss, homonymous visual field defect and general intellectual deterioration). The common cause of this is infarction of the territory supplied by the left middle cerebral artery. The prognosis for recovery is poor.

Record 4

The patient has difficulty naming objects though he knows what they are (e.g. Hold up some keys: 'What is this?'—Patient does not answer. 'Is this a spoon?'—'No'. 'Is it a pen?'—'No'. 'Is it keys?'— 'Yes'). Despite this, comprehension and other aspects of speech production are relatively normal.

This is *nominal dysphasia* (uncommon in its pure form—usually part of a wider dysphasia). The underlying brain damage is believed to be in the most posterior part of the superior temporal gyrus and the adjacent inferior parietal lobule.

---

* The left hemisphere is dominant in right-handed and in 50% of left-handed people.

† **Paraphasia:** An incorrect syllable in a word (usually there is some phonemic relationship to the original word, e.g. 'tooth spooth' for 'toothbrush') or an incorrect word in a phrase (often with a semantic relationship to the correct word, e.g. 'hand' for 'foot').

Neologism: Paraphasia with slight or no relationship to the original syllable/word.

97 / Ehlers–Danlos syndrome

Frequency in survey: 1% of attempts at MRCP short cases.

Record

The patient (may be wearing glasses; myopia common) has *epicanthal folds*, a *flat nasal bridge* and prominent ears which point downwards. There is *hyperextensibility* of the skin which is *elastic* and *very thin*. There is evidence of *poor healing* with *thin scars* (the skin tears with minor injury, usually over the knees and elbows, producing *fish-mouth* wounds). *Purpura* is present and there are (commonly) *pseudotumours* over the knees and elbows (trauma→haematoma which organizes→fatty degeneration→calcification). The joints are (remarkably) *hyperextensible* and the patient has kyphoscoliosis, genu recurvatum and flat feet.

The diagnosis is Ehlers–Danlos syndrome.

There are at least seven distinct types which vary from mild to severe and show different patterns of inheritance (dominant, recessive, X-linked).

Complications

Bleeding (mostly from the gut)
Poor healing which makes surgery difficult
Recurrent dislocations of patellae, shoulders, hips, etc.
Recurrent hydrarthrosis
Repeated falls (poor control due to hypermobile joints)
Diaphragmatic herniae
Diverticulae of the gastrointestinal and respiratory tracts
Spontaneous pneumothorax
Dissecting aneurysms
Spontaneous rupture of large arteries
Mitral valve prolapse (p. 196)

Other causes of hypermobile joints

Osteogenesis imperfecta* (p. 298)
Marfan's syndrome (tall, long bones, dislocated lens, etc. p. 244)
Turner's syndrome (p. 302)
Noonan's syndrome (males and females; short stature, webbed neck, etc., p. 302)
Down's syndrome (p. 287)
Pseudoxanthoma elasticum (p. 270)
Familial tendency in otherwise normal patients

Cutis laxa: In this condition the skin may also be hyperextensible, but in contrast to Ehlers–Danlos syndrome it has decreased elasticity, and hangs in loose folds. Late in Ehlers–Danlos, the skin in localized areas may resemble that seen in cutis laxa.

* Blue sclerae often occur in Ehlers–Danlos also.

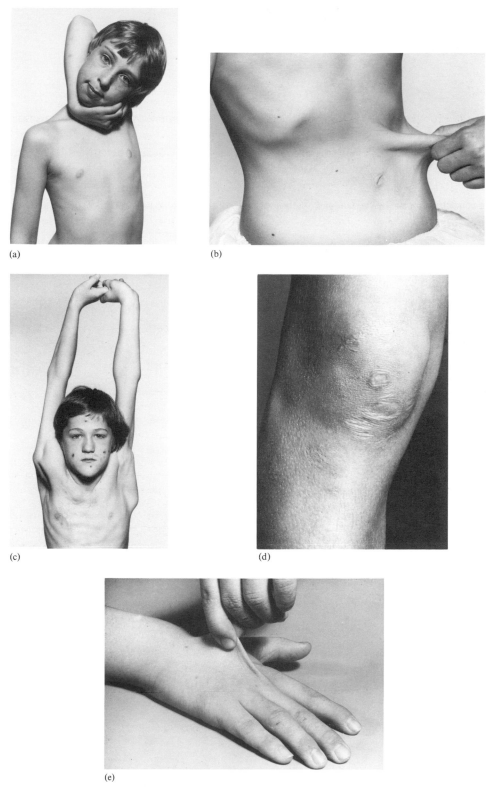

(a)

(b)

(c)

(d)

(e)

Fig. 3.97. (a), (b), (c), (d), (e) Ehlers–Danlos syndrome.

98 / Erythema ab igne

Frequency in survey: 1% of attempts at MRCP short cases

Record

There is a *reticular pigmented rash* on the . . . (describe the site—usually lateral aspect of one *leg*).

It is characteristic of erythema ab igne. (The patient obviously feels the cold. Look at the face and feel the pulse—?hypothyroidism.)

Other conditions which show a reticuloid pattern in the skin

Livedo reticularis (arborescent pattern of reddish-blue erythema or pigmentary change which may be associated with an underlying condition such as a collagen vascular disease—especially polyarteritis nodosa, cryoglobulinaemia, or a hyperviscosity syndrome)

Cutis marmorata (a physiological reaction to cold seen in 50% of normal children and many adults)

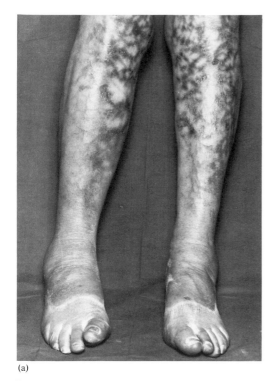
(a)

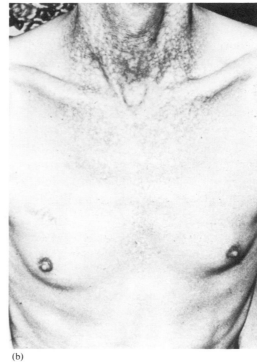
(b)

Fig. 3.98. (a) Erythema ab igne. (b) Livedo reticularis visible on the neck (SLE).

99 / Marfan's syndrome

Frequency in survey: 1% of attempts at MRCP short cases.

Record

The patient is *tall* with disproportionately *long extremities* (pubis–sole > pubis–vertex) and elongated fingers and toes (*arachnodactyly*). He has a *high-arched palate* (gothic), long narrow face and his span is greater than his height. His musculature is underdeveloped and hypotonic (and he may have a funnel or pigeon chest, pectus excavatum, kyphoscoliosis, flat feet, genu recurvatum, hyperextensibility of joints and recurrent dislocations). The tremor of the iris (*iridodonesis*) is evidence of *lens dislocation* (50–70% of patients;—a slit lamp may be needed for detection in minor cases). He has (may have) a collapsing pulse (ausculte if allowed) suggestive of *aortic incompetence* (cystic necrosis of the aortic media leading to steadily progressive dilatation of the aorta; aortic dissection can occur).

The diagnosis is Marfan's syndrome.

Autosomal dominant.

Other features which may occur in Marfan's syndrome

Heterochromia of the iris
Blue sclerae
Myopia
Undue liability to retinal detachment
Cystic disease of the lungs (tendency to spontaneous pneumothorax)
Mitral valve prolapse (p. 196—common; severe mitral incompetence may occur)
Coarctation of the aorta
Bacterial endocarditis even on valves with only minor abnormalities

Inguinal or femoral herniae
Decreased subcutaneous fat
Miescher's elastoma (small nodules or papules in the skin of the neck)
Death due to cardiovascular component (average age is mid-40s)

NB *Homocystinuria* (autosomal recessive) may produce a similar clinical picture to Marfan's except in addition mental retardation, a malar flush and osteoporosis are common and ocular lens dislocation is downwards (in Marfan's it is upwards). Homocystine can be detected in the urine by the cyanide-nitroprusside test.

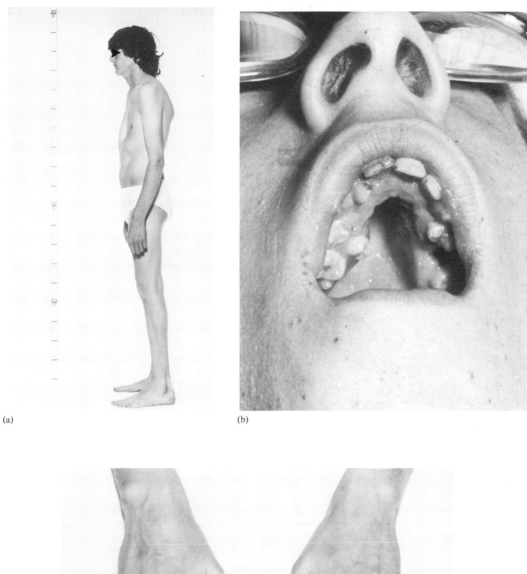

(a)

(b)

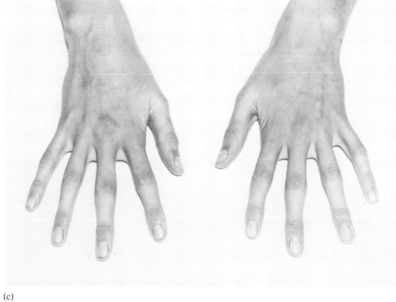

(c)

Fig. 3.99. (a), (b), (c) Marfan's syndrome.

Frequency in survey: Main focus of a short case in 1% of attempts at MRCP short cases. Additional feature in a further 1%.

Record

There is *ptosis* (one or both sides) accentuated by upward gaze, *variable strabismus* (with *diplopia*) and when she tries to screw her eyes up tight, the eyelashes are not buried. The face shows a *lack of expression*, the mouth is slack and there is generalized *facial weakness*. The patient *snarls* when she tries to smile, she cannot whistle, and her *voice* is *weak* and *nasal* (if you ask the patient to count aloud, speech may become progressively less distinct and more nasal). There is *proximal muscle weakness*. Repetitive movements cause an increase in the muscle weakness (myasthenia = abnormal muscular fatiguability).

The diagnosis is myasthenia gravis. A tensilon test will confirm it.

Males:Females = 1:2.

Other features of myasthenia gravis

Difficulty with swallowing, chewing and nasal regurgitation

Symptoms worsen as the day progresses

Tendon reflexes are normal or exaggerated (cf. Eaton–Lambert syndrome)

Antiacetylcholine receptor antibodies are present in 90%

In long-standing cases there may be an element of permanent irreversible myopathic change

Breathlessness is a sinister symptom requiring urgent attention (respiratory deterioration may develop rapidly and should be watched for by monitoring the peak flow rate)

Pathological changes are present in the thymus in 70–80% and some patients are improved by thymectomy; thymomas occur in 10–20% (mostly males) and give a worse prognosis

Associated immune disorders include thyrotoxicosis (5% of patients), hypothyroidism, rheumatoid arthritis, diabetes mellitus, polymyositis, SLE, pernicious anaemia, Sjögren's syndrome, pemphigus and sarcoidosis.

Crisis Signs of *cholinergic crisis* are collapse, confusion, abdominal pain and vomiting, sweating, salivation, lachrymation, miosis and pallor. The features which distinguish *myasthenic crisis* are response to edrophonium and absence of cholinergic phenomena. Occasionally it is exceptionally difficult to determine whether the collapsed myasthenic has been under- or over-treated. Temporary withdrawal of all drugs and assisted positive pressure respiration is then indicated.

Myasthenic crisis may be provoked by:
  Infection
  Emotional upset
  Undue exertion*
  Drugs (streptomycin, gentamicin, kanamycin, neomycin, viomycin, polymyxin, colistin, curare, quinine, quinidine, procainamide)

Eaton–Lambert syndrome (myasthenic-myopathic syndrome): This is often associated with oat-cell carcinoma of the bronchus. There is proximal muscle wasting, weakness and fatiguability. Often, however, power is initially increased by brief exercise (reversed myasthenic effect). The tendon reflexes are depressed (but increased soon after activity). The electromyographic response to ulnar nerve stimulation shows a characteristic increase in amplitude (it declines in myasthenia gravis). Cholinergic drugs have no effect. Weakness and fatiguability may be greatly improved by guanidine hydrochloride.

* Childbirth requires careful management.

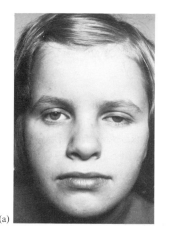

(a)

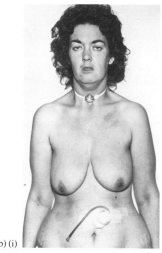

(b) (i)

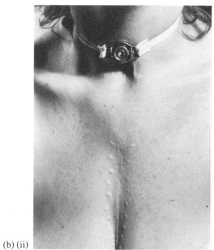

(b) (ii)

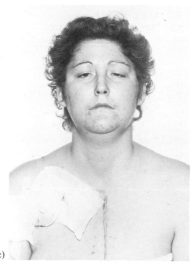

(c)

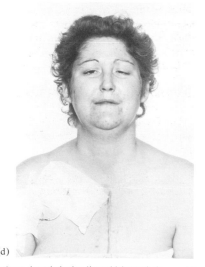

(d)

Fig. 3.100. (a) A mild case with unilateral ptosis. (b): (i) & (ii) A severe case (note myasthenic facies, thymectomy scar, gastrostomy feeding tube and tracheostomy). (c) Myasthenic facies (note the subclavian line which was being used for plasmapherisis). (d) 'Smile'.

Frequency in survey: 1% of attempts at MRCP short cases.

Record

There are *Heberden's nodes* present at the bases of the distal phalanges (and less commonly Bouchard's nodes at the proximal interphalangeal joints). There is a 'square hand' deformity due to subluxation of the base of the first metacarpal. There is swelling and deformity of the knee joints with development of varus (or valgus) deformity. There is crepitus in these joints. There is wasting and weakness of the quadriceps and glutei, and there is downward tilting of the pelvis when the patient stands on the affected leg (Trendelenberg's sign).

This patient has osteoarthrosis.

Complications

Pain
Deformity
Ankylosis

Entrapment of nerves (e.g. ulnar nerve palsy or carpal tunnel syndrome)
Cervical spondylosis

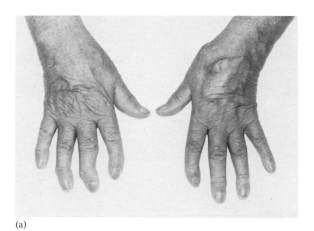

(a)

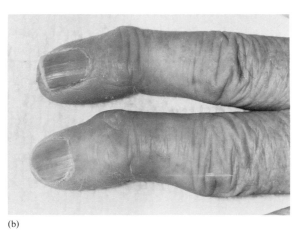

(b)

Fig. 3.101. (a), (b) Note the square hand deformity and Heberden's nodes.

Frequency in survey: Main focus of a short case in 1% of attempts at MRCP short cases. Additional feature in many others.

Record

The JVP is elevated (measure) at . . . cm above the sternal angle (look for individual waves and time against the opposite carotid artery). The predominant wave is the systolic *v* wave which reaches the ear lobes. (If there is no oscillation of the blood column, sit the patient up to find the upper level. Make sure that there is no superior vena caval obstruction with the congestion of the face and neck, and prominent veins on the upper chest—p. 224.) The carotid pulsation is irregularly irregular and the rhythm is atrial fibrillation (look for the evidence of CCF: ankle and sacral oedema, hepatomegaly, which may be pulsatile in tricuspid incompetence).

The large *v* wave suggests tricuspid incompetence either organic or due to congestive cardiac failure (see also p. 201).

Causes of a raised JVP (if venous obstruction is excluded)

Congestive cardiac failure (ischaemic heart disease, valvular heart disease, hypertensive heart disease, cardiomyopathy)

Cor pulmonale (?signs of chronic small airways obstruction, cyanosis, etc.—p. 228)

Pulmonary hypertension (large *a* wave in the JVP;—primary [young females] and secondary to mitral valve disease or thrombo-obliterative disease)

103 / Pretibial myxoedema

Frequency in survey: Main focus of a short case in 1% of attempts at MRCP short cases. Additional feature in a further 3%.

Record

There are *elevated symmetrical* skin lesions over the anterolateral aspects of the *shins* (may spread onto the feet; may affect other parts of the body, e.g. the face). The lesions are coarse, *purplish-red* (may be skin colour pink, or rarely, brown) in colour and raised with *well-defined* serpiginous *margins*. The skin is *shiny* and has an *orange peel appearance*. The hairs in the affected areas are coarse and the lesions are *tender* (and itch). The patient has *exophthalmos* (*?thyroid acropachy*) and is likely to have been rendered *euthyroid* (?pulse, etc.) by surgery (*?thyroidectomy scar*) or, more particularly, with *radioactive iodine*.

The diagnosis is pretibial myxoedema (occurs in about 5% of patients with Graves' disease).

The superficial layer of the skin is infiltrated with the mucopolysaccharide, hyaluronic acid. Biopsy scars of the area almost invariably develop keloid.

The latent interval between the treatment for hyperthyroidism and the clinical onset of pretibial myxoedema varies from four to thirty-two months with a mean time of one year.

For colour photograph see p. 380.

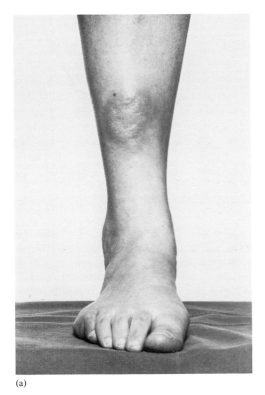

(a)

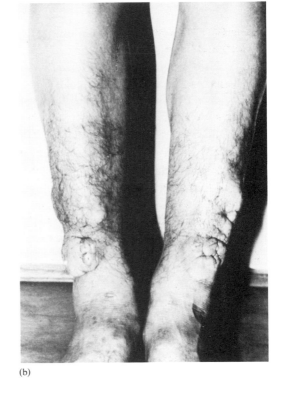

(b)

Fig. 3.103. (a), (b) Pretibial myxoedema.

104 / Retinal artery occlusion

Frequency in survey: 1% of attempts at MRCP short cases.

Survey note: Reported to have occurred as the underlying cause of optic atrophy with attenuated retinal arteries, and as a retinal artery branch occlusion causing a quadrantic field defect. No cherry-red spots were reported!

Record

The eye is blind, the *fundus* is *pale*, the *arterioles* are *thin* and *scanty* and there is a *cherry-red spot* at the macula (because the underlying choroidal circulation is intact).

The diagnosis is central retinal artery occlusion.

In the acute phase the whole fundus (except for the cherry-red spot) is milky white due to retinal oedema. By the time the retinal oedema has faded optic atrophy is generally apparent. The cherry-red spot is usually only seen for about 5–10 days. In retinal artery branch occlusion the fundoscopic appearances of thin arterioles and pale retina are limited to one area and there is a corresponding field defect (e.g. an inferior temporal field defect due to infarction of the superior nasal fundus).

The condition occurs most commonly in the elderly arteriosclerotic patient. It may be due to thrombosis, embolus (?carotid bruits, atrial fibrillation, heart murmurs) or spasm. Transient retinal artery occlusions associated with contralateral hemiparesis may occur from recurrent carotid emboli.

Occlusion of the central retinal artery may also follow giant-cell arteritis involving the arterioles around the optic disc (?headaches and temporal artery tenderness).

For colour photograph see p. 373.

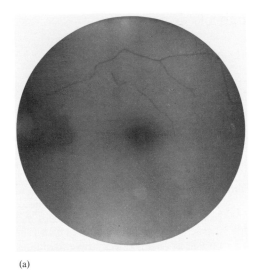
(a)

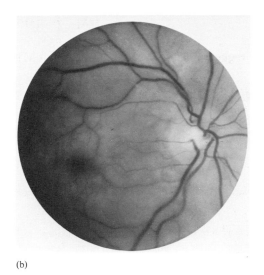
(b)

Fig. 3.104. (a), (b) Retinal artery occlusion. Note macular cherry-red spots. The milky-white fundus due to retinal oedema is very pronounced in (a).

Frequency in survey: 1% of attempts at MRCP short cases.

Record

There are *areas* of *depigmentation* around the eyes, mouth, on the knees, and on the dorsum of the feet (the hands, axillae, groins and genitalia are the other commonly affected areas).
   The patient has vitiligo.

Sites subject to friction and trauma are often affected and Koebner's phenomenon (a lesion appearing at the site of skin damage) is common. Vitiligo is usually symmetrical but occasionally the depigmentation can be unilateral and follow the pattern of a dermatome. It is inherited as a dominant trait and individuals are usually otherwise healthy. Halo naevi (hypopigmented rings surrounding dark naevi), leucotrichia, premature greying of the hair and alopecia areata as well as vitiligo may all be associated with any of the **organ-specific autoimmune diseases**:

   Myxoedema (?pulse, ankle jerks, facies—p. 138)
   Hashimoto's disease (?goitre—p. 138)
   Graves' disease (?exophthalmos, fidgety, goitre, tachychardia, etc.—p. 108)
   Pernicious anaemia (?pallor, spleen, SACD)
   Atrophic gastritis associated with iron deficiency anaemia
   Addison's disease (?buccal, skin crease, scar and general pigmentation, hypotension, etc.—p. 216)

For colour photograph see p. 377.

Idiopathic hypoparathyroidism (Chvostek's and Trousseau's signs, tetany, paraesthesiae and cramps, cataracts, ectodermal changes, moniliasis, mental retardation, psychiatric disturbances, bradykinetic rigid syndrome, epilepsy)
Premature ovarian failure
Diabetes mellitus (?fundi)
Renal tubular acidosis
Fibrosing alveolitis (?basal crepitations)
Chronic active hepatitis (?icterus, etc.)
Primary biliary cirrhosis (?xanthelasma, pigmentation, icterus, scratch marks, etc.—p. 208)

Vitiligo, the cutaneous marker of organ-specific autoimmune disease, may occur in the non-organ-specific autoimmune disease systemic sclerosis.* Other disorders associated with vitiligo are morphoea and malignant melanoma.

---

* Rarely there is an overlap between the organ-specific and non-organ-specific autoimmune diseases. Sjögren's syndrome occupies an intermediate position being associated with rheumatoid arthritis on the one hand and autoimmune thyroiditis on the other. Primary biliary cirrhosis is another condition which bridges the gap. It is associated with Sjögren's syndrome, Hashimoto's thyroiditis and renal tubular acidosis on the one hand, and systemic sclerosis, CRST syndrome, rheumatoid arthritis, coeliac disease, dermatomyositis and mixed connective tissue disease, on the other.

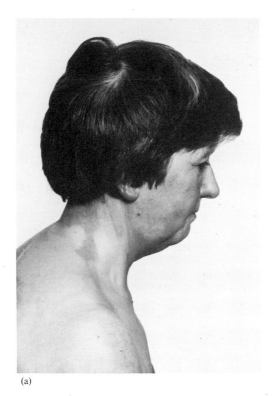

(a)

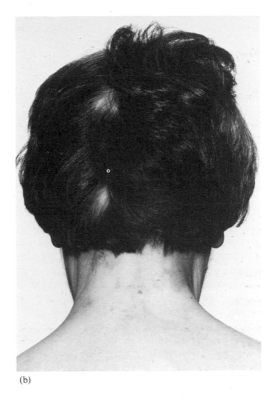

(b)

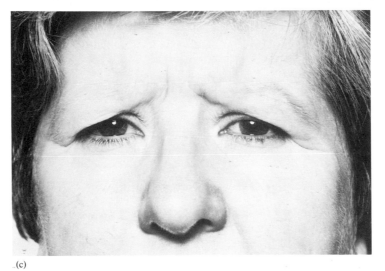

(c)

Fig. 3.105. (a), (b), (c) Note the areas of vitiligo and alopecia areata including loss of eyelashes (especially left upper lid) in this patient with diabetes mellitus.

Frequency in survey: 1% of attempts at MRCP short cases.

Record

There is *asymmetrical swelling* affecting the *small joints* of the *hands* and feet with *tophi* formation (in the periarticular tissues). These joints are (occasionally) severely *deformed*. There are tophi on the *helix* of the *ear* and in some of the tendon sheaths (especially the ulnar surface of forearm, olecranon bursa, the Achilles tendon, and other pressure points).

This patient has chronic tophaceous gout.

Chronic tophaceous gout results from recurrent acute attacks. Tophus formation is proportional to the severity and duration of the disease. However, patients with severe tophaceous disease appear to have milder and less frequent acute attacks than non-tophaceous patients. Large tophi may have areas of necrotic skin overlying them and may exude chalky or pasty material containing monosodium urate crystals. Sinuses may form. Tophi may resolve slowly with effective treatment of hyperuricaemia. Effective antihyperuricaemic therapy has reduced the incidence and severity of the tophaceous disease. A major complication is renal disease (urolithiasis, urate nephropathy). Carpal tunnel syndrome may occur.

Associations include obesity, type IV hyperlipidae-mia, and hypertension. These associations may be the cause of an association which has also been recognized between gout and two other conditions—diabetes mellitus and ischaemic heart disease.

Secondary hyperuricaemia may occur in many situations including:
  Diuretics (especially thiazides)
  Myeloproliferative and lymphoproliferative disorders (and other conditions with increased turnover of preformed purines)
  Chronic renal failure

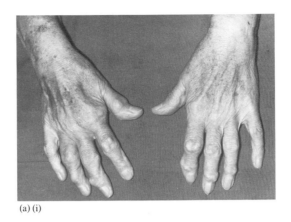

(a) (i)

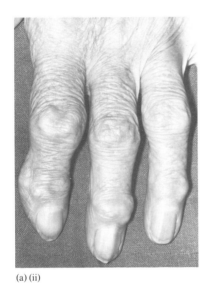

(a) (ii)

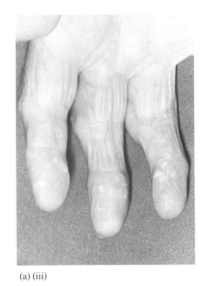

(a) (iii)

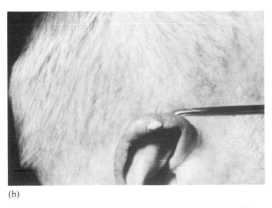

(b)

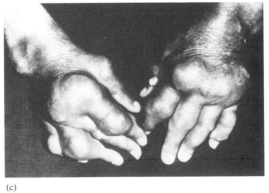

(c)

Fig. 3.106. (a): (i), (ii), (iii) Gouty tophi and arthropathy. (b) A tophus on the helix of the ear. (c) An extreme case of tophaceous gout.

107 / Fallot's tetralogy with a Blalock shunt

Frequency in survey: 1% of attempts at MRCP short cases.

Survey note: The cases of Fallot's tetralogy in our survey all had a Blalock shunt.

Record

There is a thoracotomy scar. There is *central cyanosis* and *clubbing* of the fingers. The pulse is regular (give rate) and the *left pulse is weaker than the right*. The venous pressure is normal. The apex beat is (may be) palpable (say where), there is a *left parasternal heave* and a *systolic thrill* is palpable in the pulmonary area. There is a loud *ejection systolic murmur* (unless the stenosis is so severe that virtually no blood traverses it) in the *pulmonary area*.

It is likely that this patient has had a Blalock shunt* for Fallot's tetralogy (pulmonary stenosis, ventricular septal defect, right ventricular hypertrophy and overriding aorta).

The features which may be helpful in differentiating Fallot's tetralogy from Eisenmenger's are shown in Table 3.65 (p. 193).

---

* Anastomosis of the subclavian artery to the pulmonary artery. This operation is not often performed nowadays as total correction on cardiopulmonary bypass is usually the treatment of choice.

Frequency in survey: Main focus of a short case in 1% of attempts at MRCP short cases. Additional feature in a further 1%.

Record

The pulse rate is regular at 40 per min (irregularly irregular pulse with beat-to-beat variation may be slow atrial fibrillation) and there is *no increase* in the rate on *standing* (complete heart block; mostly in older patients). The JVP is not elevated (unless there is heart failure) but just visible, and there is a complete dissociation of *a* and *v* waves with frequent *cannon waves* (flicking *a* waves occurring during ventricular systole).

This patient has complete heart block.

Other causes of bradycardia

Beta-blocker therapy: about 2% of patients receiving beta-blockers have excessive bradycardia (heart rate increases by a few beats on standing and during exercise)

Slow atrial fibrillation: the patient may be on beta-blockers and/or digoxin

Hypothyroidism (?facies, ankle jerks, etc.—p. 138)

Sino-atrial disease: bradycardia-tachycardia syndrome

Digitalis overdose

Cardiac pacing in complete heart block:

Temporary pacing for cardiovascular decompensation (fall in BP, acute left ventricular failure)

Permanent pacing for heart failure and syncope (Stokes–Adams attacks)

Demand pacing for bradycardia-tachycardia or intermittent heart block

Fixed rate pacing at 72/min in cases of persistent bradycardia

Frequency in survey: 0.9% of attempts at MRCP short cases.

Record

There is a *heliotrope* rash* around the *eyes* and the *backs* of the *hands*, especially around the *knuckles* and *fingernails*. It is also present (may be) over the extensor surfaces of the elbows and knees. There is subcutaneous oedema (mainly around the eyes and due to a transient increase in capillary permeability). There is *proximal muscle weakness* and (may be) tenderness.

    The diagnosis is dermatomyositis.

Males:Females = 2:1.

Other features of dermatomyositis

Features and associations similar to polymyositis (p. 280)

Association with malignancy (in up to 25% of adults; association much stronger after age 50)

Overlap with rheumatic fever, rheumatoid arthritis, scleroderma, lupus erythematosus and other connective tissue diseases may occur (steroid responsiveness more likely)

Signs of other connective tissue diseases commoner than in pure polymyositis

Dysphagia due to upper oesophageal involvement

Raynaud's and arthralgia are frequent

Helpful investigations include serum muscle enzymes, urinary creatinine, EMG (fibrillation, polyphasic action potentials and in some patients high frequency bizarre repetitive discharges) and muscle biopsy. The ESR is often normal despite active disease

The mainstay of treatment is steroids (initially in high doses)

There is a juvenile form occurring in the first decade. Myopathy is severe, healing occurs with contractures and calcification in the skin and muscles, but Raynaud's is rare. There is no association with malignancy

For colour photographs see p. 374.

---

* From the shrub *heliotropium* which has fragrant purple flowers. The characteristic rash is a purple/violet/lilac colour. The skin changes may be subtle and easily overlooked. The classical heliotrope rash is diagnostic of the condition and, though it is most commonly seen in the childhood form, it also occurs in the adult form. Other skin manifestations include *local and diffuse erythema, erythema nodosum like lesions, eczema, exfoliating dermatitis, blisters and scaling*, and *maculopapular eruptions*. The skin lesions may occasionally ulcerate.

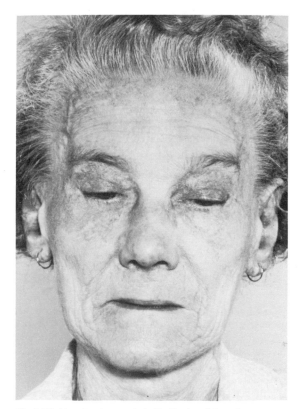

Fig. 3.109. Note the characteristic distribution of the rash.

Frequency in survey: Main focus of a short case in 0.9% of attempts at MRCP short cases. Additional feature in a further 0.6%

Record

The patient's *skin* is *soft, wrinkled* and *pale* with a *yellow tint* (the pallor is due to a combination of MSH lack and anaemia—marrow hypofunction). The areolae of the breasts are (may be) depigmented. *Pubic, axillary, facial* and *body hair is reduced* (and the *genitals* and *breasts* are *atrophied*).

These features suggest hypopituitarism (now check for a bitemporal visual field defect).

With progressing hypopituitarism gonadotrophin secretion is usually impaired first, followed by GH, TSH, ACTH* and ADH, in that order. With the onset of thyroid failure the features of hypothyroidism (p. 138) are superimposed on those in the above *record*. Lassitude, cold intolerance, dryness of skin and prolongation of tendon reflexes occur though swelling of the subcutaneous tissues is usually less prominent. The insidious onset of asthenia, nausea, vomiting, postural hypotension, hypoglycaemia, collapse and coma mark progressive ACTH lack. Diabetes insipidus develops with ADH lack, though impaired glomerular filtration caused by cortisol deficiency may mask the symptoms.

The main causes of adult panhypopituitarism (male:female = 1:2) are:

Sheehan's syndrome (following severe obstetric haemorrhage or shock—much less common nowadays with good obstetric practice)

Pituitary tumour (especially chromophobe adenoma)

Craniopharyngioma

Pituitary granulomatous lesion (tuberculoma, sarcoidosis, Hand–Schüller–Christian disease, syphilitic gumma)

Iatrogenic (hypophysectomy, yttrium or gold seed implantation)

Head injury

The factors that lead to coma in hypopituitarism include hypoglycaemia, sodium depletion, water intoxication, cerebral anoxia, hypothyroidism, hypothermia and pressure on the midbrain or hypothalamus.

---

* Pituitary hypothyroidism may protect the patient from the effects of failing ACTH secretion. In this situation misdiagnosing the cause of hypothyroidism and waking the patient from hibernation with thyroxine alone may precipitate Addisonian crisis.

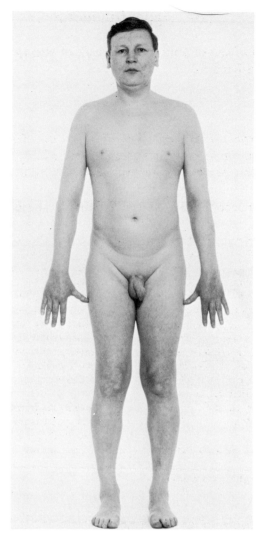

Fig. 3.110. Hypopituitarism (eight years after removal of
pituitary adenoma).

111 / Swollen knee

Frequency in survey: Main focus of a short case in 0.9% of attempts at MRCP short cases. Additional feature in a further 1.5%.

Survey note: Half of the cases were due to rheumatoid arthritis.

Record

There is generalized *swelling* of the R/L *knee joint* obscuring the lateral dimples. The *patellar tap sign** is *positive* suggesting the presence of fluid in the synovial cavity. The swelling does not extend to the back in the popliteal fossa (always check).† The joint is *painful* to move and it is *warm*.

There is an *effusion* in the knee joint. (Now look at the hands for evidence of rheumatoid arthritis—p. 68.)

Causes of a swollen knee

Rheumatoid arthritis (the swelling may be due to synovial thickening—synovium palpable as boggy tissue around the joint margin)

Osteoarthritis (osteophytes on X-ray)

Rupture of a Baker's cyst (rheumatoid arthritis)

Pseudogout (calcified menisci; birefringent calcium pyrophosphate crystals; associated with a large variety of conditions including hyperparathyroidism, haemochromatosis, acromegaly, diabetes mellitus, Wilson's disease, hypothyroidism, alkaptonuria and gout; there are also idiopathic and hereditary varieties)

Septic arthritis (purulent fluid, organisms in a smear)

Gout (urate crystals)

Trauma

Charcot's knee (painless, ?tabes dorsalis—p. 310)

Haemarthrosis of haemophilia

Oedematous states (congestive cardiac failure, nephrotic syndrome)

* With one hand above the knee joint, exert pressure to drive fluid from the suprapatellar pouch into the knee joint proper. With the index finger of the other hand, depress the patella with a sharp jerky movement. If the patella rebounds this is definite evidence of fluid in the knee joint. The sign may not be positive if there is too much or too little fluid. To test for a small amount of fluid in the knee joint, displace fluid by depressing one of the obliterated hollows on either side of the ligamentum patellae. The hollow will slowly refill.

† Swelling in the popliteal fossa extending down to the upper third of the calf in cases of ruptured Baker's cyst.

112 / Pseudobulbar palsy

Frequency in survey: 0.9% of attempts at MRCP short cases.

Record

There is monotonous, slurred, high-pitched, 'Donald Duck' *dysarthria* and the patient *dribbles persistently* from the mouth (he has dysphagia and may have nasal regurgitation). He *cannot protrude his tongue* which lies on the floor of the mouth and is *small and tight*. *Palatal movement* is *absent*, the *jaw jerk* is *exaggerated* and he is *emotionally labile*.

The diagnosis is pseudobulbar palsy (?bilateral generalized spasticity and extensor plantar responses).

The commonest cause

Bilateral CVAs of the internal capsule

Other causes

Multiple sclerosis
Motor neurone disease
High brain-stem tumours

113 / Pemphigus/pemphigoid

Frequency in survey: 0.9% of attempts at MRCP short cases.

Record 1

This middle-aged (or elderly) patient has flaccid *thin-roofed blisters* (usually over the axillae and trunk), which vary in size (usually 1–2 cm in diameter). Most of the blisters have *burst* leaving *red* and *exuding areas* (which are extremely tender). There are also (not always) red denuded patches in the *mouth* (the first site involved in up to 50%), *pharynx* and *eyes*.

The patient has pemphigus.

Record 2

This elderly patient has *tense blisters* varying in size from a few millimetres to a few centimetres in diameter involving . . . (describe where—usually it is the limbs but it can be widespread). There are also *reddened* and *urticarial* (sometimes eczematous) *patches* surrounding and separate from the blisters. There are no lesions in the mouth (they do occur but are uncommon).

The diagnosis is pemphigoid.

Pemphigus vulgaris: This condition occurs most commonly in Jewish people. The site of the blister is in the epidermis. Occasionally lesions may occur without initial blister formation. The mucous membranes never have blisters, only denuded patches. It is a progressive and fatal condition if not treated with corticosteroids in very high doses (initially 100–200 mg daily of prednisolone). Azathioprine may reduce the maintenance dose of steroid. It can be caused by penicillamine, phenylbutazone and rifampicin. There is an increased incidence in patients with thymoma and myasthenia gravis. *Acantholysis* is a characteristic histological feature. Nikolsky's sign* is invariably present.

Pemphigoid: The site of the blisters is at the basement membrane between the epidermis and the dermis; therefore the blister is thicker and less likely to rupture than in pemphigus. Mucosal lesions are less common in pemphigoid. Though it is self-limiting (2 years) systemic steroids are usually given (initially 60–80mg/day) and azathioprine may reduce the maintenance dose. It does not have a high mortality like pemphigus. It has been alleged that it is sometimes a manifestation of underlying malig-

nancy but this point is not proven. It can be caused by frusemide, clonidine and PUVA.

Other bullous disorders

Dermatitis herpetiformis (groups of blisters on the elbows, knees and buttocks; associated with coeliac disease—p. 306)

Epidermolysis bullosa congenita (congenital blistering disorders usually of hands and feet; genetically determined; range from simple blisters to severe scarring with contractures; teeth and nails abnormal in some forms)

Epidermolysis bullosa acquisita (associated with inflammatory bowel disease, amyloidosis and internal malignancy)

Herpes gestationis (pregnancy or early puerperium, erythematous/urticarial lesions with blistering—hands usually; no relation to herpes virus; resolves in a few weeks; may require steroids; recurs with increased severity in subsequent pregnancies)

Hailey–Hailey disease (benign familial pemphigus, onset age 10–30 years; unrelated to pemphigus)

For colour photograph see p. 375.

---

* Firm pressure on apparently normal skin causes it to slide off. Nikolsky's sign may also occur in other severe bullous eruptions, such as those due to dermatitis herpetiformis, epidermolysis bullosa or drugs.

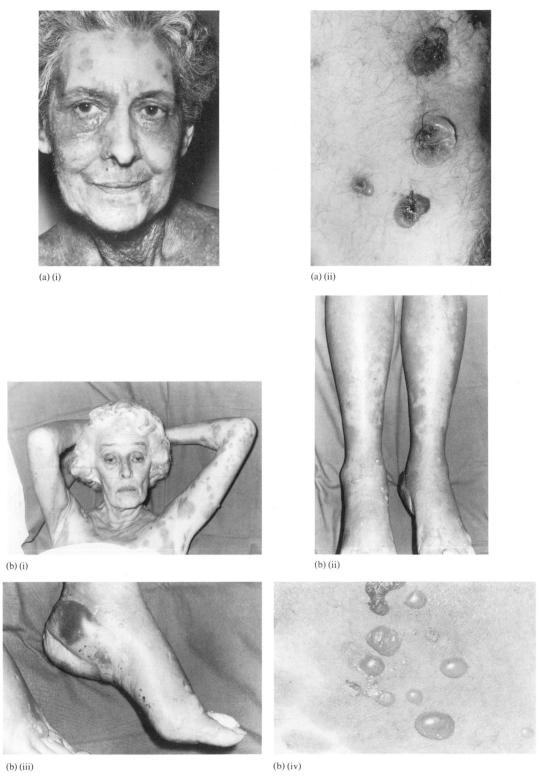

(a) (i)

(a) (ii)

(b) (i)

(b) (ii)

(b) (iii)

(b) (iv)

Fig. 3.113. (a): (i), (ii) pemphigus. Note denuded areas and ruptured blisters. (b): (i), (ii), (iii), (iv) pemphigoid. Note the tense blisters.

114 / Syringomyelia

Frequency in survey: 0.9% of attempts at MRCP short cases.

Record

This patient (with *kyphoscoliosis*) shows *wasting* and weakness of the *small muscles* of the *hands* (sometimes there is curling of the fingers), flattening of the muscles of the ulnar border of the forearm and the upper limb *reflexes* are *absent* (conspicuous fasciculation is uncommon). There is *dissociated sensory loss** over (one or both of) the upper limbs and the upper chest† and there are *scars* (from painless burns and cuts) on the hands. The lower limb reflexes are exaggerated and the plantars are extensor. A *Horner's syndrome* is (may be) present (involvement of sympathetic neurones especially at C8/T1).

These findings suggest syringomyelia (*?nystagmus*, which may occur with lesions from C5 upwards—i.e. involving the medial longitudinal bundle—see Fig. 3.48, p. 157)

Syringobulbia Syrinxes may involve upper cervical and bulbar segments (usually an extension of syringomyelia but the syrinx may begin in the brainstem) and cause:

Nystagmus

Ataxia

Facial dissociated sensory loss (initially onion skin loss over the outer part of the face, from involvement of the lower part of the Vth nucleus in the cord, may occur before the syrinx reaches the medulla)

Bulbar palsy (wasted fasciculating tongue, palatal paralysis, nasal dysarthria, dysphagia, weakness of sternomastoids and trapezius from XIth nerve involvement, etc.—p. 236)

Trophic and vasomotor disturbances are common in syringomyelia, e.g.:

Areas of loss of, or excessive, sweating

La main succulente (ugly, cold, puffy, cyanosed hands with stumpy fingers and podgy soft palms)

Coarse, thickened skin over the hands with callosities over the knuckles and scars from old injuries

Slow healing and indolent ulceration of digits

Charcot's joints may occur, usually at the elbow or shoulder. Tabes dorsalis (knees, hips) and diabetes mellitus (toes, ankles) are the other causes of Charcot's joints (see also p. 154).

Skeletal abnormalities which may be associated with syringomyelia

(Kypho-) scoliosis (mild, very common)

Short neck (e.g. fusion of the cervical vertebrae; Klippel–Feil syndrome)

Asymmetrical thorax

Sternal depression or prominence

Cervical ribs (may cause diagnostic difficulty)

---

* Analgesia and thermoanaesthesia but light touch and proprioception intact. In the early stages cold stimuli may be perceived but not warm.

† Due to destruction by the syrinx of crossing axons carrying pain and temperature sensation. The area affected depends on the length of the syrinx—e.g. lower cervical and upper thoracic. Separate from this effect on crossing axons, the syrinx may also involve one or both spinothalamic tracts producing dissociated sensory loss in one or both lower limbs.

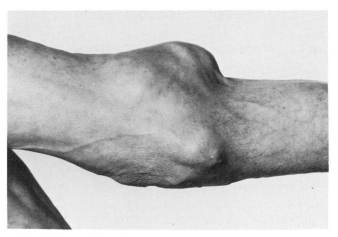
Fig. 3.114. Charcot's joint at the elbow.

115 / Pseudoxanthoma elasticum

Frequency in survey: 0.8% of attempts at MRCP short cases.

Record

There is *loose skin* mainly over the *neck, axillae, antecubital fossae* and *groins,* in which there are seen (1–3 mm) *yellow pseudoxanthomatous plaques* (there may be *redundant folds of lax skin*). There is a '*chicken-skin*' appearance because of the clear margins around the hair follicles.

This patient has pseudoxanthoma elasticum.

It is due to an inherited defect of elastin. There are four main types (two are recessive and two are dominant). An occlusive arteriopathy is the major cause of symptoms. Steroids should be avoided and the diagnosis is confirmed by skin biopsy.

Other features which may occur

Angioid streaks* in the retina (60% have eye changes)
Blue sclerae

Loose jointedness
Hypertension due to renovascular disease (50%)
Gastrointestinal (10%), genito-urinary or respiratory haemorrhage
Coronary artery disease
Peripheral vascular disease (weak or absent pulses, claudication, often vascular calcification)
Mitral incompetence
Hypothyroidism (?due to involvement of thyroid vasculature)

For colour photographs see p. 382.

* The triad of skin lesions, angioid streaks of the retinae and vascular abnormalities is called the Grönblad–Strandberg syndrome. Other causes of angioid streaks include Ehlers– Danlos syndrome, Paget's disease of the bone and sickle-cell anaemia.

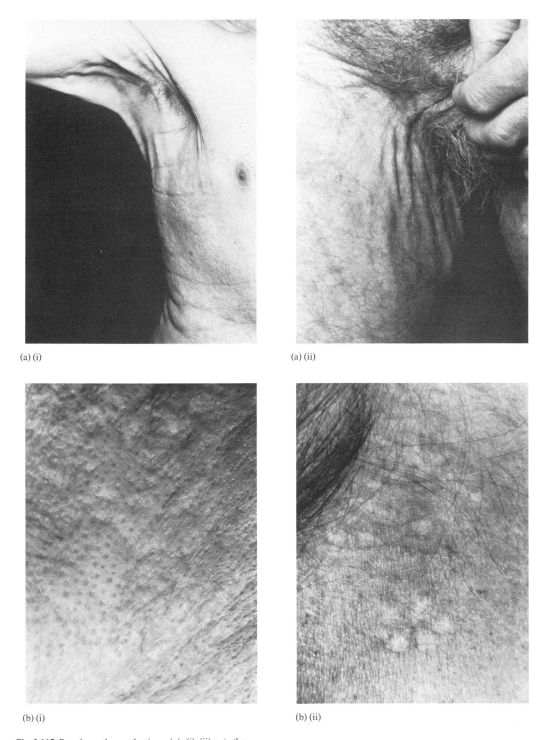

(a) (i)

(a) (ii)

(b) (i)

(b) (ii)

Fig. 3.115. Pseudoxanthoma elasticum (a): (i), (ii) note the loose skin. (b): (i), (ii) Plucked chicken-skin appearance.

116 / Radiation burn on the chest

Frequency in survey: Main focus of a short case in 0.8% of attempts at MRCP short cases. Additional feature in a further 4%.

Survey note: Usually one of many physical signs in a patient with carcinoma of the bronchus (see experience 1, p. 327), sometimes causing superior vena cava obstruction. Rarely other intrathoracic malignancy. Occasionally the main focus of a short case.

Record

There is an area of *erythema* on the *chest* wall. The chest has been marked (radiotherapy *field markings* or 'Red Indian' marks) for deep X-ray therapy and this (or the signs of *intrathoracic malignancy*) suggests that it is due to a radiotherapy burn (see p. 132).

For colour photograph see p. 379.

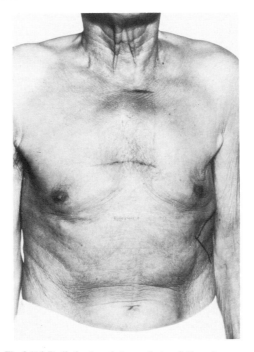

Fig. 3.116. Radiation burn between the two field marks over the chest, and marks over the left lower chest wall (carcinoma of the lung).

Frequency in survey: Main focus of a short case in 0.8% of attempts at MRCP short cases. Additional feature in a further 0.4%.

Record

There is (in this patient who may complain of burning paraesthesiae in the feet) loss of *light touch, vibration* and *joint position* sensation over the feet (*stocking*, may also be *glove*), and *Romberg's* sign is positive. The legs are (may be) weak, and though the knee (may be brisk) and *ankle jerks* are *lost* (due to peripheral neuropathy) the *plantar responses are extensor*.

The pupils are normal, there are no cerebellar signs or pes cavus (p. 290) and though the patient is not (may not be) clinically anaemic* (having checked conjunctival mucous membranes) and the tongue and complexion are normal (glossitis and classical 'lemon yellow' pallor are now rarely seen in SACD), these findings suggest the diagnosis of subacute combined degeneration of the cord. (Findings in the abdomen might be splenomegaly, carcinoma of the stomach as this is commoner in pernicious anaemia, or a laparotomy scar from a previous gastrectomy.)

Though vitamin B_{12} neuropathy usually starts with peripheral neuropathy followed by posterior column signs, and signs of pyramidal disturbances are seldom marked in the early stages (progressive spasticity may occur), vitamin B_{12} deficiency should always be excluded in a patient in whom any of the following are unexplained:

Peripheral sensory neuropathy

Spinal cord disease

Optic atrophy (rare)

Dementia (frank dementia rare; progressive enfeeblement of intellect and memory, or episodes of confusion or paranoia may be seen; more commonly the patient is simply difficult and uncooperative).

Causes of severe vitamin B_{12} deficiency

Addisonian pernicious anaemia (NB associated organ-specific autoimmune diseases especially autoimmune thyroid disease, diabetes mellitus, Addison's, vitiligo and hypoparathyroidism—see also p. 254)

Partial or total gastrectomy

Stagnant loop syndrome

Ileal resection or Crohn's disease

Vegan diet

Fish tapeworm

Chronic tropical sprue

Congenital intrinsic factor deficiency

Lhermittes phenomenon: The patient describes a 'tingling' or 'electric feeling' or 'funny sensation' which passes down his spine, and perhaps into lower limbs, when he bends his head forward. The most common cause is multiple sclerosis but it can also occur in cervical cord tumour, cervical spondylosis and subacute combined degeneration of the cord.

* Though the patient may be anaemic, vitamin B_{12} neuropathy may develop without anaemia and with normal blood film and bone marrow. Serum vitamin B_{12} level may be required to confirm the diagnosis.

Frequency in survey: 0.8% of attempts at MRCP short cases.

Record

This young lady has a unilateral *dilated pupil* which *fails* (or almost fails) *to react to light*. There is no ptosis or diplopia and eye movements are otherwise normal (i.e. not IIIrd nerve palsy).

The patient has a myotonic pupil. Her tendon reflexes may be lost (check if allowed).

If exposed to light for prolonged periods the pupil may constrict slowly. If then exposed to darkness for a long period it will again dilate very slowly. During accommodation–convergence, after a delay which may last several minutes, the abnormal pupil constricts slowly until it may become smaller than the normal pupil. The reaction to mydriatics is normal (Argyll Robertson pupil dilates poorly with mydriatics) and the pupil may be hyper-reactive to cholinergic substances.

The condition is usually chronic and symptomless but in some cases onset is acute with associated blurring of vision and photophobia. Syphilitic serology will be negative. Differential diagnosis from neurosyphilis may be difficult in the chronic stages of this disorder, when the pupil may be chronically constricted, and especially when both pupils are affected (bilateral involvement rare with Holmes–Adie pupils but invariable with syphilitic Argyll Robertson pupils).

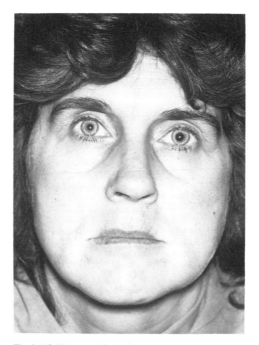

Fig. 3.118. Holmes–Adie pupil.

119 / Nephrotic syndrome

Frequency in survey: 0.7% of attempts at MRCP short cases.

Record

There is *extensive oedema* affecting the ankles, lower legs and periorbital tissues (especially in the morning) of this (may be young*) patient. The skin is pale (oedema in the skin). There are (may be) white bands across the nails (from chronic hypoalbuminaemia). There are (may be) bilateral *pleural effusions* and *ascites*.

This patient's extensive oedema could be due to nephrotic syndrome.†

Commonest cause

Glomerulonephritis (77%—usually minimal change in childhood but membranous in adults)

Other common causes in the UK

Systemic lupus erythematosus (?characteristic rash, arthropathy, etc.—p. 222)
Diabetic nephropathy (?medic-alert bracelet, fundi)
Renal amyloidosis (usually secondary amyloidosis; ?evidence of rheumatoid arthritis or other chronic disease, etc.—see footnote p. 65)
Renal vein thrombosis

Malaria due to *Plasmodium malariae* is an important cause in areas where it is endemic. There are about 70 rare causes.

Investigations for nephrotic syndrome

Urine microscopy (?red cells, casts, lipid deposits)
24 h urinary protein
Urinary protein selectivity (clearance ratio of IgG to tranferrin below 0.15 in minimal change disease, which carries a good prognosis)
Creatinine clearance (GFR)
Specific tests for the causal diseases (glucose, ANF, etc.)
Renal biopsy

Complications

Thrombosis (DVT, arterial, pulmonary, renal vein)
Malnutrition (high protein diet unless marked uraemia)
Atheroma and ischaemic heart disease (hypercholesterolaemia)
Infection

---

*The oedema of the acute poststreptococcal glomerulonephritis (proteinuria, haematuria, oliguria, oedema, hypertension, renal failure) which mainly affects children and young adults, is usually due to salt and water retention. Only in a small proportion does heavier proteinuria leading to nephrotic syndrome develop.

†Defined as proteinuria > 3.5 g per 1.75 m^2 of body surface per 24 h, hypoalbuminaemia and oedema. Hypercholesterolaemia is often present.

Frequency in survey: 0.7% of attempts at MRCP short cases.

Record

The patient has an *absent gag reflex* on the R/L side (and will have ipsilateral impaired taste over the posterior third of the tongue). *Palatal movements* on that side are *reduced* and the *uvula* is *drawn* to the *opposite side*. The R/L *sternomastoid* muscle is *wasted* and there is weakness in rotating the head to the opposite side. The *shoulder* is *flattened* and there is weakness of elevation of that shoulder.

There is therefore a lesion affecting the *IXth, Xth and XIth cranial nerves* on the R/L side.

This suggests a jugular foramen syndrome (check carefully for evidence of ipsilateral wasting, fasciculation and deviation of the tongue—XIIth nerve, ipsilateral Horner's and, if allowed, for evidence of brain-stem compression, e.g. spastic paraparesis).

An isolated lesion of the glossopharyngeal nerve is rare. It is usually damaged with the vagus and accessory nerves near the jugular foramen which all three nerves traverse (Fig. 3.120). A lesion inside the skull is more likely to cause a syndrome restricted to the IXth, Xth and XIth nerves only (syndrome of Vernet). An internal lesion may cause brain-stem compression*. A lesion outside the skull is more likely to involve the XIIth nerve as well (syndrome of Collet–Sicard)—this nerve exits through the hypoglossal foramen near the external opening of the jugular foramen. An external lesion may also involve the cervical sympathetic* (syndrome of Villaret). Other combinations of associated lower cranial lesions are vagus and accessory (syndrome of Schmidt), and vagus, accessory and hypoglossal (syndrome of Hughlings Jackson).

Causes of jugular foramen syndromes

Neurofibroma of IXth, Xth or XIIth nerves (especially left XIIth in young females)
Meningiomas
Epidermoid tumours (cholesteatomas)
Glomus or carotid body tumours
Metastases
Cerebello-pontine angle lesions (p. 285—may also extend down and involve the last four cranial nerves in numerical order)
Infection from the middle ear spreading into the posterior fossa
Granulomatous meningitis

---

*Intrinsic brain-stem disease may cause lower cranial nerve palsies and Horner's syndrome (e.g. pp. 268 and 320), but when the pathology is in the brain-stem there is nearly always spinothalamic sensory loss on the opposite side of the body to the lesion.

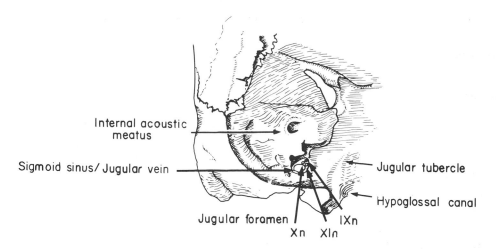

Internal acoustic meatus

Sigmoid sinus/Jugular vein

Jugular tubercle

Hypoglossal canal

Jugular foramen

Xn   XIn   IXn

Fig. 3.120. The posterior aspect of the posterior cranial fossa (after removal of the squamous part of the occipital bone) showing the jugular foramen and the nerves passing through it (note the position of the hypoglossal canal which conducts the XIIth nerve).

Frequency in survey: Main focus of a short case in 0.7% of attempts at MRCP short cases. Additional feature in a further 2%.

Record

This elderly (or middle-aged) patient has a *vesicular rash* in the *area supplied by the . . . nerve* (say which/where).* The lesions are in *clusters* at different stages of development (the stages each cluster goes through is papule → vesicle → [pustule, sometimes haemorrhagic] → crusting → scar). The regional lymph nodes are enlarged.

The diagnosis is herpes zoster.

Complications

Cranial nerve palsy (especially facial nerve palsy which may occur not only with lesions of the external auditory meatus [Ramsay Hunt syndrome], but also with trigeminal zoster and zoster of the head, neck and mouth†)

Peripheral motor palsy (LMN deficit from involvement of motor root—sometimes permanent)

Post-herpetic neuralgia (10%; commoner in the elderly; can be very severe and difficult to treat)

Eye damage (ophthalmic zoster)

For colour photograph see p. 375.

Zoster sine herpete (typical pain, etc. but no rash—serological evidence confirms)

Other complications include visceral nerve involvement (pain or dysfunction in an organ), myelitis (transverse or ascending—rare), disseminated encephalitis (rare), cerebellar ataxia (rare) and diffuse polyneuritis (rare).

Generalized herpes zoster is usually associated with an underlying reticulosis (especially Hodgkin's), leukaemia, or carcinoma (especially bronchogenic).

*The commonest is a thoracic dermatome. Cranial nerve involvement is next in frequency. The ophthalmic division of the trigeminal nerve is the commonest cranial nerve. With cranial nerve involvement there are often signs of meningeal irritation and sometimes mucous membranes are affected.

†In true Ramsay Hunt (see p. 184) the zoster is probably of the geniculate ganglion. In other cases there may be multiple cranial ganglia involvement (see anecdote 24, p. 343) and an associated localized encephalitis and neuronitis. Eighth nerve involvement (vertigo and deafness) is a particularly common association with facial palsy due to herpes zoster.

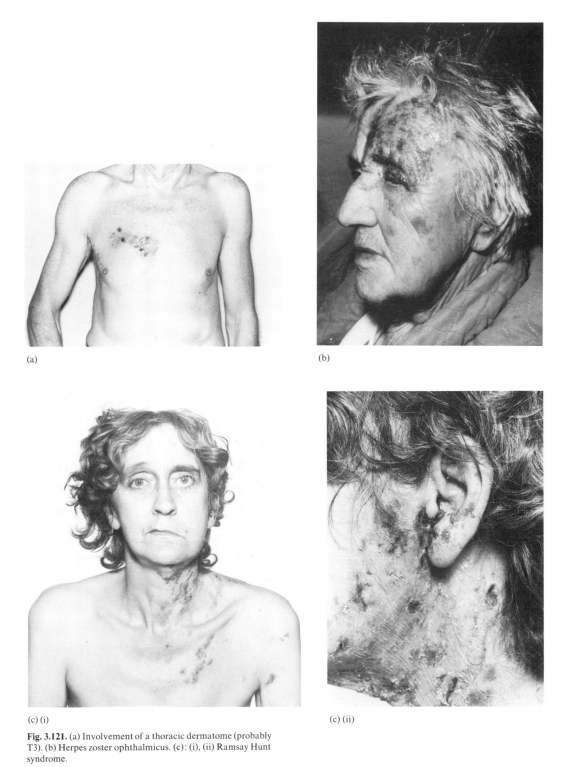

(a)

(b)

(c) (i)

(c) (ii)

Fig. 3.121. (a) Involvement of a thoracic dermatome (probably T3). (b) Herpes zoster ophthalmicus. (c): (i), (ii) Ramsay Hunt syndrome.

122 / Polymyositis

Frequency in survey: 0.6% of attempts at MRCP short cases.

Record

There is *symmetrical,** *proximal* muscle *weakness* (the patient may be unable to sit up from lying or stand up from squatting position) with associated muscle *wasting*. The muscles are *tender* (in 50% of cases—suggesting an inflammatory myopathy). The tendon reflexes are present though reduced.† There is (may be) dysphonia (and/or dysphagia) due to involvement of the bulbar muscles.

The diagnosis is polymyositis.

Males: Females = 1 : 2.

Features of polymyositis

A rash may occur (dermatomyositis—p. 260)
Features and associations similar to dermatomyositis (p. 260)
Association with malignancy (8%)
Onset of muscle weakness is usually insidious (with difficulty in running, climbing stairs, getting up from a chair, and combing hair)
Lower limb-girdle more often affected than shoulder-girdle
Ocular involvement is rare (if present, think of myasthenia gravis)
Respiratory muscle weakness can lead to respiratory failure—monitor peak flow rate and vital capacity
Cardiac muscle may be involved

Other causes of proximal muscle weakness

Carcinomatous neuromyopathy (including Eaton–Lambert syndrome—see p. 246)
Diabetic amyotrophy (?fundi, peripheral neuropathy)
Muscular dystrophies (?long-standing, familial—p. 212)
Dystrophia myotonica (?frontal balding, cataracts, myotonia, etc.—p. 144)
Alcoholism
Thyrotoxicosis (?eye signs, hypermobile, goitre, etc.—p. 108)
Corticosteroid treatment (?Cushingoid facies, underlying disorder, etc.—p. 218)
Familial periodic paralysis
Osteomalacia
Hyperparathyroidism
Insulinoma

Polymyalgia rheumatica is characterized by pain and stiffness of proximal muscles, especially shoulder girdle, in a patient who is usually elderly. The ESR is high. Significant objective weakness is not common. There is a relationship with temporal arteritis.

---

*In general, if muscle weakness is symmetrical it suggests myopathic disease, and if asymmetrical neurogenic disease.

†If very reduced or absent it suggests underlying carcinoma causing polyneuropathy and polymyositis.

123 / Argyll Robertson pupils

Frequency in survey: 0.5% of attempts at MRCP short cases. Additional feature in a further 0.4%.

Record

The pupils are *small* and *irregular* and react to *accommodation but not to light.**

The likely diagnosis is tabes dorsalis (?wrinkled forehead with ptosis, stamping ataxia, Romberg's test positive, loss of joint position and vibration sense, absent ankle jerks, Charcot's knee joint and aortic incompetence—p. 310).

The exact site of the lesion is not known. It is generally believed to be in the tectum of the midbrain proximal to the oculomotor nuclei. The classical Argyll Robertson pupil is very small. However, pupils affected by neurosyphilis are not always small and may even be dilated. They may be unequal in size. Though the signs may be more advanced in one eye than the other, pupillary abnormalities occurring in neurosyphilis are invariably bilateral. Argyll Robertson-like pupils occasionally occur in diabetes mellitus.

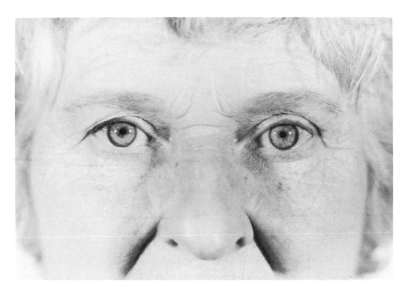

Fig. 3.123. Argyll Roberston pupils in a diabetic patient. Her serology was negative.

*The light reflex may become sluggish before it disappears, but the accommodation reflex is always brisker than the light.

Frequency in survey: 0.5% of attempts at MRCP short cases.

Record

There is flattening of the bridge of the nose (*saddle-nose*), the superior maxilla is underdeveloped which makes the mandible appear prominent (*bull-dog jaw*), and there is frontal bossing. There are *rhagades* at the corners of the mouth and there are *Hutchinson's teeth* (widely spaced peg-shaped upper incisors with a crescentic notch at the cutting edge) and *Moon's molars* (dome-shaped deformity of the first lower molars with underdeveloped cusps). The *tibiae are sabre-shaped*.

The diagnosis is congenital syphilis.

Other manifestations of late* congenital syphilis

VIIIth nerve deafness
Clutton's joints (effusions into the knee joints with no pain or difficulty with joint movement)
Interstitial keratitis (acute attacks;† may eventually lead to corneal opacities—ground-glass appearance of cornea)

Old choroidoretinitis (peripheral and bilateral—'Salt and pepper fundus'
Optic atrophy
Perforations of the palate or nasal septum
Collapse of the nasal cartilage

---

*Early congenital syphilis in the first few months of life resembles severe secondary syphilis in the adult. Features include rhinitis, a mucocutaneous rash, osteochondritis, dactylitis, hepatosplenomegaly, lymphadenopathy, anaemia, jaundice, thrombocytopenia and leucocytosis. Nephrotic syndrome may occur.
†May be due to hypersensitivity. Corticosteroids may sometimes help.

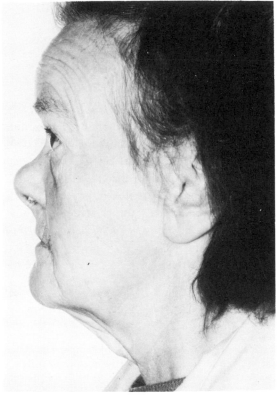

(a)

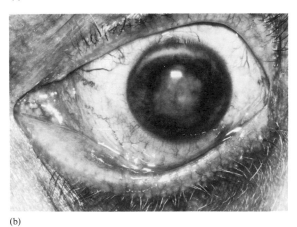

(b)

Fig. 3.124. Congenital syphilis. (a) Note the saddle nose. (b) Interstitial keratitis has led to corneal opacification.

Frequency in survey: Main focus of a short case in 0.5% of attempts at MRCP short cases. Additional feature in a further 0.8%.

Record

There is (in this ?stout, ?middle-aged lady who complains of pain, numbness or paraesthesiae in the palm and fingers which are particularly bad in the night*) *sensory loss* over the *palmar* aspects of the *first three and a half fingers* and *wasting* of the *thenar eminence*. There is weakness of *abduction, flexion* and *opposition* of the *thumb*.

The diagnosis is median nerve palsy. The non-involvement of the flexor muscles of the forearm suggests that the cause is carpal tunnel syndrome (now check the facies for underlying *acromegaly* or *myxoedema*; underlying *rheumatoid arthritis* should be obvious). *Tinel's sign*† is positive to confirm this.

Though in early cases there may be no abnormal physical signs, usually some impairment of sensation over the affected fingers can be detected. Tenderness on compression of the nerve at the wrist† and thenar atrophy are relatively rare. If the story is characteristic the absence of physical signs should not deter one from advising treatment with intracarpal tunnel steroid injection or carpal tunnel decompression.

Causes of carpal tunnel syndrome

Idiopathic (almost entirely females, middle-aged, often obese; or younger women with excessive use of hands; may occur in males after unaccustomed hand use—e.g. house painting)

Pregnancy

Contraceptive pill

Myxoedema (?facies, hoarse croaking voice, pulse, ankle jerks, etc—p. 138)

Acromegaly (?facies, large spade-shaped hands, bitemporal hemianopia, etc.—p. 104)

Rheumatoid arthritis of the wrists (?spindling of the fingers, ulnar deviation, nodules, etc.—p. 68)

Osteoarthrosis of carpus (perhaps related to an old fracture)

Tuberculous tenosynovitis

Primary amyloidosis (?peripheral neuropathy, thick nerves, autonomic neuropathy; heart, joint and gut [rectal biopsy] involvement may occur—see also footnote p. 126)

Tophaceous gout (p. 256).

---

*The nocturnal discomfort may be referred to the whole forearm with paraesthesiae extending beyond the cutaneous distribution of the median nerve in the hand. The sensory *signs* however, are confined to the classical median nerve distribution (Fig. 2.1, p. 24).

†*Tinel's sign* is tingling in the distribution of a nerve produced by percussion of that nerve. Percussion over the carpal tunnel sometimes produces a positive Tinel's sign in carpal tunnel syndrome. Other signs are *Phalen's sign* (the patient flexes both wrists for 60 sec and this produces a prompt exacerbation of paraesthesia which is rapidly relieved when the flexion is discontinued) which is positive in half the patients, and the *tourniquet test* (a sphygmomanometer is pumped above systolic pressure for 2 min and this produces the paraesthesiae). Symptoms may sometimes be induced by *hyperextension* at the wrist.

Frequency in survey: 0.5% of attempts at MRCP short cases.

Record

On the R/L side there is evidence of *fifth* (may be absent corneal reflex only), *sixth* (p. 110) and *seventh cranial nerve impairment* (both may be minimal), *perceptive deafness* (*eighth nerve*—the patient usually has tinnitus but may complain of vague unsteadiness or giddiness*), and *cerebellar* impairment (may be slightly impaired rapid alternate motion of the hands only). There is *nystagmus* (again may be just a few beats intermittently; it may be cerebellar and/or vestibular in origin).

These findings suggest a lesion at the cerebello-pontine angle, *acoustic neuroma*† being the commonest cause (X-ray for evidence of expansion of the internal auditory meatus).

The CSF protein is elevated (may be >3 g l^{-1}). Caloric testing almost invariably reveals a dead labyrinth. The IXth and Xth cranial nerves may be involved and dysphagia and dysphonia may occur.

In severe cases, with large tumours, there may be signs of raised intracranial pressure (?papilloedema) in addition to ipsilateral cerebellar involvement.

---

*Rotational vertigo in acoustic neuroma seldom occurs in the discrete attacks that are found in Menière's syndrome.

†Meningioma can give a similar picture (normal auditory meatus on X-ray).

Frequency in survey: 0.5% of attempts at MRCP short cases.

Record

The pulse is regular (give rate) and of good volume. The jugular venous pressure is not raised. The apex beat is *not palpable on the left side*, but can be felt in the fifth *right* intercostal space in the midclavicular line.

This patient has dextrocardia.* (If allowed, listen to the lung fields—Kartagener's syndrome—and feel the abdomen to see which side the liver is on—situs inversus.)

If situs inversus is present the patient is usually otherwise normal. Dextrocardia without situs inversus is usually associated with cardiac malformation. Dextrocardia may occur in Turner's syndrome.

Kartagener's syndrome: Dextrocardia, bronchiectasis, situs inversus, infertility, dysplasia of frontal sinuses, sinusitis and otitis media. Patients have ciliary immotility.

---

*Consider the possibility of this diagnosis if you cannot feel the apex beat and then have difficulty hearing the heart sounds. As you gradually move the stethoscope towards the right side of the chest, they get louder.

128 / Down's syndrome

Frequency in survey: Main focus of a short case in 0.5% of attempts at MRCP short cases. Additional feature in a further 0.6%.

Record

This short-statured patient has *low-set ears*, a *flattened nasal bridge*, *slanting eyes*, *epicanthus*, white *'Brushfield spots'* in the iris and a small *mouth which hangs open* revealing a large heavily fissured tongue. There is an over-rolled helix of each ear. There is a single *transverse palmar crease* (not pathognomonic) and a short inward curving little finger. The axial triradius is situated towards the centre of the palm (normally should be near the wrist). There is generalized hypotonia and hyperextensibility of the joints.

The patient has Down's syndrome.

Trisomy 21 (occasionally translocation between 21 and 14).

Other features which may occur

Congenital heart lesions (septal defects, Fallot's tetralogy)

Lenticular opacities
Mental retardation which varies from very mild (author of an autobiography) to very severe
Dementia of Alzheimer type

Frequency in survey: Main focus of a short case in 0.5% of attempts at MRCP short cases. Additional feature in a further 1.6%.

Survey note: All cases were due to either drugs or cirrhosis.

Record

There is gynaecomastia (it may be unilateral). This is confirmed on palpation by the presence of *increased glandular tissue.* (Now look for signs of *cirrhosis, heart failure* [spironolactone], *atrial fibrillation* [digoxin], *clubbing and cachexia* [carcinoma of the lung], *absence of body hair* [hypogonadism, oestrogen therapy] or evidence of an *endocrine disorder—see below.*)

There may be feminization of the nipples and tenderness of the breasts. Gynaecomastia must be differentiated from tumours of the breast and simple adiposity.

Causes of gynaecomastia

Pubertal (very common—due to transient dominance of circulating oestradiol over testosterone)

Senile (normal rise in oestrogens and fall in androgens with age)

Cirrhosis of the liver (?stigmata—p. 78)

Thyrotoxicosis (?exophthalmos, goitre, etc.—p. 108)

Hypothyroidism (?facies, pulse, ankle jerks, etc.—p. 138)

Carcinoma of the lung (5% of patients; sometimes with hypertrophic pulmonary osteoarthropathy)

Klinefelter's syndrome (47 XXY, small testes, mental deficiency, incomplete virilization, raised LH and FSH)

Pituitary disease,* i.e. acromegaly, hypopituitarism

(?visual field defect; abnormal skull X-ray)

Isolated gonadotrophin deficiency (e.g. Kallman's syndrome—hypogonadotrophic hypogonadism and anosmia, often with harelip or cleft palate)

Testicular tumours

Addison's disease (?pigmentation—buccal and scar;—p. 118)

Adrenal carcinoma

Testicular feminization (androgen insensitivity)

Drug-induced:†

Oestrogen therapy (carcinoma of the prostate)

Digoxin

Griseofulvin

Alkylating agents (cause testicular damage)

Antiandrogens (including cyproterone acetate, spironolactone and possibly cimetidine)

Other drugs include phenothiazines, reserpine, tricyclics, methyldopa, isoniazid, amphetamines, androgens, anabolic steroids, and adrenocortical steroids.

*NB Prolactin excess in the absence of oestrogens produces galactorrhoea rather than gynaecomastia.

†The letters of the word MADRAS form a useful mnemonic: methyldopa, aldactone, digoxin, reserpine, alkylating agents, stilboestrol.

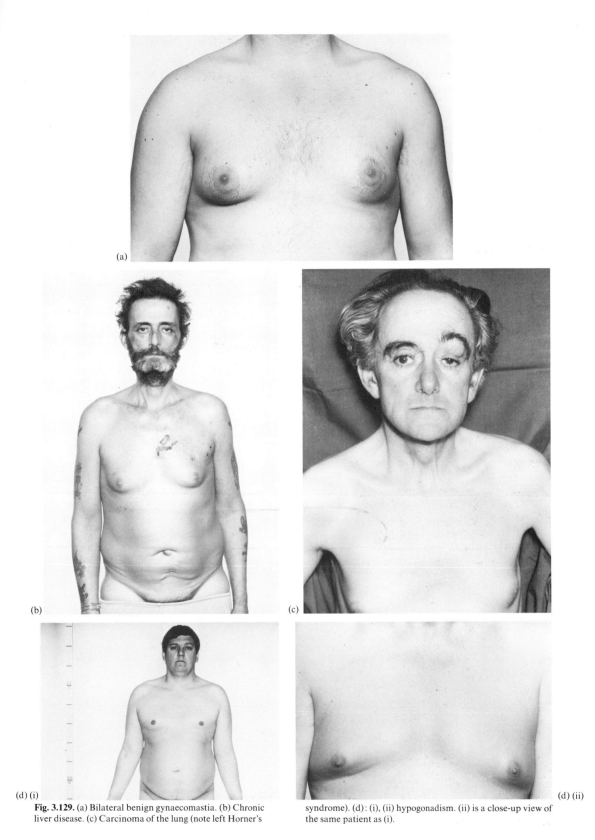

(a)

(b)

(c)

(d) (i)

(d) (ii)

Fig. 3.129. (a) Bilateral benign gynaecomastia. (b) Chronic liver disease. (c) Carcinoma of the lung (note left Horner's syndrome). (d): (i), (ii) hypogonadism. (ii) is a close-up view of the same patient as (i).

Frequency in survey: Main focus of a short case in 0.5% of attempts at MRCP short cases. Additional feature in a further 1%.

Record

The knee and *ankle jerks are absent* and the *plantar responses are extensor*.

Possible causes

1 Subacute combined degeneration of the cord (?posterior column signs, Rombergism, clinical anaemia, splenomegaly, etc.—p. 273).
2 Syphilitic taboparesis (?Argyll Robertson pupils, ptosis and wrinkled forehead, posterior column signs, Rombergism, etc.—p. 310).
3 Friedreich's ataxia (?pes cavus, [kypho-]scoliosis, nystagmus, cerebellar ataxia, scanning speech, etc.—p. 220).
4 Motor neurone disease (?fasciculation, absence of sensory signs, etc.—p. 116)
5 Common conditions in combination (e.g. an elderly person with diabetes and cervical myelopathy—see experience 56, p. 338).

131 / Lichen planus

Frequency in survey: 0.5% of attempts at MRCP short cases.

Record

This young (or middle-aged) patient has *flat-topped, polygonal*, shiny, slightly scaly, violaceous *papules* on the wrists (and other flexor surfaces usually, though it may affect any part of the skin). Fine white streaks (*Wickham's striae*) are seen on the surface of the lesions which also show *central umbilication*. The *Koebner phenomenon* is present (i.e. lesions appear in a linear pattern along a scratch mark). There are also lesions in the *buccal mucosa* (in 50% of cases—white, lacy pattern).

This patient has lichen planus (itching is usual and may be quite severe).

Males: Females = 1 : 1.

Lichen planus usually resolves in 6–24 months but it may recur. Steroids (systemic, local or intralesional) may be required if pruritus is severe and in the hypertrophic variety (see below). A deficiency of glucose-6-phosphate dehydrogenase has been found in lichen planus skin. Eruptions may be induced by heavy metals, colour photograph developers, streptomycin, methyldopa, chloroquine, mepacrine and PAS.

Other sites for lichen planus

Scalp (atrophy of the skin with patchy, permanent alopecia)

Nails (dystrophy of nail plate with longitudinal streaking of the nail; if it is severe there may be complete loss of the nail plate)

Palms and soles

Other forms

Hypertrophic lichen planus (plaque-like lesions with a thick, warty surface on the front of the legs)

Erosive lichen planus

Bullous lichen planus

For colour photographs see p. 378.

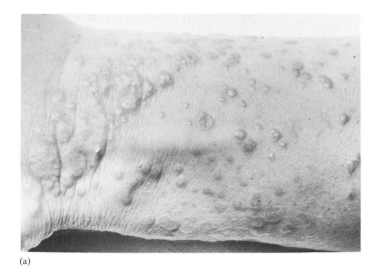

(a)

(b)

Fig. 3.131. (a) Lichen planus of the wrist. (b) The left buccal mucosa is exposed to show the characteristic lacy, white pattern.

132 / Lateral popliteal nerve palsy

Frequency in survey: 0.5% of attempts at MRCP short cases.

Record

There is *wasting* of the *anterior tibial* and *peroneal* group of *muscles*, the patient *cannot dorsiflex* or *evert* the R/L foot, and there is *impairment* of *sensation* over the *outer side* of the *calf*. He cannot stand on the R/L heel and the gait is altered as a result of *foot drop* (there is an audible 'clop' of the foot as he walks).

The diagnosis is lateral popliteal (common peroneal) nerve palsy.

Injury to the nerve is usually at the head of the fibula where it can be involved in fractures or compressed by splints, tourniquets or bandages. Some individuals are particularly susceptible to temporary pressure palsy of this nerve (and in some cases other nerves such as the radial and ulnar as well), experiencing symptoms induced by crossing knees or unusual physical activity.

The nerve has two branches—the superficial and deep peroneal nerves. The superficial supplies sensation to the lateral calf and dorsum of the foot supplying the peroneus longus and brevis muscles. The deep branch supplies sensation to a triangular area of skin between the first and second toes dorsally and it innervates the anterior tibial muscles, the long extensors of the toes and the peroneus tertius muscle.

133 / Ptosis

Frequency in survey: Main focus of a short case in 0.5% of attempts at MRCP short cases. Additional feature in at least a further 5%.

Record 1

There is *unilateral* ptosis.*

Possible causes

1   Third nerve palsy (?dilated ipsilateral pupil, divergent strabismus, etc.—p. 110).
2   Horner's syndrome (?ipsilateral small pupil, etc.—p. 164).
3   Myasthenia gravis (may be the only sign of this condition; ?induced or worsened by upward gaze; variable strabismus, facial and proximal muscle weakness, weak nasal voice, all of which may worsen with repetition, etc.—p. 246).
4   Congenital/idiopathic† (may increase with age; there may be an associated superior rectus palsy).
5   Dystrophia myotonica (usually bilateral).

Record 2

There is *bilateral* ptosis.*

Possible causes

1   Myasthenia gravis.
2   Dystrophia myotonica (?myopathic facies, frontal balding, wasting of facial muscles and sternomastoids, cataracts, myotonia, etc.—p. 144).
3   Tabes dorsalis (?Argyll Robertson pupils, etc.—p. 310).
4   Congenital† (may increase with age).
5   Bilateral Horner's (e.g. syringomyelia—?wasting of small muscles of the hand, dissociated sensory loss, scars, extensor plantars, etc.—p. 268).
6   Ocular myopathy‡ (?absence of soft tissue in the lids and periorbital region, ophthalmoplegia, mild facial and neck weakness).
7   Oculopharangeal muscular dystrophy (similar to ocular myopathy but late onset and dysphagia prominent).

Other causes of ptosis

Pseudoptosis (following recurrent inflammation or extreme thinning of lids after repeated angioneurotic oedema)
Voluntary ptosis (to suppress diplopia)

Apraxia of the eyelids (the patient may need to pull down the lower eyelids, tilt back the head or open the mouth to enable the eyes to be opened; there is usually evidence of basal ganglia involvement)

---

*NB Overaction of frontalis with wrinkling of the forehead tends to be associated with ptosis due to non-myopathic conditions.
†The tensilon test should be negative before this diagnosis is accepted.

‡Many of the ocular myopathies are associated with characteristic morphological features ('ragged red fibres') and a variety of biochemical mitochondrial defects and are now referred to as chronic progressive external ophthalmoplegia (CPEO).

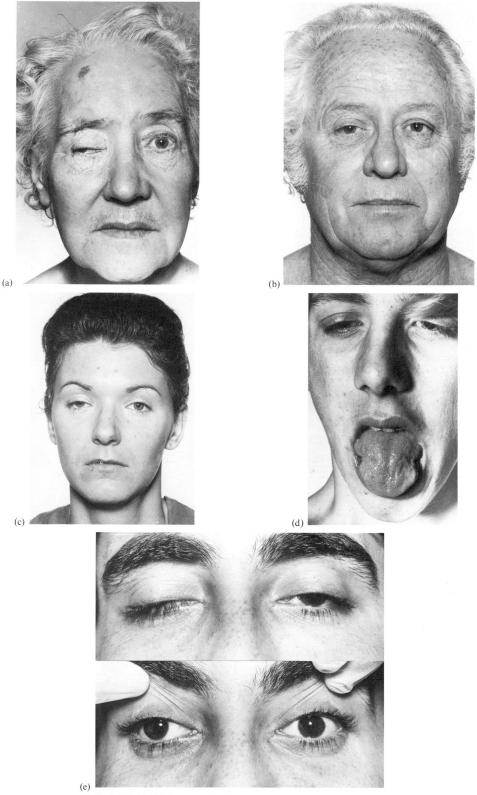

Fig. 3.133. (a) Third nerve palsy. (b) Right Horner's syndrome.
(c) Myasthenia gravis. (d) Dystrophia myotonica. (e) Ocular
myopathy.

Frequency in survey: 0.5% of attempts at MRCP short cases.

Record

The *sclerae* are *slaty-blue*. (Look for evidence of *deformity* from poor fracture healing; ask the patient if he has been particularly prone to *fractures* in the past.)

The diagnosis is osteogenesis imperfecta (the patient may be deaf due to *otosclerosis*).

In the adult the diagnosis is likely to be the milder tarda type* (usually dominant). In this type the sclerae are more likely to be blue and the fragile bones of childhood become stronger after adolescence though they remain abnormal. The blueness is due to the thin sclerae allowing choroid pigment to show through. Though blue sclerae are not always present, some patients manifest only blue sclerae or otosclerosis without clinical bone disease. Deafness from otosclerosis does not usually develop before the third decade and may occur even later still. Laxity of ligaments, hypotonia of muscles and muscle wasting (partly disuse atrophy) are other features which may occur. Serum alkaline and acid phosphatases are often elevated and the urine often contains hydroxyproline, pyrophosphate and glycosoaminoglycans. Though no specific treatment is known, favourable responses to calcitonin have been reported. Osteogenesis imperfecta may be confused with idiopathic juvenile osteoporosis but in the latter condition osteoporosis is typically confined to the vertebral column, there is no family history of fractures and the sclerae are normal in colour.

Other conditions in which blue sclerae may occur

Marfan's syndrome (p. 244)
Ehlers–Danlos syndrome (p. 240)
Pseudoxanthoma elasticum (p. 270)

For colour photograph see p. 378.

---

*Other types are:
(i) The severe prenatal type which causes intrauterine death or life for only a few days after birth.
(ii) The severe type in which the baby survives but is extremely susceptible to fractures. The bones are soft as well as brittle and may therefore bow. Deformities are common and walking may induce fractures. Blue sclerae are less common.

135 / Pulmonary stenosis

Frequency in survey: 0.5% of attempts at MRCP short cases.

Record

The pulse is regular and the JVP is not elevated (prominent *a* wave in severe cases). The cardiac apex is not palpable but there is (may be) a *left parasternal heave*. A *systolic thrill* is palpable over the left second and third interspaces. An *ejection click* and a *systolic murmur* (and maybe also a fourth heart sound) are heard over the *pulmonary area*. The murmur is louder during inspiration and radiates to the suprasternal notch. The second sound is (may be) split (the pulmonary component is soft).

The diagnosis is pulmonary stenosis.

Poststenotic dilatation of the pulmonary arteries may be seen on the chest X-ray and, in the severe case, right ventricular hypertrophy and diminution of pulmonary vascular markings. A minor degree of pulmonary stenosis is compatible with a normal life span. Surgical relief is required in symptomatic cases or if there is a gradient of more than 50 mmHg across the pulmonary valve. If surgery is delayed too long in severe pulmonary stenosis an irreversible fibrotic change can take place in the hypertrophied right ventricle.

Frequency in survey: Main focus of a short case in 0.5% of attempts at MRCP short cases. Additional feature in a further 2%.

Record

The *fingers* are *cold* and *cyanosed** with (may be) *atrophy* of the *finger pulps* (and in severe cases gangrene of the fingertips).

The patient is likely to have Raynaud's phenomenon (now look for features of underlying connective tissue diseases, especially systemic sclerosis).

Causes of Raynaud's phenomenon

1   Idiopathic Raynaud's disease* (common, especially young females, thumbs often spared, starts in childhood, usually benign).
2   Vibrating tools (e.g. pneumatic drills, polishing tools).
3   Systemic sclerosis (Raynaud's may be the first symptom; ?smooth, tight, shiny skin on the hands and face, typical mask-like facies, telangiectasia, etc.—p. 90).
4   Other connective tissue disorders (especially mixed connective tissue disease but also SLE, polymyositis, Sjögren's syndrome and rheumatoid arthritis).
5   Cervical rib (?supraclavicular bruit, ipsilateral diminished radial pulse especially during a Raynaud's attack, wasting of the small muscles of the hand and C8/T1 sensory impairment though neurological signs of cervical rib are often minimal if vascular signs are prominent).

Other causes

Cold agglutinins
Cryoglobulinaemia
Hypothyroidism
Heavy metal poisoning

Women who develop toxaemia of pregnancy are more likely to have a history of Raynaud's disease (suggesting an abnormal vascular reactivity or unidentified humoral agent underlying both conditions).

---

*In idiopathic Raynaud's disease the arteries show an exaggerated physiological response to cold and go into intense spasm to produce numb, dead-white fingers. With rewarming the classical colour sequence is white to blue (cyanosis) then blue to red (rebound hyperaemia which is painful). The patient (usually with systemic sclerosis) in whom Raynaud's is discussed in the MRCP examination is likely to have chronically impaired arterial circulation leading to cyanosis even in the warm hospital environment.

Frequency in survey: 0.5% of attempts at MRCP short cases.

Record

The patient (who probably presented with primary amenorrhoea) is *short* (usually less than 1.5 m) with a *short webbed neck** (only found in 54%) and shows *cubitus valgus* deformity. She has a *shield-like chest* (and may have widely separated nipples). The *nails are hypoplastic* and she has *short 4th metacarpals* (other metacarpals may also be short). The *hairline is low*, she has a *high-arched palate* and there are *numerous naevi*. The secondary sexual characteristics are underdeveloped (unless the patient has been treated with oestrogens).

The diagnosis is Turner's syndrome. (If allowed: examine the cardiovascular system—abnormal in 20%; especially coarctation of the aorta—p. 235—but also ASD, VSD and AS.)

The patient with Turner's syndrome is likely to have streak gonads and a chromosome constitution which is mostly 45, XO. Red–green colour blindness (an X-linked recessive character) occurs as frequently in Turner's as it does in normal males, and other X-linked conditions may occur.

Other features which sometimes occur

Lymphoedema
Genito-urinary abnormality (e.g. horseshoe kidney)
Hypertelorism
Epicanthal fold
Mental retardation (only 12%)

Strabismus
Ptosis
Intestinal telangiectasia
Premature osteoporosis
Premature ageing in appearance
Higher incidence of diabetes mellitus and Hashimoto's thyroiditis

Noonan's syndrome: May affect both sexes. Females have Turner's phenotype but normal 46 XX, normal ovarian function and normal fertility. Noonan's are more likely to have right-sided cardiac lesions (especially pulmonary stenosis) whereas Turner's are more likely to have left-sided lesions.

*A pathognomonic feature.

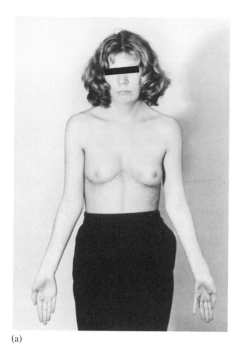

(a)

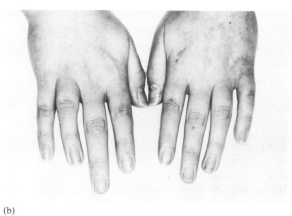

(b)

Fig. 3.137. (a) XO/XX mosaic. Note the webbed neck, increased carrying angle and scar under the breasts (special incision for ASD repair). (b) The hands of another patient.

Frequency in survey: 0.5% of attempts at MRCP short cases.

Record

There are (in this middle-aged or elderly patient) erythematous, *thickened, indurated, plaque-like lesions* (which itch) over . . . (describe the site; can be on any part of the body). There are also (may be) raised ulcerated nodules.

The appearances are suggestive of mycosis fungoides (cutaneous lymphoma).

Males > Females.

Mycosis fungoides is a T-cell tumour of the skin which usually shows no evidence of visceral involvement for several years. The initial lesions may be confused with psoriasis, eczema or contact dermatitis. They usually progress very slowly to nodules which may ulcerate. Diffuse exfoliative erythroderma may develop. Extracutaneous involvement (especially lung, liver and spleen) does not usually become manifest for many years (though it can be found in two-thirds of patients at autopsy). Lymph node involvement suggests the likelihood of further extracutaneous spread. Treatment includes steroids, cytotoxic agents, PUVA and radiotherapy.

Other reticuloses, for example Hodgkin's disease and leukaemia, may present as infiltrative papules or plaques in the skin diagnosed by skin biopsy.

For colour photograph see p. 378.

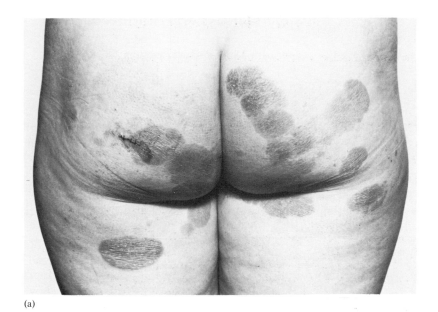

(a)

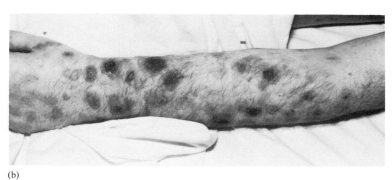

(b)

Fig. 3.138. (a) Early lesions of mycosis fungoides showing well-demarcated, scaly, atrophic, erythematous patches. (b) Mycosis fungoides showing early ulceration of plaques.

139 / Dermatitis herpetiformis

Frequency in survey: 0.3% of attempts at MRCP short cases.

Record

This middle-aged (or elderly) patient has groups of *erythematous papules* and *excoriations* on the *elbows, knees, buttocks, scalp, upper back* and at *pressure points* (very occasionally it is generalized). There are (may be) *vesicles* which have (usually) a raised, reddened background (vesicles may be present but have usually been ruptured by scratching—the lesions are intensely *pruritic*).

The diagnosis is dermatitis herpetiformis and this is nearly always associated with a gluten-sensitive enteropathy (*coeliac disease*).

Males: Females = 2 : 1.
About 85% of patients are HLA–B8/DRw3.

Dermatitis herpetiformis can occur at any stage of adult life (rare in childhood). Once developed it is persistent. It is treated with a gluten-free diet and/or dapsone (side effects include rashes, haemolysis and agranulocytosis). The differential diagnosis is from pemphigus, pemphigoid and other bullous disorders (p. 266). Involvement of the oral mucosa is uncommon. There may be a higher incidence of developing malignancies than in the general population.

For colour photograph see p. 378.

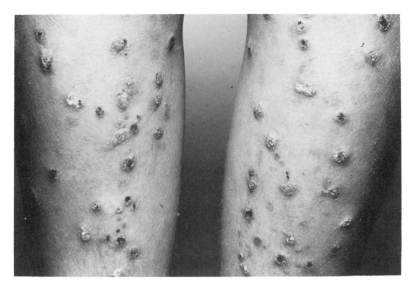

Fig. 3.139. Dermatitis herpetiformis.

140 / Urticaria pigmentosa (mastocytosis)

Frequency in survey: 0.3% of attempts at MRCP short cases.

Record

There are *multiple*, small, discrete, round (or oval), reddish-brown (or yellowish-brown) *pigmented macules* (and/or papules). After *friction, urticarial wheals* develop (due to histamine release from the mast cells—Darier's sign).

The diagnosis is urticaria pigmentosa.

The adult variety is thought to be a form of reticulosis. If involvement is extensive, a hot bath followed by vigorous drying may lead to flushing, hypotension, bronchospasm and diarrhoea. In a minority, systemic involvement may occur with involvement of the liver, spleen and bone marrow. Bowel involvement may lead to malabsorption. A small percentage of patients develop leukaemia which can be, but is not usually, mast-cell leukaemia.

For colour photogaphs see p. 380.

141 / Pneumothorax

Frequency in survey: 0.3% of attempts at MRCP short cases.

Record

The R/L *side* of the chest (of this tall, thin, young adult male—old patients are usually bronchitic) *expands poorly* compared with the other side. Though the *percussion note* on the R/L side is *hyperresonant*, the tactile fremitus, vocal resonance and *breath sounds* are all *diminished* (large pneumothorax of one side may push the *trachea* and apex beat to the opposite side).

These findings suggest a pneumothorax of the R/L side.

Males: Females = 6:1.

A 'crunching' sound in keeping with the heart beat may be heard when the pneumothorax is small.

Treatment is not required in a healthy individual with a small pneumothorax (i.e. if only a quarter of one side is affected). An intercostal tube attached to an underwater seal is indicated for:

Larger pneumothorax associated with dyspnoea, increasing in size or not resolving after one week

Tension pneumothorax

Pneumothorax complicating underlying severe chronic bronchitis with emphysema

Pneumothorax exacerbating acute severe asthma (hence chest X-ray mandatory in acute severe asthma)

Recurrent spontaneous pneumothorax is treated by obliteration of the pleural space (pleurectomy; application of irritating substances into the pleural cavity; scarification of the pleura followed by intrapleural suction).

Frequency in survey: Main focus of a short case in 0.3% of attempts at MRCP short cases. Additional feature in a further 0.8%.

Record 1

There are (in this underweight patient who appears older than his years) *Argyll Robertson pupils* (p. 281). There is bilateral *ptosis* with *wrinkling* of the *forehead* due to compensatory overaction of the frontalis, there is loss of *vibration* and *joint position* sense, loss of *deep pain* in the Achilles tendon, hypotonia, *absent reflexes* and plantar responses; the gait is ataxic and *Romberg's* test is *positive*.

The diagnosis is *tabes dorsalis.** The patient may have *optic atrophy* (may antedate other manifestations; centre of vision may be the last to be affected) and is at risk of developing a *Charcot's* neuropathic hip, knee, or ankle joint.

Record 2

As appropriate from the above plus: The *plantars* are *extensor* (with or without other pyramidal signs and other signs of GPI— see below).

The diagnosis is *taboparesis*.

Other features of tabes dorsalis, though well known, are rarely seen now; features such as:

Wide-based, high, stepping gait

Zones of cutaneous analgesia with delayed perception of pain

Ligament laxity allowing extreme degrees of lower limb movement

Perforating foot ulcers

Lightening pains (a good reliable history is virtually pathognomonic and may antedate other symptoms)

Bladder insensitivity

Other forms of neurosyphilis

General paresis of the insane† (dementia which classically progresses to euphoria and delusions of grandeur though this is less common than simple dementia, epileptic fits, tremor of the hands, lips and tongue ['trombone' tremor], spastic paraparesis of cortical origin)

Meningovascular syphilis‡ (may present in a wide variety of ways including: isolated cranial nerve palsies especially IIIrd and VIth, cerebral or spinal stroke, meningism, epilepsy. Rare syndromes include meningomyelitis, pachymeningitis, acute transverse myelitis, Erb's spastic paraplegia, syphilitic amyotrophy which resembles motor neurone disease)

---

*Tabes dorsalis occurs 10–35 years after infection and the prognosis is poor. There is atrophy of the posterior nerve root and (probably secondary) degeneration of the posterior columns (lumbosacral and lower thoracic worst affected).

†GPI occurs 10–15 years after infection and the prognosis is good if it is treated before the development of cortical atrophy (initially the patient may present simply with a change of temperament, slight pupillary abnormalities and brisk reflexes).

There is meningeal thickening and degeneration of the cerebral cortex (especially frontal).

‡Meningovascular syphilis (only 3% of syphilitic patients) occurs in the first 4 years after infection and shows a good response to treatment except where cerebral or spinal cord infarction has occurred. Fibrosed meninges may nip cranial nerves and endarteritis may produce areas of ischaemic necrosis.

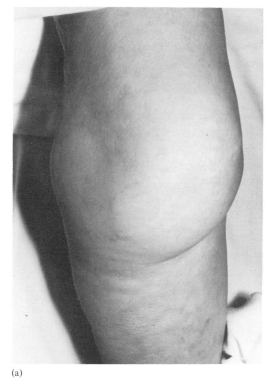

(a)

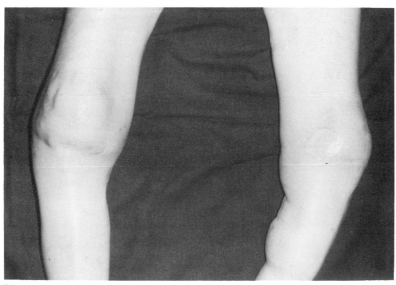

(b)

Fig. 3.142. (a) (b) Charcot's knee joints.

143 / Atrial septal defect

Frequency in survey: 0.1% of attempts at MRCP short cases.

Record

The pulse in this middle-aged female is irregularly irregular (onset of atrial fibrillation is usually the cause of symptoms after the third or fourth decade, otherwise asymptomatic). The JVP is not elevated (unless in right heart failure). The apex beat is just palpable and not displaced and there is a *left parasternal heave* (there may be a systolic thrill over the pulmonary area in large left to right shunts). The second heart sound is widely split (the first may also be split with a loud tricuspid component), and the two-component split is not influenced by respiration (*fixed splitting*). There is an *ejection systolic murmur* (due to high flow across the pulmonary valve) over the pulmonary area. (Occasionally there may be a harsh, explosive and brief early diastolic murmur—pulmonary incompetence—and an ejection click, both due to pulmonary artery dilatation. A mid-diastolic rumble over the tricuspid area suggests a large shunt.)

The diagnosis is atrial septal defect (ASD).

Males : Females = 1 : 3.

Other features of ASD

Ostium secundum defect is the commonest type

rSR in the right precordial leads on ECG. Right-axis deviation is associated with an ostium secundum defect, left-axis deviation suggests an ostium primum defect

Dilated proximal pulmonary arteries and an enlarged right heart with pulmonary plethora* on chest X-ray. The peripheral pulmonary vascularity is replaced by clear lung fields with the advent of pulmonary hypertension. The superior vena cava is enlarged in the sinus venosus type

Paradoxical (anterior) septal movement during systole and right ventricular dilatation on echocardiography

Diagnosis confirmed by catheterization; the catheter lands in the *left* atrium. The shunt can be assessed by serial oxygen saturations from the left to the right atrium

Surgical closure for ostium secundum defect is recommended if the pulmonary to systemic flow ratio is 2 : 1 or more

Patients with pulmonary hypertension are cyanosed and may have clubbing of the fingers (Eisenmenger's syndrome—p. 192). The systolic murmur becomes faint and an early diastolic murmur with a loud P_2 appears. Operative repair is contraindicated

Usual causes of death: right heart failure, arrhythmias, pulmonary embolism, brain abscess, rupture of pulmonary artery

May be associated with acquired mitral stenosis (Lutembacher's syndrome)

---

*The main differential diagnosis of *pulmonary plethora* due to a left to right shunt is ASD, VSD (p. 182), PDA (p. 200). It may be possible to differentiate these on chest X-ray by looking at the left atrium and aorta. Small left atrium and normal aorta suggests ASD, large left atrium and normal aorta suggests VSD, large left atrium and large or abnormal aorta suggests PDA.

Frequency in survey: 0.1% of attempts at MRCP short cases.

Record

There are large *necrotic ulcers* with *ragged* bluish-red *overhanging edges* together with areas containing erythematous plaques with pustules. They are situated . . . (describe site—can occur anywhere on the body).

The appearances are suggestive of pyoderma gangrenosum. The patient may have *ulcerative colitis* or Crohn's disease.

It may also be associated with rheumatoid arthritis and myeloproliferative disorders. Fifty per cent of patients with pyoderma gangrenosum have ulcerative colitis. It is frequently an indicator of the severity of the disease. Healing often parallels that of the colitis and colectomy may allow this to be rapid. Topical steroids often help. The histopathological findings are non-specific.

Other skin manifestations of ulcerative colitis

Aphthous ulcers
Erythema nodosum
Erythema multiforme
Perianal fistulae and abscess formation
Purpura

Other causes of leg ulcers

Venous ulceration (only 50% have superficial varices)
Ischaemic arterial ulceration (usually anterior or lateral lower leg, pain, cold pulseless cyanotic feet, shiny hairless lower legs)
Diabetes mellitus (see p. 154)
Vasculitis (rheumatoid arthritis or other connective tissue disorder)
Infection (acute pyogenic, tuberculous, syphilitic, cutaneous leishmaniasis)
Tumour (squamous cell, basal cell, melanoma)
Haematological (sickle-cell, thalassaemia, acholuric jaundice, paroxysmal nocturnal haemoglobinuria)
Neurological (diabetes, tabes dorsalis, leprosy, syringomyelia)

For colour photographs see p. 381.

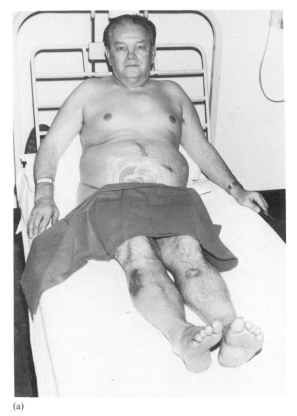

(a)

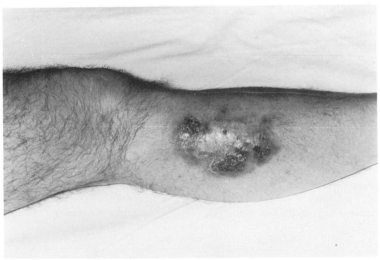

(b)

Fig. 3.144. (a) Note scarred abdomen and ileostomy bag this patient with inflammatory bowel disease. (b) Pyoderma gangrenosum on the leg of the same patient.

Frequency in survey: Did not occur as the main focus of a short case. It was however considered to be the underlying cause of a short case in at least 16% of attempts at MRCP short cases.

Record 1

The patient (?a young adult) has *ataxic nystagmus* (p. 156), *internuclear ophthalmoplegia* (p. 112), *temporal pallor of the discs* (p. 76), and *slurred speech* (p. 238) with *ataxia* (p. 170) and widespread *cerebellar* signs (p. 130). There are *pyramidal* signs and *dorsal column* signs.

The likely diagnosis is demyelinating disease* (a useful euphemism for multiple sclerosis).

Record 2

The legs of this (?middle-aged) patient have increased tone, they are bilaterally spastic and weak. There is bilateral *ankle clonus* and patellar clonus and the *plantars* are *extensor*. The *abdominal reflexes* are absent. The heel-shin test suggested some *ataxia* in the legs and there is slight *impairment of rapid alternate motion* in the upper limbs.

These features suggest that this *spastic paraplegia* is due to demyelinating disease. An examination of the fundi may show involvement of the discs.†

Male : Female = 2 : 3.

Features of multiple sclerosis (MS)

Rare in tropical climates

Euphoria despite severe disability (not invariable—the patient may be depressed)

Unpredictable course

May present acutely, subacutely, remittently or insidiously

Relapses and remissions (occurring in two-thirds of patients) are often a useful diagnostic pointer

May very closely imitate other neurological conditions (including neurosis)

Fatigue or a rise in temperature may exacerbate symptoms (the patient may be able to get into, but not out of, a hot bath)

Paroxysmal symptoms (e.g. trigeminal neuralgia) may occur and may respond to carbamazepine

Lhermitte's phenomenon may occur (see p. 273)

Benign course more likely if
—early age of onset
—relapses and remissions
—onset with optic neuritis, or sensory or motor symptoms—in contrast to those of brain-stem or cerebellar lesions

The visual evoked response (VER) test is useful in a patient with an isolated lesion which may be due to MS—e.g. spastic paraparesis†, VIth nerve palsy, trigeminal neuralgia, facial palsy, postural vertigo

CSF examination may show an increase in total protein up to 1 g l⁻¹ or an increase in lymphocytes up to 50/mm³ in 50% of patients. The IgG proportion of the total protein is increased in two-thirds of patients

*The features in this *record* are some of those which are commonly seen in a case of MS. There are, of course, few neurological signs which it may not produce.

†MS may present in middle-age with insidious spastic paraplegia mimicking cord compression. Signs above the level of the cord lesion may point clinically to demyelination as the cause.

In this case the slight cerebellar signs are highly suggestive of MS. However, a tumour at the foramen magnum could also be the cause. If the diagnosis is of a tumour there may be papilloedema. If the diagnosis is MS the discs may show global or temporal pallor (and the VERs may be delayed—even if, as is often the case, the discs are normal).

146 / Felty's syndrome

Frequency in survey: Did not occur as the main focus of a short case. It was however considered to be present in a short case in 1% of attempts at MRCP short cases.

Record

There is a *symmetrical deforming arthropathy* with *spindling* and *ulnar deviation* of the fingers, and *nodules* at the elbows. The *spleen* is enlarged at . . . cm. (Check for anaemia.)

If *neutropenia* is present (?evidence of secondary infection) this, in combination with rheumatoid arthritis and splenomegaly, would constitute Felty's syndrome.

Occurs in older patients with long-standing rheumatoid disease (5%).

Other signs and features of Felty's syndrome

Lymphadenopathy
Skin pigmentation
Vasculitic leg ulceration
Keratoconjunctivitis sicca
Thrombocytopenia
Haemolytic anaemia
Lack of relationship between the degree of haematological abnormality and the size of spleen
Tests for antinuclear factor and LE cells are often positive as well as rheumatoid factor which is invariably positive

147 / Hypertrophic obstructive cardiomyopathy

Frequency in survey: Did not occur in MRCP survey.*

Record

The pulse is regular and of normal volume (in severe cases it has a *'jerky'* character) and the JVP is not elevated (may show a prominent *a* wave). The cardiac apex is forceful in the left fifth intercostal space just outside the midclavicular line, there is (may be) a strong *presystolic impulse* (*double apical impulse* caused by atrial systole), and a *systolic thrill* is palpable over the left sternal border. There is a *fourth heart sound*, and an *ejection systolic murmur* (may be harsh) over the left third interspace, which radiates widely to the base and to the axilla (perhaps because it merges with the pansystolic murmur of mitral incompetence which frequently accompanies HOCM).

The findings suggest hypertrophic obstructive cardiomyopathy (HOCM).

Other features of HOCM

Patients may be asymptomatic. Severe cases are marked by symptoms such as dyspnoea, palpitations, angina, dizziness and syncope (often postural in nature or produced after cessation of exercise, cf. aortic stenosis where syncope usually occurs during exercise)

The systolic murmur may be increased by exercise, nitroglycerine and digoxin, and decreased by beta-blockers and squatting

ECG: Normal in 25%. ST-T and T wave changes, tall QRS in mid-precordial leads. Q wave in inferior and lateral precordial leads (due to septal hypertrophy). Sometimes left-axis deviation

Chest X-ray may be normal, or it may show left atrial enlargement

Echocardiography characteristically shows asymmetrical septal hypertrophy, and may show systolic anterior motion of the anterior mitral valve leaflet

Angiocardiography may show marked thickening of the ventricular septum and left ventricular free wall, small left ventricular cavity, and narrow outflow tract (an hour-glass appearance). Anterior movement of the anterior mitral valve leaflet is commonly seen. In the borderline case vigorous contraction of the left ventricle may be the only suggestive feature

---

*A case of HOCM was included in one mock Membership examination. One of the examiners commented to us that none of his prospective candidates got the correct diagnosis. It is of course possible that conditions such as HOCM did occur in the exam sittings covered by our survey, but the candidates concerned did not get, or even suspect, the diagnoses and were not enlightened by their examiners.

Frequency in survey: Did not occur in MRCP survey.

Record

There is *wrist drop* and sensory loss over the first dorsal interosseous.*

    The diagnosis is radial nerve palsy.

The hand hangs limply and the patient is unable to lift it at the wrist or to straighten out the fingers. If the wrist is passively extended he is able to straighten the fingers at the interphalangeal joints (because the interossei and lumbricals still work) but not at the metacarpophalangeal joints where the fingers remain flexed. The patient may feel that his grasp is weak in the affected hand because of lack of the wrist extension necessary for powerful grip. If the wrist is passively extended the power of grip improves. Abduction and adduction of the fingers may appear weak in radial nerve palsy unless they are tested with the hand resting flat on the table with the fingers extended.

The commonest cause (of this rare condition) is 'Saturday night paralysis' in which the patient, heavily sedated with alcohol, falls asleep with his arm hanging over the back of a chair. The nerve is compressed against the middle third of the humerus, and brachioradialis (flexion of the arm against resistance—with the arm midway between supination and pronation) and supinator are also paralysed as well as the forearm extensor muscles. Muscle wasting does not usually occur and complete recovery in a matter of weeks† is usual. If the nerve is injured by a wound in the axilla paralysis involves triceps so that extension at the elbow is lost as is the triceps reflex.

---

*Though the cutaneous area supplied by the radial nerve is more extensive than this (Fig. 2.1, p. 24) an overlap in supply by both median and ulnar nerves usually means that only this small area over the first dorsal interosseus has detectable impaired sensation.

†Usually damage occurs to the myelin sheath only and the Schwann cells will repair the nerve rapidly. If the pressure is prolonged and causes axonal degeneration then the peripheral nerve regeneration rate is about 1 mm/day (from the undamaged proximal nerve).

149 / Lateral medullary syndrome (Wallenberg's syndrome)

Frequency in survey: Did not occur in MRCP survey.

Record

(Assumes a lesion affecting the artery on the right.) On the right of the patient (who presented with acute vertigo*) there is (*ipsilateral*):

Horner's syndrome (descending sympathetic tract).

Cerebellar signs (cerebellum and its connections).

Palatal paralysis and diminished gag reflex (may be dysphagia and hoarseness due to a vocal cord paralysis—IXth and Xth nerves).

Decreased *trigeminal* pain and temperature sensation (descending tract and nucleus of the Vth nerve).

On the left of the patient the trunk and limbs (and sometimes the face) show (*contralateral*) decreased *pain and temperature* sensation† (spinothalamic tract).

The patient has a lateral medullary syndrome (produced by infarction of a small wedge of lateral medulla posterior to the inferior olivary nucleus—see Fig. 3.149) classically due to a lesion of the right *posterior inferior cerebellar artery*.‡

Involvement of the nucleus and tractus solitarius may cause loss of taste. Hiccup may occur. When occlusion of the posterior inferior cerebellar artery is isolated the pyramidal pathways escape and there is no hemiplegia. In the majority of cases of lateral medullary syndrome there is also an occlusion of the vertebral artery and pyramidal signs are present. Rarely, occlusion of the lower basilar artery, vertebral artery, or one of its medial branches produces the *medial medullary syndrome* (contralateral hemiplegia which spares the face, contralateral loss of vibration and joint position sense and ipsilateral paralysis and wasting of the tongue).

Other eponymous brain-stem infarction syndromes

Weber's syndrome (*midbrain*; ipsilateral IIIrd nerve palsy and contralateral hemiparesis)

Nothnagel's syndrome (*midbrain*; ipsilateral IIIrd nerve palsy and cerebellar ataxia)

Millard–Gubler syndrome (*pons*; ipsilateral VIth nerve palsy and facial weakness with contralateral hemiplegia)

Foville's syndrome (*pons*; as Millard–Gubler but with lateral conjugate gaze palsy)

These and a number of other eponymous brain-stem syndromes (e.g. Claude, Benedict, Raymond–Cestau) were, in their classic descriptions, mostly related to tumours and other non-vascular diseases. The diagnosis of brain-stem vascular disorders is facilitated more by knowledge of the neuro-anatomy of the brain-stem than of these eponyms. In one analysis of 50 patients (Cornell–Bellevue series) with brain-stem infarction, only two fitted into these syndromes as originally described. The rest had an extensive mixture of signs and symptoms indicating an overlap in the areas believed to be infarcted by occlusions in specific arteries.

*Vestibular involvement may produce nystagmus, diplopia, oscillopsia, vertigo, nausea and vomiting.
†Involvement of the cuneate and gracile nuclei may cause numbness of the ipsilateral (right in this case) arm.
‡Occlusion of any one of five vessels may be responsible— vertebral, posterior inferior cerebellar, superior, middle, or inferior lateral medullary arteries. The resulting clinical picture is variable and the rehabilitating patient may not show all features.

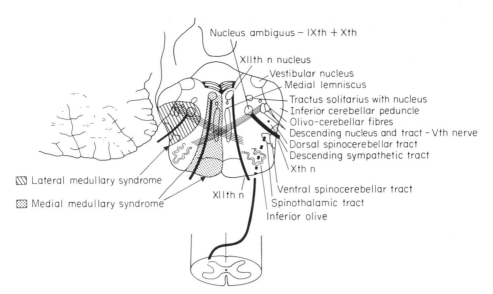

Nucleus ambiguus – IXth + Xth
XIIth n nucleus
Vestibular nucleus
Medial lemniscus
Tractus solitarius with nucleus
Inferior cerebellar peduncle
Olivo-cerebellar fibres
Descending nucleus and tract – Vth nerve
Dorsal spinocerebellar tract
Descending sympathetic tract
Xth n
Ventral spinocerebellar tract
Spinothalamic tract
Inferior olive
XIIth n

Lateral medullary syndrome

Medial medullary syndrome

Fig. 3.149. A cross-section through the medulla at the level of the inferior olivary nucleus showing the area infarcted in the lateral and medial medullary syndromes respectively.

(Adapted from Mohr, J.P. *et al.* in Harrison's *Principles of Internal Medicine*, 10th ed, p. 2037, by kind permission of the publishers McGraw-Hill.)

From the survey it is clear that the commonest reason for finding no abnormality is missing the physical signs which are present (probably anecdote 5 below and possibly anecdote 4; see also experience 50, p. 336). Nevertheless, short cases have occurred in which it seems that there was no abnormality and 'normal' was the correct diagnosis. The three or four from the survey are detailed below. We have learned from an invigilator who was responsible for the organization at one centre recently, that he was told by the College that patients without physical signs could be included in the short cases. Despite this we feel that it is likely that most cases of 'normal' will be either because the physical signs are no longer present by the time the patient comes to the examination (anecdote 1 below), or that the examiners and candidate disagree with the selectors of the cases about the presence of physical signs (may have happened in anecdote 2 below; see also experience 68, p. 339).

Anecdote 1

A candidate was asked to examine a patient's eye movements. He found no abnormality and said so. He reports that this was confirmed by the examiners and he passed. Apparently the patient had been included in the exam because she had had internuclear ophthalmoplegia, but this was no longer present at the time of this exam.

Anecdote 2

A candidate was asked to examine the fundi. He found no abnormality and diagnosed a normal fundus. He reports that the patient had multiple sclerosis and that he knows one of the examiners who has since confirmed that her fundi were considered to be normal. He passed the examination but he felt he would have failed if he had said 'bitemporal pallor'.

Anecdote 3

A candidate was asked to examine the abdomen. She could find no abnormality and told the examiner she thought the abdomen was normal. She was asked to demonstrate the 'tests' for splenic enlargement. She passed the examination and in retrospect she still feels that it was a normal abdomen.

Anecdote 4

A candidate was asked to examine a man's abdomen. He could find no abnormality and diagnosed a normal abdomen. In retrospect he is not sure if he missed something. Though he failed the clinical he felt he had passed the short case section.

Anecdote 5

A candidate was asked to examine the heart. He could find no abnormality and said so because he thought he had to be honest. He has no idea what the diagnosis was. He failed.

Section 4
Experiences, Anecdotes, Tips, Facts and Figures, Quotations

'I know 'cos I was there'*

*MAX BOYCE

This section starts with a hundred MRCP short-case *experiences* and *anecdotes* (taken from the large number recounted to us by the candidates in our survey and also including a few from those brought to us by some flies on the walls!). Because of limited space only a few full accounts are given; the remainder are extracts. Though most occurred at the recent examination sittings which we surveyed, some are taken from exam sittings spanning the last 10 years (including when the exam was only 20 minutes long). The tragedies and triumphs do not seem to change with time.

We have placed the extracts into specific groups. If an examiner spots a weakness, such as poor observation or examination technique, he is likely to explore this further before deciding whether to pass or fail a candidate. Consequently, some of the experiences are grouped according to which aspect of the candidate's clinical competence the examiner might have been probing most. A miscellaneous group of anecdotes follow the experiences. Though the outcome was not necessarily decided by the particular short case(s) in question, for additional information we have indicated with each experience and anecdote whether the candidate passed or failed. A standard list of useful *tips* is given, before some further *facts and figures* which were gleaned from the survey. The section finishes with a selection of *quotations* from successful MRCP candidates. At the end of the questionnaire, the candidates in our survey were asked if there were any comments they would like passed on to the candidates of the future. We felt the consistencies and occasional discrepancies in the advice of such a large number of 'authorities' might be of interest to some candidates and so we present here a selection from the large number received. In order not to distort the force and intentions contained in these advisory comments, we have tended to offer them verbatim. Inevitably some of the quotations are contradictory in their opinions—as with all examinations, individuals have different experiences and offer differing advice. Our views on these discrepancies are reflected throughout the book as far as they could be dealt with*. Ultimately you will have to come to your own conclusion depending upon the circumstances of a particular case.

Experiences

1   In his first case (first attempt) a candidate was asked: 'Examine this man's heart'. He found a short systolic murmur in a hypertensive patient and diagnosed aortic sclerosis. He did not look for radio-femoral delay because he had been asked to examine the heart and not the cardiovascular system. The examiners let him realize that he had missed coarctation of the aorta. Filled with anger and dismay at this injustice he was taken to the next case where he was asked to listen to the *back* of a woman's chest. He had a quick look at the *front* (was not asked to) and spotted the radiation marks (he felt that the examiners were trying to hide

---

*For example, the discrepancies of quotations under the heading: 'Listen, obey and do not stray'—in general we support extending the examination beyond the examiner's instruction, whenever necessary, so long as this is done with intelligence and discrimination.

this clue from him). He looked purposefully at the back and noted pleural aspiration marks. He therefore suspected a pleural effusion and performed the relevant clinical steps to confirm this impression. He was asked the probable cause and without hesitation gave the diagnosis of bronchial carcinoma along with the supportive evidence. He was then asked to examine a man's cranial nerves. He performed a rapid, efficient screen and reported left VIth, VIIth, XIIth nerve palsies and left lateral nystagmus but he was not asked for a diagnosis. For his fourth case he was asked to look at a man and he gave the spot diagnosis of acromegaly. When asked how to diagnose the condition he suggested an X-ray of the pituitary fossa, serum growth hormone levels, GTT, etc. Next he was asked to look at a patient's arm and he instantly recognized the 'plucked chicken skin' appearance of pseudoxanthoma elasticum in the antecubital fossa. Finally he was asked to look at a woman's face where he saw nothing obvious until he spotted a small left pupil and slight ptosis. He immediately diagnosed a left Horner's syndrome and was asked for, and gave, the possible causes. Though his performance in all but the first case had been impeccable he was convinced, until the result arrived, that he had failed because of that first case. In retrospect his reaction to the first case may have had a positive effect on the subsequent performance. Instead of going to pieces (e.g. experience 2 and quotations 39 and 40, p. 350) he felt anger at being asked to examine the heart when the key finding was at the femoral pulse. He conducted the rest of the exam with ruthless efficiency and avenged himself by looking for more than he was asked to. The parting words of the examiner were: 'You'll never miss radio-femoral delay again will you?' (Pass)

2 On his second attempt another candidate was asked first to 'Examine the abdomen'. Without looking anywhere he coned down and felt the liver edge. After a long time, and some persuasion, he noticed the palmar erythema, anaemia, gynaecomastia and decreased body hair. These signs, in particular the gynaecomastia, together with the diagnosis of cirrhosis had to be dragged out of him by the examiners. The candidate had been nervous before the start and now, realizing that he had performed badly on the first case through lack of proper inspection, was already becoming engulfed in the 'downward spiral syndrome'. At the second case the examiner said: 'We haven't much time so just quickly feel the pulse and listen over the apex and base'. He was confused as he did not know where the base was so he listened at the lower left sternal edge and the apex. He did not look at the neck or at the praecordium. He felt a collapsing pulse, heard a systolic murmur and diagnosed mitral incompetence. In retrospect he thought that he must have missed mixed aortic valve disease. On the next case he was asked to examine the legs. He realized that things were going very badly and that he had to score highly from then on. He looked down on two thin legs, imagined two inverted champagne bottles and, before he could stop himself, heard himself saying 'Charcot–Marie–Tooth disease'. The examiner, who was apparently becoming increasingly doubtful about the candidate's capability at performing a competent clinical examination, had to drag a hesitant, unstructured examination out of him which revealed spastic paraparesis. A discussion followed on the possible causes. In the next case the candidate looked at a fundus with whiteness around the disc and diagnosed myelinated nerve fibres. In his last case he examined a patient's hands with swollen metacarpophalangeal and proximal interphalangeal joints, tapered fingers, wasted intrinsic muscles and papery thin skin. With his morale gone, it took a long time before he saw any of the abnormalities and longer still to suggest rheumatoid arthritis (?on steroids). (Fail)

3 After an indifferent start in the first short case, a candidate was asked to examine a man's pulse. He found it regular and the rate was 40 beats/minute. He was then asked to listen to the precordium but he failed to comment on the variable intensity of the first heart sound which could have led him to the diagnosis of complete heart block. He was next asked to look at a woman's face. There was perioral tethering and telangiectasis, but since he had not performed a *visual survey* and his presentation was loose, he was side-tracked into saying that she could have hereditary haemorrhagic telangiectasia. It became obvious to him (he was asked to look at the hands—sclerodactyly) that the patient had scleroderma! The examiner then asked him: 'On which part of the tongue would you say the telangiectasiae would most likely be found in hereditary haemorrhagic telangiectasia, if you were teaching a class of medical students!' Having been unable to impress the examiners so far, he was asked to look at a man's neck. (The bell went almost immediately signalling the end of the exam.) The patient was lying down and his neck movements were completely restricted. The candidate diagnosed cervical spondylosis. The typical 'question mark' posture of ankylosing spondylitis only became recognizable when the patient sat up!

In his second attempt, this candidate was asked to examine a middle-aged woman with a goitre—he felt it was really quite straightforward. The goitre was asymmetrical but he annoyed one examiner by using the term 'slightly asymmetrical'. He also let out the word 'tumour' in front of the patient when asked to discuss management. (Fail)

4 A candidate on his first attempt was asked to look at a man's legs (the examiner pulled the pyjamas to the lower end of the patella, leaving a lateral scar covered—which the candidate did not see until the end). He found a swollen, warm left leg and diagnosed a deep venous thrombosis. He was asked for other possibilities and said ruptured Baker's cyst. The examiner said he would not ask who Baker was but wanted an explanation of the term. The examiners probed for further possibilities such as cellulitis, muscle rupture and also asked about ruptured plantaris muscle. On his next case he was asked to look at some hands and describe them. He diagnosed rheumatoid arthritis and was asked to explain the reasons for ulnar deviation, subluxation and boutonnière deformity. The examiner asked: 'Why is it called boutonnière? Have you ever seen a button hook? Why is the wrist like that? What are the important functions of the hand?' He was then asked to look at the knees of the same patient. He found a swollen, painful right knee which he thought was due to synovial swelling. He said he had been about to say: 'Charcot's joint' but realized it was painful. He diagnosed rheumatoid arthritis of the knee and was then asked how he knew it was synovial swelling. At the next patient the examiners said: 'I think we would be interested in this lady's precordium'. During the examination he was interrupted at various times: 'What do you think of the pulse?'; 'What do you think of the JVP?'; and in fact they stopped him before he had finished and asked for the findings. He diagnosed mixed mitral valve disease but had missed the mitral valvotomy scar. The examiner then handed him an ophthalmoscope and said: 'We would like you to use this on the next patient'. The candidate noticed that this patient showed some incoordination and a spastic leg so he expected to find optic atrophy. When he mentioned this diagnosis the examiner asked him if he knew what sort of visual field defect he would expect and then asked him to test the visual fields. On the last case he was asked to feel the abdomen. He found an inguinal hernia, a palpable aorta and a palpable liver edge at about 2 cm below the right costal margin. He said he did not think it was hepatomegaly. The examiners asked what signs he would look for if the patient did have hepatomegaly! (Pass)

In the following examples the examiner seems to be probing the power and range of the candidate's observations

5   A candidate, in her first attempt, was somewhat uncertain about her performance in the first two short cases. She was then asked to examine the motor system of a man's legs. She found global weakness, wasting and loss of reflexes. She gave a differential diagnosis of lower motor neurone paralysis which included a disc lesion, spinal canal problems, degenerative disorders and motor neurone disease. The examiners asked her to look at the patient's tongue—it was fasciculating. She was then able to narrow the differential diagnosis to the last-mentioned possibility. (Pass)

6   A candidate was asked: 'Look at this man's chest and then examine his respiratory system'. The patient had a right mastectomy scar and the skin changes of previous radiotherapy. There was dullness to percussion and reduced breath sounds at the right base. The candidate diagnosed carcinoma of the breast and a right pleural effusion. (Pass)

7   Taken to her first short case, a candidate was asked only to listen to a patient's heart. No other CVS examination was expected. She found the features of mitral stenosis but did not notice the valvotomy scar. This was pointed out to her by the examiner. (Pass)

8   After rapid progress through the first three short cases, a candidate was asked to look at a woman's hands. He found the changes of rheumatoid arthritis. A description was not wanted, only the diagnosis. The examiner then asked him: 'Why is she wearing a cervical collar?' The candidate, who had noticed but not mentioned it, said that it could be due to atlanto-axial subluxation. (Pass)

9   After mistaking a malar flush for SLE in a patient who had mitral stenosis, a candidate was asked to examine a woman's hands. She diagnosed acromegaly. Although the patient had wasting of the thenar eminence, she missed this and the diagnosis of carpal tunnel syndrome, until the examiner told her about the patient's symptoms. The candidate diagnosed optic atrophy, splenomegaly and hepatosplenomegaly successively in three other short cases and was then shown a patient and asked: 'On general appearance what is wrong with this man?' She thought that he had a myopathic facies and diagnosed dystrophia myotonica. The examiner asked why she thought he had a hearing aid. She looked at the head again and realized that the patient had an enlarged cranium, rather than wasted facial muscles, and diagnosed Paget's disease. (Fail)

10   At her next attempt this candidate gave a better account of herself in four short cases but missed a nodule at the elbow in a patient with rheumatoid arthritis. She was then asked to examine a man's abdomen. She found an enlarged and knobbly liver and diagnosed secondaries in the liver, but forgot to test for ascites. She was asked if there was any free peritoneal fluid. The examiners watched intently as she demonstrated the presence of ascites. (Pass)

11   A candidate was asked to examine the abdomen. He found bilateral masses in the loins and diagnosed polycystic kidneys. The patient also had a craniotomy scar for a ruptured berry aneurysm. On another case he was able to diagnose hypothyroidism by looking at a woman's face. The examiner asked why she was in a surgical ward and he suggested severe constipation as a reason. (Pass)

12   In his second attempt a candidate was asked: 'Examine this lady's cardiovascular system, commenting as you go'. He diagnosed mixed mitral valve disease but missed (cardiac) cachexia and a left mastectomy scar. The examiners wanted him to comment that she was very ill and to suggest why. They also asked for comments as to whether the mitral stenosis or mitral incompetence was dominant. (Fail)

13   A candidate was asked: 'Comment on this patient's appearance. Pretend he is sitting opposite you on the underground train and perform one clinical test'. The candidate noted frontal bossing, bilateral ptosis, deafness, missing fingers on the right hand and a saddle-shaped nose. Initially the candidate thought he had congenital syphilis and wanted to do a Romberg's test. The examiner manipulated the discussion and got him round to thinking about dystrophia myotonica. After this the candidate suggested a handshake as the one clinical test. He was then asked to examine the abdomen of the next patient. He found bilateral enlarged and 'lumpy' kidneys which were easily palpable and he diagnosed polycystic kidneys. The candidate was then shown the patient's left forearm and, having worked on a renal unit, he immediately recognized the presence of an arteriovenous fistula for haemodialysis. The examiners seemed quite impressed with this. (Pass)

14   Another candidate was shown the same patient with dystrophia myotonica and asked: 'What observations do you make?' He commented on bilateral ptosis, wasted sternomastoid and temporalis muscles, and after demonstrating myotonia in the hands was able to make the diagnosis. There then followed a brief viva on cardiomyopathy in dystrophia myotonica! (Pass)

15   After failing to palpate polycystic kidneys, a candidate was asked to listen to a patient's heart. He found mitral incompetence and noted that the patient's face looked acromegalic. However, he did not mention the acromegaly until he was directly asked about it. (Fail)

16   A candidate was taken to a patient with a recent laparotomy scar and asked to examine his neck. He noticed a biopsy scar and on palpation found matted glands. He diagnosed Hodgkin's disease and the examiner asked him for a differential diagnosis. (Pass)

17   In his fourth attempt a candidate was asked to make some observations on a patient with a goitre, then on his next case to feel the pulse and suggest what had happened to that patient (he had atrial fibrillation, exophthalmos and a right hemiplegia). He was then taken to the foot of the next patient's bed and asked: 'Look at this patient from here. What would you like to do now?' He noticed a man with long extremities, muscle wasting, a pustular rash, paronychia, nicotine-stained fingers and pectus excavatum. He had to be prompted to the diagnosis of Marfan's syndrome. He was then asked to look into the patient's mouth (high-arched palate) and to listen to his heart (aortic incompetence). He found both of these but did not mention the hyperextensible joints. (Pass)

18 'This lady is breathless—listen to her heart' was the opening instruction to a candidate who was appearing for the first time. He diagnosed mitral stenosis but the examiners pointed out that he had not noticed that the lady had rheumatoid arthritis as well. He was taken to his next case and told: 'This patient is breathless—examine the respiratory system'. He found crepitations and basal dullness so he diagnosed pulmonary fibrosis and pleural effusion. Having learned from the previous case, he was able to relate both to the rheumatoid arthritis which he had already observed in this patient. (Pass)

19 After having difficulty deciding whether a patient had diabetic or hypertensive retinopathy, a candidate was asked to examine another patient's neck. He diagnosed a small multinodular goitre but the examiners remained dissatisfied. They asked if the patient was thyrotoxic or not. While he examined for a tremor he noticed the gross rheumatoid arthritis in the hands. He reported that the examiners were looking for the diagnosis of autoimmune thyroid disease. (Fail)

20 A candidate was invited to look at a patient's face. The face was normal when looking straight ahead but on further examination he discovered weakness of the lower part of the right side of the face and he diagnosed a right upper motor neurone VIIth nerve palsy. He missed the surgical scar just below the jaw on the right side and, in retrospect, felt it was a partial right lower motor neurone VIIth nerve palsy. (Fail)

21 A candidate was asked to look at a patient's face. He said: 'Acromegaly'. The examiner asked if he was happy with that. The candidate realized that he should have looked for more physical signs so at once he said he would like to look for complications such as bitemporal hemianopia, hypertension, cardiomegaly, or evidence of treatment already given. The patient did, in fact, have a hemianopia. (Pass)

In the experiences that follow the spotlight seems to be on the candidate's examination technique

22 After diagnosing psoriasis and lupus pernio in fairly quick succession, a candidate was asked to examine a patient's legs neurologically. He found bilateral upper motor neurone signs and was then asked the level of the lesion. The candidate proceeded to examine the arms and found upper motor neurone signs in one arm. He next tested the jaw jerk which was normal. No further questions were asked. (Pass)

23 A candidate was asked to examine a patient's abdomen. He found an enlarged organ in the left hypochondrium and thought that it was a polycystic kidney but he admits that his examination was 'cack-handed'. In retrospect he believes it was a spleen. He was later asked to look at a patient's fundi. He diagnosed choroiditis but in retrospect he feels that it was probably a diabetic retinopathy with laser burns. (Fail)

24 After an opening case of a Ramsay Hunt syndrome a candidate was asked to examine a woman's fundi, to look for pyramidal signs in her hands, and to elicit her plantar responses.

He found early papilloedema on the left and an increased finger jerk and supernator jerk on the right, and an extensor plantar on the right. He admitted that he had made a mess of doing the finger jerks and did not know the two ways of eliciting these; in fact the examiner had to demonstrate the tests. He was about to test the plantar response with the end of the patella hammer when he was stopped by the examiner who gave him a thin wooden orange stick! (Pass)

25 Having spoiled the first two short cases a candidate was asked to look at, and then examine, the legs of a man who complained of unsteadiness. He found ataxia, pyramidal weakness with clonus in both legs and bilateral extensor plantar responses and he diagnosed multiple sclerosis. However, the examiner was not at all happy with his neurological examination technique and, in fact, showed him how to do it! (Fail)

26 In his third attempt, a candidate missed something in two of the first four short cases (diabetic maculopathy, calcinosis in scleroderma). He was then asked to watch a patient walk and to examine his lower limbs. He could see bilateral foot drop with wasted anterior compartments but did not make the diagnosis of Charcot–Marie–Tooth disease. The examiners criticized the way he examined the reflexes. (Fail)

27 A candidate was told: 'This man has gone off his feet. Examine the legs and say why'. He found gross wasting, fasciculation, absent ankle jerks and flexor plantar responses and he diagnosed progressive muscular atrophy (motor neurone disease). He commented to us that he had had to wait for what seemed to be three to four minutes before any fasciculation was seen, though when it did come it was very obvious. (Pass)

28 A candidate was asked to examine a patient's eyes. He was almost blind in the left eye with a left VIth nerve palsy. He commented that he might well have failed the examination had he not tested visual acuity and thus found the explanation for the absence of diplopia. (Pass)

29 A candidate was asked to examine a man's hand neurologically. The patient had gross wasting and weakness of the small muscles of the hand. Although the candidate diagnosed a T1 lesion he admitted that he looked very confused examining the hands. A little unsettled by this experience he was asked to examine another patient's abdomen and jugular venous pressure. He found a pulsatile liver and giant v waves. He diagnosed tricuspid incompetence but admitted that he lacked confidence and this showed in the way he carried out the examination. He was then asked to examine the chest of a patient who had a thoracotomy scar, stridor and clubbing. He did not notice the stridor and also missed the pleural effusion. (Fail)

30 On being asked to examine the abdomen of a patient a candidate found bilateral subcostal masses. He gave the findings and said the diagnosis was probably polycystic kidneys. The left-sided mass could have been a small spleen moving diagonally across the abdomen from under the rib cage on inspiration but it was bimanually ballotable. He gave the findings and persevered with the diagnosis of polycystic kidneys. The examiners persisted in discussing the possibility that the mass was a spleen but the candidate stuck to his diagnosis which he thinks was right. (Pass)

31 A candidate was asked: 'Examine this man's chest. Is there anything else you would look for?' He found ankylosing spondylitis with poor expansion and excursion of the chest, but commented that he had to get the patient out of bed before he appreciated the ankylosing spondylitis. There was no evidence of aortic regurgitation or upper lobe fibrosis. (Pass)

32 A candidate examined the abdomen of a 35-year-old Negro woman and found a 6 cm spherical mass in the upper left quadrant. He commented that he was allowed to 'go through the motions'—nodes, mouth, hands, etc. He said it was not a spleen or a kidney and he explained why. He gave a brief differential diagnosis ... 'Expressionless and without comment they led me away'. (Pass)

33 A candidate had done well in his first four short cases except that he failed to demonstrate stridor in a patient with superior vena cava obstruction. He was taken to his fifth case and asked: 'Show me how you examine the reflexes in the legs'. He found absent knee and ankle jerks and extensor plantar responses. He offered the differential diagnosis of tabes dorsalis, subacute combined degeneration of the cord and hereditary neuropathy such as Freidreich's ataxia. He was asked what else he would like to examine and he suggested the pupillary reflexes. He found small regular pupils which reacted to light and accommodation, but more to accommodation. He was asked if these were Argyll Robertson pupils and he answered: 'No'. The other examiner said: 'You said that this picture in the legs may be due to tabes dorsalis. How do you explain the extensor plantars?' He answered that this indicates pyramidal tract involvement. The examiner pointed out that this is called taboparesis, not tabes dorsalis. The candidate felt that his unfamiliarity with differing manifestations of neurosyphilis let him down, and he had failed to recognize Argyll Robertson pupils. (Fail)

34 The opening short case of a candidate in his first attempt was a patient with an obvious squint and exophthalmos. He was asked to _examine_* the eyes, look at the neck and feel the pulse. He stated the obvious, but did not test the eye movements adequately and reports: 'Actually the examiner expected me to examine the eye movements properly and identify the muscle paralysed'. The examiner then explained that exophthalmos and goitre suggest thyrotoxicosis and that the normal sinus rhythm suggests that the latter has been treated. The candidate was also shown cases of clubbing of the fingers, cyanosis, and psoriatic arthropathy, all of which he could recognize, and the examiner finally took him to a patient and asked him: 'Examine the abdomen'. He found an enlarged liver of three finger-breadths and a spleen of four finger-breadths and diagnosed hepatosplenomegaly. The examiner's parting comment was: 'It is no good only making a diagnosis; there is a proper method to examine the patient!' (Fail)

35 A candidate was asked to examine the back of the chest of a young man. He diagnosed bilateral pleural effusions and he felt that these were probably due to nephrotic syndrome. The examiners agreed. However he had forgotten to test for vocal resonance or tactile vocal fremitus. (Fail)

*Our italics. The candidate was expected to do more than just look at the eyes.

36 A candidate was asked to examine a patient's heart. He went through all the correct examination steps except that he forgot to lift up the arm and feel for a collapsing pulse. He diagnosed mixed mitral valve disease. One examiner proceeded to listen to the heart while the other examiner asked if the candidate had felt for a collapsing pulse. The candidate now wonders if he missed aortic valve disease. (Fail)

37 A candidate was asked to examine the eyes of a girl aged about 20–30 years. He went comprehensively through, checking visual acuity and visual fields before testing eye movements. He felt the examiners were impatient at the delay in finding the nystagmus which was present. The examiners asked what he wanted to examine now. The candidate, thinking that the diagnosis was likely to be multiple sclerosis, said he wanted to look at the fundi. He could not understand why the examiners seemed so irritated by this. They wanted him to demonstrate the cerebellar signs which were present. The candidate felt that this was an easy case on which he had made no great errors and yet the examiners seemed to have been unimpressed by his performance. (Fail)

38 A candidate was asked to examine a patient's legs neurologically and then to ask him some questions. He found global aphasia and a profound right-sided spastic hemiparesis. He diagnosed a dominant hemisphere vascular lesion. He was asked: 'What might be the cause?—The patient is 40';—(pause)—'Feel the pulse'. He was in atrial fibrillation. 'What do you think the cause is now?' (Pass)

39 A candidate was shown a woman with a spastic paraparesis which she correctly diagnosed. After she had been taken to the next case, the examiners said: 'By the way, which side of the fire does that other lady usually sit by?' Luckily, she had noticed the erythema ab igne on the legs. (Pass)

A lack of polish and fluidity may make the examiners reflect on the clinical competence of a candidate. In the following examples, the examiners seem to be endeavouring to find the real clinical depth

40 An examiner pointed to a patient with typical rheumatoid hands and said to a candidate: 'This lady had a fit six months ago, examine her hands'. During his examination he found no skin rash or nodules. He diagnosed SLE in view of the fit. However, in retrospect, he still wonders if the diagnosis was rheumatoid arthritis. (Pass)

41 A candidate was asked to examine the CVS in a patient. He found a slow rising pulse, an ejection systolic murmur and an early diastolic murmur. He diagnosed mixed aortic valve disease with predominant aortic stenosis. The examiners asked him to guess his blood pressure. (Pass)

42 After correctly diagnosing spastic paraparesis, a candidate was asked to give the differences between upper and lower motor neurone lesions. In the next case he was asked to feel a man's pulse. He suggested slow atrial fibrillation but in retrospect he thinks it may have been complete heart block. There then followed a discussion about the differential diagnosis and the management of complete heart block with different types of pacemakers. (Fail)

43   A candidate who was taking the examination for the fourth time was taken to his first case and asked: 'Feel this patient's pulse and apex beat, and listen to the base of the heart'. He was required to give a full description of the findings and the probable diagnosis at each stage. He found pulsus bisferiens, a displaced apex, an ejection systolic and an early diastolic murmur. (Pass)

44   A candidate who was unhappy with his examination technique and the mistakes he had made in an easy first case, was asked to examine the right arm of a 40-year-old man. He reports finding a 'flail' arm with increased reflexes. He thought his method of examination was poor and he was unsure of the diagnosis. He was then asked to examine the same man's abdomen and reports finding bilateral, large, smooth, more or less symmetrical masses in the lumbar regions which he diagnosed as bilateral hydronephrotic kidneys.* (Fail)

45   A candidate was asked to 'Examine the eyes from a neurological point of view'. He found bilateral ptosis and a homonymous hemianopia and he said to the examiner that he could not explain the findings by one lesion. The examiner said: 'Examine the hands'. The candidate became preoccupied with the obvious rheumatoid arthritis and came up with the suggestion of rheumatoid arthritis associated with myasthenia gravis, which would explain the ptosis but not the hemianopia. The examiner said: 'Feel the pulse'. The candidate found an irregular pulse and diagnosed atrial fibrillation causing a cerebral embolus. (Pass)

46   A candidate examined the back of the chest of a patient and found a pleural effusion. He had to go through the full examination and was asked what he did at every move, what each finding was caused by and how he interpreted it, e.g. breath sounds, crepitations, etc. (Pass)

Common errors

47   Having done well in his first three short cases a candidate was asked to give a running commentary as he examined the cardiovascular system. He commented on a collapsing pulse and on a mitral valvotomy scar but found no murmurs. He diagnosed mitral stenosis and got involved in a long discussion on the causes of a collapsing pulse! (Fail)

48   A candidate was asked to listen to a woman's heart. He found systolic and diastolic murmurs maximal at the base of the heart, to the left of the sternum. He diagnosed mixed aortic valve disease. In retrospect he is sure that he missed the typical machinery murmur of a patent ductus arteriosus. (Fail)

49   A candidate was asked to examine a man's chest, commenting as he went along. Though he thought the patient had chronic obstructive airways disease he was not actually asked for a diagnosis, but instead became caught up in a discussion on the distinction between a wheeze and stridor. (Pass)

50   Still flustered by two of the previous three cases which had gone badly, a candidate examined a fundus of a patient whose pupil had been dilated. He could not find much wrong

*We wonder if this patient had polycystic kidneys and an old CVA (ruptured berry aneurysm/hypertension).

and wondered if there was some vascular abnormality. He made a wild guess at diabetic retinopathy and wonders in retrospect if this was a branch vein or artery occlusion. His comment was: 'I was totally lost by this time!' (Fail)

51 A candidate examined the fundi of a patient and diagnosed bilateral optic atrophy and background diabetic retinopathy. He told us he had 'blurted out my impressions before stopping and thinking'. Even in retrospect he does not know what the diagnosis was. (Fail)

52 A candidate was asked to examine the fundi of a patient (dilated pupils, dark room). He saw haemorrhages, exudates and some whiteness around the disc. He was put off by the examiners talking in the background and by his paranoia that the examiners were thinking that he was taking too long so he stopped before he had finished. He offered the diagnosis of diabetic retinopathy and myelinated nerve fibres. One examiner looked in the fundi while the other enquired if any microaneurysms had been seen. The candidate was not sure. There was then a discussion about the treatment of diabetic retinopathy and when photocoagulation was mentioned the examiner asked if there was any evidence of this. In retrospect the candidate felt diabetic retinopathy was probably right but wonders about the possibility of having missed hypertensive retinopathy and papilloedema. He felt that if only he had continued examining longer to elicit the exact findings present he would have saved himself over £200.* (Fail)

53 A candidate, nervous on his first attempt, was asked to palpate the abdomen. He found bilateral masses in the upper quadrants but states that he was interrupted before he could examine them properly. He thought they were polycystic kidneys but in the stress of the moment he found himself saying hepatosplenomegaly before he could stop himself! (Fail)

54 A candidate was asked to feel the pulse of a patient. She was unable to feel it and guessed that atrial fibrillation must be present. (She failed) Another candidate was taken to the same patient and admitted that she could feel neither the radials, brachials nor carotids (the patient was in low output cardiac failure). Afterwards she was told by the examiners at the sherry reception (Edinburgh) that they had re-examined the patient and agreed with her. (Pass)

55 A potential candidate was asked to examine the back of the chest of a patient with bronchiectasis who had appeared in the examination. During auscultation the patient, in her enthusiasm to cooperate, breathed deeply and expired forcibly, generating upper airways wheeze.† The candidate, who already had his stethoscope in his ears, was unaware of the racket the patient was making. He reported the finding of widespread wheeze (the basal crepitations were completely drowned) though there was no wheezing at all when the patient was asked to breath deeply in and out in a relaxed fashion.

---

*Correct at time of publication.
†You can generate upper airways wheeze yourself by expiring hard at the same time as voluntarily narrowing your upper airways. If in doubt in the hysterical asthmatic, ask the patient to purse his lips as he breathes. This manoeuvre will abolish factitious wheeze. Though the wheeze of such a patient may be heard down the corridor, the pulse is not significantly elevated in the absence of true severe asthma (unless the acute asthma is due to the inappropriate prescription of a β blocker!).

Double pathology

56 A candidate in her first attempt was asked to examine a woman's legs neurologically. She found absent ankle jerks, increased knee reflexes and equivocal plantars. She was told that the patient was a diabetic and she noticed that she was wearing a cervical collar. Her mind alerted to the possibility that there was a combination of a peripheral neuropathy and cervical spondylosis. (Pass)

57 After three successful cases a candidate was shown a patient and told: 'This patient has something wrong with his cardiovascular system. Find out in the most expeditious way'. She noticed exophthalmos and found a large abdominal scar and cardiac outflow tract obstruction. The patient later said that he had had a repair of a thoracic aortic aneurysm! (Pass)

58 After an easy first short case (splenomegaly) a candidate was asked to look at the face of a woman who presented with melaena. In retrospect he felt the patient had acromegaly and Peutz–Jeghers syndrome (!) but he had not spotted the latter condition quickly enough. He was asked to examine the visual fields and, having mentioned the presence of greasy skin, was drawn into a discussion on skin function. (Fail)

59 A candidate who had had a genial discussion on scleroderma and its complications, was then asked to examine the legs of a man whom he was told had diabetes mellitus. He found a peripheral neuropathy and peripheral vascular disease. He also spotted that the patient had coexistent facio-scapular dystrophy. (Pass)

60 In his second attempt, a candidate who had not done too well in the opening short case was then asked to examine the heart only of the next patient. He found mixed aortic valve disease. He also suspected mitral stenosis but did not mention it as he had not expected to find double valve pathology. (Fail)

Invigilators' diaries

61 A candidate was asked to examine the legs of a patient. He was allowed to carry out a large proportion of a full neurological examination before he became aware, with prodding from the examiner, of the large skull, hearing aid and the bowed tibiae of Paget's disease. The examiner commented that if he had *looked* at the patient first he might have saved himself the time wasted on the unnecessary neurological examination.

62 A candidate was asked to examine the eyes of a patient. He carried out most of the examination of the eye movements before he noticed the obvious blue sclerae of osteogenesis imperfecta. The examiner was irritated by this and commented that the candidate had wasted several minutes of the examiner's time by not looking at the eyes properly and noticing an obvious physical sign.

63 A candidate was asked to examine the fundi of a patient with diabetic retinopathy and laser photocoagulation scars. It was the end of the afternoon and the tropicamide drops, which had been put in that morning to dilate the pupil, had worn off. The candidate said she could see nothing and asked to take the patient into a darkened room. A side room was found but it was only semi-dark. She still said she could see nothing. The examiner was very unimpressed that she had missed what he considered to be a very easy case of diabetic retinopathy. When the invigilator tried to help save the candidate by apologizing that the drops had worn off, the examiner retorted that the pupils would not be dilated in the casualty department.

64   A patient in the examination had a 'full house' of mixed mitral and aortic valve disease. The examiner commented that candidates kept failing to hear all the murmurs. He suspected that having heard one or two loud ones, they stopped listening for the others which were less obvious.

65   A candidate was asked to look at a lady's hands. He described Heberden's nodes, spindling of the fingers and proximal joint swelling, all of which the patient had. He suggested combined osteoarthritis and rheumatoid arthritis. When the examiner asked about conditions associated with rheumatoid arthritis, the candidate looked beyond the hands and noticed the generalized pigmentation and then the palmar crease pigmentation of Addison's disease. The latter condition was the reason for the patient's inclusion in the examination— the joint changes had not been noted before.

66   A patient with a small calcified embolus in the fundus had been included amongst the patients available for one session of the examination. Before the exam, when the examiners were going around the patients by themselves, one examiner came away from this fundus and said to another examiner: 'Could you see the embolus?'. 'No', said the second. 'Neither could I', replied the first: 'I'm not going to take any of my candidates on that case'. The case was used by other examiners on just one or two candidates.

67   A patient known to have Behçet's disease was included as a fundus case with optic atrophy. On fundoscopy he had optic atrophy, choroidoretinitis and also sheathing of the vessel walls. All the examiners agreed that they had not seen a fundus like it before and that it was a 'museum' case. The underlying cause was not discussed with any of the candidates who were only expected to see what was there and describe it accurately. Calling the vessel sheathing 'silver wiring', as one candidate did, was considered unacceptable.

68   Before one examination session all the examiners gathered around a patient to be shown his signs, which were said to include splenomegaly. Two or three of the examiners felt the abdomen and agreed that they could not feel the spleen. After these had moved on, another of the examiners examined the abdomen and called the invigilator over, saying: 'Put your hand here, like this—the spleen is palpable—can you feel it?'

69   A candidate was asked to examine the heart of a patient with mitral valve prolapse. Unfortunately the backrest collapsed while he was examining and could not be repaired so the patient could only be examined lying flat or sitting upright. Though the examiners accepted that this was off-putting, they did not feel that it justified missing all the signs and getting systole and diastole the wrong way round!

70 A membership examiner was heard telling a group of students that many candidates fail to recognize atrial fibrillation. Furthermore, in his experience, about 20% of candidates cannot accurately demonstrate the second left intercostal space. He had also noticed that candidates were often poor in their technique of examining ankle jerks.

71 A candidate was asked to examine the fundi of a patient with laser-treated diabetic retinopathy. She diagnosed diabetic retinopathy but when asked if she had seen any microaneurysms or photocoagulation scars she was not sure.

72 A candidate was shown a euthyroid diabetic patient with necrobiosis lipoidica diabeticorum and was given some of the patient's historical features which were vaguely suggestive of hyperthyroidism; he was then told to assess the girl's thyroid status. Despite the normal pulse rate and lack of other supportive signs the candidate apparently managed to diagnose hyperthyroidism!

73 An examiner was watching a candidate feeling for the apex beat of a female patient. The rough handling of the patient's breast irritated the examiner who later commented: 'That sort of behaviour brings a candidate immediately to the pass/fail borderline'.

Ungentlemanly clinical methods

74 A candidate was asked to examine a patient's respiratory system. He found clubbing and basal crackles and diagnosed bronchiectasis. He confessed that he was helped along in this diagnosis because he could see it on the examiner's clipboard!

75 A candidate was asked to examine the fundi. The examiners were several yards away and as he was examining he quietly asked the patient if he was a diabetic, to which the patient answered: 'Yes'. The candidate diagnosed proliferative diabetic retinopathy with photocoagulation scars in one eye and a vitreous haemorrhage in the other. He was asked why it was difficult to see one of the fundi well and replied that it was because of the vitreous haemorrhage. (Pass)

Anecdotes

1 A candidate was unsettled by his rather mediocre performance in the first two short cases. The examiner then asked him to examine a patient's hands and knees. He found hypoplastic nails and absent patellae but admitted that he had no idea what the diagnosis was (nail-patella syndrome). (Fail)

2 A candidate was asked to examine the chest of a patient 'from the front only'. She found all the findings compatible with a left upper zone fibrosis/collapse and suggested that this could be due to previous tuberculosis. She was then allowed to inspect the patient's back which revealed a thoracoplasty scar. The candidate was told that she was correct. (Pass)

3 A candidate was asked to examine a woman's legs and found erythema ab igne. The examiners then asked for the differential diagnosis of reticulate rashes on the legs and for the different skin biopsy appearances! (Pass)

4 A candidate was shown a patient and asked to look at the skin over her knees. It was a young girl, who said: 'I am double-jointed, doctor'. The candidate found 'cigarette paper' scars over both knees and diagnosed Ehlers–Danlos syndrome. There then followed a discussion about heredity and complications. He was then shown his next short case and was told that this patient had had a car accident three weeks ago. He found a healing, abnormal scar over the left shin and he again diagnosed Ehlers–Danlos syndrome. The examiners asked if he would be surprised to learn that the patients were related—the candidate answered: 'No'. (Pass)

5 A candidate was asked to examine a patient's cardiovascular system. He found several murmurs and suggested patent ductus arteriosus but he is still not sure whether that was the correct diagnosis. He commented that the examiners were irritated because he felt the pulse first. They seemed to want him to go straight to the precordium, though they had asked for a 'cardiovascular system' examination. (Pass)

6 A candidate was asked to examine a patient's eyes and then the neck. He found unilateral proptosis and a goitre and diagnosed thyrotoxicosis. He reported that he did not notice the proptosis until he looked from above. (Pass)

7 After seeing a patient with motor neurone disease a candidate was asked to examine an abdomen. He found a palpable left kidney which he suspected to be either polycystic or hydronephrotic. There was also a mass in the right iliac fossa, which he thought was probably a transplanted kidney. (Pass)

8 After an opening case of rheumatoid hands, a candidate was asked to look at the hands of another patient. He found purple, swollen fingers with no arthritis, nail involvement or evidence of scleroderma but he noted some telangiectasis on his face and lips. He was told that he could ask the patient some questions to determine the cause. He said he thought the patient had Raynaud's disease but wondered retrospectively if this may have been a case of CRST syndrome. He reported: 'The examiners wanted the causes of Raynaud's phenomenon and for me to look for evidence of diseases such as scleroderma, SLE, etc. They wanted me to ask the patient if he worked with vibrating tools and what happened to his hands if he put them into cold water'. (Pass)

9 A candidate was told that a female patient was breathless and he was asked to examine her abdomen, and to explain her breathlessness. He found massive hepatosplenomegaly plus anaemia and instead of coming out with myelosclerosis as the diagnosis, he said sarcoidosis! At this stage the examiners, who had been very pleasant until then, began to look impatient! (Fail)

10 A candidate was asked to look at a patient's legs and found erythema nodosum. He was asked to discuss the histology of this condition which he did not know. He was then shown an ECG of another patient which showed a supraventricular tachycardia with a 2 : 1 block.* (Pass)

---

*This is the only candidate who was shown an ECG in our short cases survey.

11 A candidate who had made reasonable progress through his first five short cases, was briefly shown a patient with Parkinsonian facies who had a parenteral nutrition infusion in progress. He was asked to comment on the type of line used for feeding and to describe the procedure.* (Pass)

12 A candidate was asked to examine a patient's abdomen. He found hepatosplenomegaly. The examiners then showed him the arteriovenous shunt and asked him to re-examine the abdomen. His diagnosis then became polycystic kidneys! He was sure he had failed outright but tried to keep his head, remembering that it was possible to get by with one disaster! (Pass)

13 A candidate was asked to examine the abdomen of a woman with jaundice and hepatosplenomegaly. The examiners got annoyed when he started with examining her hands. (Pass)

14 A candidate was asked: 'Look at this rash in a 16-year-old girl'. There was a maculopapular rash on the limbs but not on the trunk. There was no involvement of the eyes, nails, joints or mouth. He was asked what the diagnosis was and if he would like to ask the patient some questions. The condition had been present for 5 years and the joints were painful. He offered the differential diagnosis of juvenile chronic arthritis or SLE. In retrospect he feels it was the former (Still's disease). (Pass)

15 Until a candidate reached his fifth short case his only blemish was that he took a minute in counting the respiratory rate of a patient with dyspnoea and clubbing. He was asked to examine the abdomen of a woman who weighed 'about 20 stone'. He found two subcostal masses and diagnosed hepatosplenomegaly. In retrospect he was sure that they were polycystic kidneys and that arguing the case for hepatosplenomegaly made matters worse and wasted a lot of time. (Fail)

16 A candidate was asked to examine a patient's left eye with the ophthalmoscope provided. He reported that he found optic atrophy, a detached retina, laser photocoagulation scars and aphakia. He suggested that the patient had had a diabetic cataract previously. The examiner asked about primary and secondary optic atrophy and then asked about the refractive error of the patient—covering the head of the ophthalmoscope with his hand as he did so! (Pass)

17 A candidate was told: 'Examine this rash but don't rub it'. He found a brownish macular rash on a young, healthy-looking woman. He had no idea what the diagnosis was. In retrospect he thinks it must have been mastocytosis. (Fail)

18 A candidate was told that a patient had a chronic cough. On examination he found right upper lobe consolidation and offered a differential diagnosis of tumour or TB. He was then shown the patient's chest X-ray which showed a cavity with a crescentic upper border and he diagnosed a mycetoma. (Pass)

---

* We presume that the patient had Steele–Richardson syndrome.

19 A candidate was asked to examine a heart and found isolated aortic incompetence. Two cases later he was asked to examine the heart in a different patient and was surprised to again find isolated aortic incompetence. (Pass)

20 In his second attempt a candidate was asked to listen to a heart. He heard a mid-diastolic murmur and came up with the diagnosis of mitral stenosis. The examiner asked him to auscultate again; on doing this he could also hear an early diastolic murmur. (Fail)

21 'Ask this lady some questions and find out what the problem is' was the instruction addressed to a candidate. He found a rather garrulous lady with senile dementia. He did not ask her questions very well and the examiner stepped in to help. The diagnosis was discussed and the examiner apparently agreed that it was difficult. Afterwards the candidate was told by the organizing registrar that they had had difficulty finding good cases—otherwise this dementia case would probably not have been included in the examination. (Pass)

22 A candidate at his fourth attempt was so nervous as he went into the viva that when the examiner asked the first question, though it was easy, he found he could not speak. After a pause both examiners started writing on their pads which further increased the tension in the atmosphere. Eventually the candidate found his voice and gave a faultless performance for the rest of the viva. At the end he was still very concerned that the exam was overshadowed by a bad start so before he left he apologized for it, saying that it was because he was so nervous. The examiners smiled and said that it was very understandable in a way which made him feel that his bad start had not had much effect on their overall judgement. He was glad he brought this up and obtained their reassurance because otherwise he feels he may still have been worrying about the viva when he went into the long and short cases. (Pass)

23 A candidate was asked to examine the pulse of a patient and found a right brachial artery aneurysm. He reports that the examiner expected him to find the right radial pulse reduced in volume compared to the left but that he could not confirm this. The possible causes he offered were traumatic, iatrogenic or mycotic and in retrospect feels that it was most likely to have been a mycotic aneurysm due to SBE many years before. (Pass)

24 A candidate was asked to look at a man's face. He found herpes zoster in the left ear and in the distribution of the mandibular division of the trigeminal nerve. He also reported a left facial nerve paralysis and wasting of the left side of the tongue with deviation of the protruded tongue to the left. He diagnosed Ramsay Hunt syndrome plus herpes affecting the Vth and XIIth cranial nerves. He was asked if such extensive involvement was possible and answered: 'It appears so'. (Pass)

25 A candidate was asked to examine the fundus of a patient. He found that the lens had been removed because of a cataract. It was very difficult to see the fundus so he guessed the diagnosis of diabetic retinopathy which he still believes was correct. (Pass)

Useful tips

1   Practise being harassed. Get some 'mock' examiners to put you under stress. Nervousness gets no credit: the examiner is more likely to think that in a real emergency you would not rise to the challenge (though see anecdote 22, p. 343).

2   In every spare moment practise talking short case *records* (not just reading them) and talking lists (not just writing them). Get the order of lists right—give the common and uncontroversial ones first. Avoid controversial causes.

3   Dress smartly and conservatively.

4   Take to the examination a pen torch, red-headed hat pin (dip a white-headed one in red paint if necessary), a tape measure and some cotton wool.

5   Be polite to the patient and the examiners; say 'Please' and 'Thank you'. The occasional use of 'Sir' will not do any harm.

6   Do not repeat the examiner's questions.

7   Do not hurt the patient, especially during the abdominal examination. Look at the patient's face during deep palpation.

8   Make sure that during the examination of the patient you let the examiner see that you are doing the correct things—as one does in a driving test (which in many ways is similar to the short case examination).

9   Think *whilst* you are examining. Extend the end of the examination by a few seconds, if necessary, to give you time to put the findings together, and to prepare what you are going to say to the examiner.

10   Do not let your tie or hair dangle in the patient's face. When you have finished be sure to leave the patient adequately covered up.

11   Look at the examiner rather than at the patient or the floor when answering, and speak clearly and fluently (do not mumble).

12   Be aware that the stress of the examination can cause you to 'blurt out' things you do not really mean (anecdote 9, p. 341 and experiences 2, 4, 51, 53, pp. 328, 329, 337). Keep calm and think before you speak.

13   Remember common things are common. Beware of thinking that because it's MRCP it's likely to be something rare. Study the frequencies we have provided and start at the top of the list not the bottom.

14   Present cases to the examiner as if you are speaking to an equal about an easy case.

15   Do not talk while the examiner is talking and be wary of arguing with him. If you make a mistake be prepared to say: 'I withdraw that', rather than try to defend it. Remind yourself that the examiner is the judge and the jury!

16   Do not try to pull the wool over the examiner's eyes. He is eminent and intelligent or he would not be an examiner, and he will resent it if you treat him as a fool.

17   Do not guess or waffle. Cut your losses and admit if you do not know.

18   Avoid strange mannerisms of speech and action including using your hands excessively when speaking. Avoid 'ers' in your speech as much as possible.

19   Be confident—but not over-confident. A supercilious attitude is fatal.

20   Do not be casual. Say 'myocardial infarction' rather than 'heart attack' or 'MI'; stand properly without leaning on the bed or putting your hands in your pockets.

21   Avoid using drug trade names—always use the proper pharmacological name.

22   Do not mention dubious or 'slight' physical signs (e.g. starting your presentation on a case of mitral stenosis with: 'The pulse is slightly collapsing').

23   At the end say: 'Thank you', in a sincere manner.

Facts and figures

1 It is often said that the more short cases you see the better. For what it is worth, the average number of 'main focus' short cases seen in our survey* on a

Pass attempt was 6.1 (range 4–10)

Fail attempt was 5.5 (range 3–8)

It is possible that part of this difference was due to some candidates in the survey forgetting some of their fail attempt short cases because of the time lapse between the exam sitting and filling in the questionnaire.

2 It is often said that if you are going to pass MRCP Part II, you are much more likely to do so on your first attempt. In our survey the percentage of successful candidates by number of attempts was:

65% passed on their first attempt

16% passed on their second attempt

12% passed on their third attempt

5% passed on their fourth attempt

$\frac{1}{2}$% passed on their fifth attempt

$\frac{1}{2}$% passed on their sixth attempt

These figures have to be interpreted with caution because (i) the participants in the survey were self-selected (e.g. candidates who endured the exam several times may have been less inclined to recall unpleasant experiences and fill in a larger number of questionnaires), and (ii) we have no information on the numbers who fail and never sit again at each attempt (e.g. we do not know whether the 5% who passed on their fourth attempt were the vast majority or the tiny minority of those sitting the examination for the fourth time).

3 According to our survey, as you enter the examination room on any one attempt at the short case, you have an:

86% chance of meeting *mitral* and/or *aortic* valve disease

86% chance of meeting either palpable *kidney*(s) or *liver* and/or *spleen*

80% chance of meeting one of the following six conditions which you may be able to spot at once:

Exophthalmos

Chronic liver disease

Paget's disease

Systemic sclerosis

Hemiparesis

Acromegaly

74% chance of meeting one of:

Diabetic retinopathy

Optic atrophy

Hypertensive retinopathy

Retinitis pigmentosa

Papilloedema

*Since 1981 when the length of the exam increased to 30 minutes.

Choroidoretinitis
68% chance of meeting one of:
    Rheumatoid hands
    Wasting of the small muscles of the hand
    Systemic sclerosis
    Psoriasis/psoriatic arthropathy
    Ulnar nerve palsy
57% chance of meeting one of:
    Pleural effusion
    Fibrosing alveolitis
    Old tuberculosis
    Carcinoma of the lung
    Chronic bronchitis and emphysema
    Bronchiectasis
33% chance of meeting thyroid disease

4 Candidates are not often asked to look at investigations such as X-rays during the short cases, as such skills are tested in the written section of the examination. Nevertheless 6% of candidates in our survey were shown an X-ray or ECG. This broke down approximately into:
    Chest X-ray 4.5% (pleural effusion, bilateral hilar lymphadenopathy, hilar shadow, pulmonary hypertension, mycetoma)
    X-ray of legs 0.5% (Paget's)
    CT scan 0.5% (occipital infarct)
    ECG 0.5% (SVT with 2:1 block)

Quotations

Adopt good bedside manners

1 The examination is the same as the final MB but with no help or encouragement from the examiners. Your approach to the patient is *very* important.

2 Don't panic; don't let them hassle you; be kind to the patient.

3 Always introduce yourself by name to the patient and explain what you are going to do (in lay terms!). Position the patient correctly and check whether the part is painful. Do not be afraid to ask the examiner if you can examine a 'remote' part if you consider this necessary (he can always say no).

4 For women I would like to suggest that you wear something comfortable which will accommodate your stethoscope, and leave your handbag in a cloakroom. There is enough stress without worrying if your buttons are undone!

5 Remember to suggest moving away from the patient when having to use words like 'tumour' or 'multiple sclerosis'.

Practise clinical examination and presentation

6 Don't try the MRCP too soon. See as much as possible—'cushy' jobs are not helpful in the end.

7 My theoretical knowledge was good enough but I lacked short-case practice (failed attempt).

8 Go to as many clinical courses for Membership as possible. Work out the best method for the examination of each system and practise it until it is second nature to you. Be as direct and positive in your answers as possible (even if they are wrong!)

9 I know I passed the written and the viva but I failed badly on the short cases. Don't take the examination unless you can properly prepare for it. I was very anxious and was not thinking while I was examining. I kept imagining that the cases were supposed to be difficult, rare or complex.

10 Talk through as many short cases as possible before the examination with someone who has been through it recently, or with someone who is used to teaching, and preferably do this on a one-to-one basis.

11 Practising the technique of examination is essential so that it becomes second nature under stress. Persuade colleagues to grill you mercilessly on cases and differential diagnoses. Certain 'favourite' topics seem to recur so make sure you know these. Also don't make any statements unless you can back them up.

12 The most important point is to look professional—as if you have done it quickly and thoroughly a hundred times before. You do not need to know much. Take your own equipment as you know how it works and you don't have to ask for it and wait.

13 Before the examination I spent 6 weeks getting registrars to take me on short cases and then questioning me under examination conditions. Be meticulous about examination technique and don't be fooled by the apparent relaxed nature of the examiners—examine everything properly. Don't listen to nonsense from tutors about one mistake making a failed exam.

14 The more practice at presenting short cases the better.

15 I had a lot of practice presenting short cases to a 'hawk' of an SR. This experience was invaluable.

16 Adopt a systematic approach to the examination of all the major systems and have the features of the common clinical states at your finger tips, e.g. upper and lower motor neurone lesions, the auscultatory findings of various valvular lesions, etc. There is a need for a well integrated, comprehensive system for presenting the findings to examiners. Do not rush the presentation thereby omitting important points.

17 It's important to have a method for examining each system. I don't think the examiners necessarily want you to make a diagnosis but just to describe the signs.

18 Be very professional in your presentation. I agree it's an easy exam—it's easy to fail!

Get it right

19 Do not rush a case—they were very keen to stop me once they considered that I had enough information to make a diagnosis.

20 If you are unsure of the diagnosis then describe the findings and give a differential diagnosis.

21 Do not be afraid to allow a few seconds of silence to pass before answering a question whilst you collect and organize your thoughts.

22 Know the diagnosis before you leave the patient and state it confidently. Be prepared for further questions on the physical signs and the management of the disease.

23 When examining fundi don't stop until you have finished and have thought of what to say.

24 Don't pass comments that cannot be substantiated. Everything will be challenged if you are on the borderline.

25 The examiners already had in their mind what answers they would accept and they kept on until they got the actual wording they wanted.

26 Try not to be obtuse in the short cases or to pick on unimportant details, as the examiners may then draw you into a frustrating and often irrelevant discussion as to what you mean or sidetrack you from the main issue.

Listen, obey and do not stray

27 Just stick to what they ask, don't mess around. For example, don't start checking the temperature just because you hear a murmur. It seems to irritate them.

28 Do only what is asked of you. Give positive and concise answers to questions, unless a differential diagnosis is requested.

29 Always do a full examination of the system asked—show off your technique. Do not be put off by 'dead-pan' examiners. The result comes as a particular shock when you have been sitting exams for many years *without* failing them.

30 I think I passed (third attempt) because I could carry the examiner's instructions one step further, i.e. feeling the pulse of someone who has a dysphasia. Perhaps that is the secret!

31   They may ask you just to listen to the heart so that you cannot get clues from the pulse and palpation.

32   I suspect that they liked the way I examined the first patient (a neurological case in which I extended the examination beyond the legs) and then decided that I was probably competent. From then on they seemed to be on my side. Most of the time I didn't get asked for a diagnosis, just for the signs, and they didn't then continue to corner me. All was surprisingly amiable!

33   Perform the examination and answer questions as requested. Try asking patients as much as possible; my examiners made *no* attempt to stop me. For example, I asked the patient in whom I had to look at the fundus, if he was a diabetic. I was left with the impression that the examination, although difficult, was fundamentally *fair*.

One wrong does not make one fail

34   Treat each short case individually and put your apparent disasters behind you.

35   Don't be put off by messing up one short case; keep trying! Be sure you understand whether a full system examination, or only part of an examination, is required. The examiners may appear irritable and unsympathetic—don't worry!

36   Don't be put off if you get a few things wrong. I made a lot of mistakes (that I know of!) and still passed.

37   Do not be distracted by mistakes made (or imagined) in preceding cases or by the examiners' mannerisms or approach.

38   The old adage is: 'Be generally observant'. Being very nervous does not necessarily fail you; one bad case should not put you off.

39   I was put off right from the beginning after they stopped me during the examination of the first case—a vague, non-specific instruction was given and I had not found enough to be sure of. I was on the downward slope from then on. I might have passed had I pulled myself together and put the experience of Case 1 behind me.

If you say less they want more

40   After the first case there was a long silence as if they were waiting for me to say more— I went to pieces after this.

41   Be prepared for supplementary questions and for examiners who disagree or argue with your comments.

42   Be complete in your examination—examine everything even if it doesn't seem relevant. For example, all hearts need to be listened to for early diastolic and mid-diastolic murmurs even if you think you already have the diagnosis. Every possible aspect of eyes needs to be looked at if asked to examine the eyes, unless something in the instruction suggests otherwise.

If you know it—say it

43 When you know the diagnosis—say it.

44 Offer a diagnosis if you are reasonably confident of it—this way you can save time from having to discuss a differential diagnosis and you will get through more cases. Try not to let the examiners rush you from case to case, thus forcing you to take short cuts in your examination technique.

45 Have a system for examining. Think, don't rush and don't say more than you have to.

46 Mention all the things you notice especially if they are obvious—even if asked about something else.

Humility is more persuasive than selfrighteousness

47 Be kind and confident but humble in the short cases.

48 Don't argue your case too strongly. Beware of polycystic kidneys in obese ladies! (anecdote 15, p. 342).

49 By far the major problem was keeping my head and holding my ground *politely* when we disagreed.

50 Learn good examination techniques for all systems. Do not argue with the examiners and be polite to the patients.

51 If you know you have made a glaring error retract the remark and start again—if you're right (or at least think you are) stick to your answer.

Keep cool: agitation generates aggression

52 'Panic not'. This is greatly helped if you have practised a lot of short cases under stress and seen most things before.

53 A good start is a great help. It's like skating on thin ice—if you keep going and don't fall through, you make it.

54 The most off-putting aspect of each case is the lack of feedback from the examiners as to whether you are right or wrong. This is much more disconcerting than criticism.

55 Stay calm and talk sensibly even when the diagnosis appears unclear (easy to say—difficult to do!)

Simple explanations raise simple questions

56 Very simple, straightforward answers seem to prompt straightforward questions.

57 They appear to want simple basic signs and physical examination but I am sure they penalize heavily if obvious signs are missed. They seemed quite happy for me to ask the patient questions. It is also a great relief when the answers are what you want (also gives one time to think when the patient is answering).

58 The examiners seem to be impressed by short definitive answers and not with long lists of differential diagnoses. I think it is best to answer questions as directly as possible and get on to the next case.

59 Don't be clever—give simple answers to simple questions. The examination is unfortunately an extremely unfair lottery—there is no substitute for luck.

60 Always be honest—it pays in the end (experience 54, p. 337).

Think straight, look smart and speak convincingly

61 If the diagnosis is obvious focus down and elicit all relevant signs regardless of the generality of the instruction. If the diagnosis is not immediately obvious, examine the relevant parts systematically and hope for the best. Do not be put off by mistakes or be paranoid about your performance (I was, and suffered for it).

62 Beware of dual pathology. Don't wait for the examiners to tell you what to do, just go ahead and do it. Shake hands with the patient and introduce yourself; this gives you a chance to exclude finger clubbing, etc. and to see whether the patient is deaf or disorientated.

63 Be definite about the positive findings, i.e. do not hedge your answer with 'possibly', 'almost', 'perhaps'. If there is no obvious first-choice answer then give a sensible and relevant differential diagnosis.

64 I think I failed because of hesitancy; I gave no impression of confidence and blurted out statements without thinking.

65 You must be quick and comprehensive in your examination; it looks bad if you need to go back to do something which you forgot.

You have seen it all before

66 My cases were more straightforward than I had been led to expect. In fact nothing was particularly rare.

67 It is easy to be daunted by the feeling that there will be conditions you have never heard of and that the cases will be difficult and rare. In fact after my experience in these four attempts it seems that in most cases the same old conditions keep recurring and they are mostly straightforward if you can only keep calm.

Use your eyes first and most

68 One of the short cases—pretibial myxoedema—was given away by the eyes. I think from talking to other people that there is often an obvious 'clue' in the short cases.

69 Spend at least 10–15 seconds just looking at the patient before even attempting an examination. Speak slowly and clearly and look the examiners in the eye.

70 Always look at the patient as well as the part in question. In one case (skin lesions in a Negro) my first impulse was to suspect a tropical disease (?cutaneous leishmaniasis!) but the presence of exophthalmos gave me the diagnosis (pretibial myxoedema). Don't be put off by examiners who are (as mine were) totally noncommital.

71 Do exactly what is asked but give yourself a second or two to look at the whole patient from the end of the bed.

Examiners are different

72 The examiners were very pleasant and wanted to see how confident I was when faced with a problem. They could have failed me on many things but appeared to be wanting to see how my mind worked. They like you to be slick, thorough, and to present your findings precisely without dithering. I am sure they assess you very quickly on the first two cases and decide whether they would like you to be in charge of their patients. Stay relaxed and be honest.

73 Don't get flustered. If you say something silly retract it quickly and continue to talk. They are aggressive and try to hurry you. Don't let them! Look smart and be nice to the patients.

74 Try to be calm and imagine that you are seeing the cases in a clinic and carrying out a routine examination. The examiners made me very nervous especially with their comments which, in retrospect, I should have tried to ignore as they were only trying to test my knowledge and physiological comprehension of the physical signs I had elicited.

75 There was nothing difficult. The examiners were polite, unobtrusive, to the point and clear with their instructions. They were also amazingly expressionless throughout.

76 Don't be bullied by the examiners. There is no substitute for experience. You can pass even if you make a mess of one short case.

77 Don't let them rattle you. Never think you have failed until you get the letter.

78 The examiners kept asking me if I was sure of my findings as though they were trying to put me off. I wish I was this good always!

Appendices

1 / Checklists

1 / Heart

1 *Visual survey*
  (a) Breathlessness
  (b) *Cyanosis*
  (c) Pallor
  (d) *Malar flush*
  (e) Carotids
  (f) Jugulars
  (g) *Valvotomy scar*. midline scar
  (h) Ankle oedema
  (i) Clubbing; splinter haemorrhages.
2 Pulse (rate and rhythm).
3 Lift up the arm (?collapsing).
4 Radio-femoral delay.
5 Brachials and carotids (?slow rising).
6 Venous pressure.
7 Apex beat.
8 Tapping impulse.
9 Right ventricular lift.
10 Other pulsations, thrills, palpable sounds.
11 Auscultation (time heart sounds etc.; turn patient onto left side; lean patient forwards).
12 Sacral oedema (?ankle oedema).
13 Lung bases.
14 Liver.
15 Blood pressure.

2 / Abdomen

1 *Visual survey* (pallor, jaundice, spider naevi, etc).
2 Pigmentation.
3 Hands (Dupuytren's contracture, clubbing, leuconychia, palmar erythema, flapping tremor).
4 Eyes (anaemia, icterus, xanthelasma).
5 Mouth (cyanosis, etc.).
6 Cervical lymph nodes.
7 Gynaecomastia.
8 Spider naevi.
9 Scratch marks.
10 Body hair.
11 Look at the abdomen (pulsation, distention, swelling, distended abdominal veins).
12 Palpation (light palpation, internal organs, inguinal lymph nodes).
13 Percussion.
14 Shifting dullness.
15 Auscultation.
16 Genitalia.
17 Rectal.

3 / Fundi

Observe
1 *Visual survey* (Medic-alert bracelet, etc.)
  Ophthalmoscopy.
2 Lens.
3 Vitreous.
4 Disc (optic atrophy, papillitis, papilloedema, myelinated nerve fibres, new vessels).
5 Arterioles and venules (a-v nipping, silver wiring).
6 Each quadrant and macula (haemorrhages, microaneurysms, exudates, new vessels, photo-coagulation scars, choroidoretinitis, retinitis pigmentosa).
7 Do not stop until you have finished and are ready.

4 / Hands

Observe
1 Face (*systemic sclerosis*, Cushing's, acromegaly, arcus senilis, icterus and spider naevi, exophthalmos).
2 Inspect the hands (rheumatoid, sclerodactyly, wasting, psoriasis, claw hand, clubbing).
3 The joints (swelling, deformity, Heberden's nodes).
4 The nails (pitting, onycholysis, clubbing, nail fold infarcts).
5 The skin (colour, consistency, lesions).
6 The muscles (wasting, fasciculation).
Palpate and test
7 Hands (Dupuytren's contracture, nodules, calcinosis, xanthomata, Heberden's nodes, tophi).
8 Sensation (light touch, pinprick, vibration, joint position).
9 Tone.
10 Power.
11 Pulses.
12 Elbows.

5 / Legs

Observe

1 *Visual survey (Paget's disease,* hemiparesis, exophthalmos, nystagmus, thyroid acropachy, rheumatoid hands, nicotine-stained fingers, wasted hands, muscle fasciculation).
2 Obvious lesion (see Group 1 diagnoses).
3 Bowing of the tibia.
4 Pes cavus.
5 One leg smaller than the other.
6 Muscle bulk.
7 Fasciculation.

Test

8 Tone.
9 Power
  (i) Lift your leg up (L1, 2)
  (ii) Bend your knee (L5, S1, 2)
  (iii) Straighten your leg (L3, 4)
  (iv) Bend your foot down (S1)
  (v) Cock up your foot (L4, 5) y.
10 Coordination (heel-shin).
11 Tendon reflexes (clonus).
12 Plantar response.
13 Sensation (light touch, pinprick, vibration, joint position).
14 Gait (ordinary walk, heel-to-toe, on toes, on heels).
15 Rombergism.

6 / Chest

1 *Visual survey*—general appearance (cachexia, superior vena cava obstruction, systemic sclerosis, lupus pernio, kyphoscoliosis, *ankylosing spondylitis*).
2 Dyspnoea.
3 Lip pursing.
4 Cyanosis.
5 Accessory muscles.
6 Indrawing (intercostal muscles, supraclavicular fossae, lower ribs).
7 Chest wall (upward movement, asymmetry, scars, radiotherapy stigmata).
8 Clubbing (tobacco staining, coal dust tattoos, rheumatoid deformity, systemic sclerosis).
9 Pulse (flapping tremor).
10 Venous pressure.
11 Trachea (deviation, tug, notch-cricoid distance).
12 Lymphadenopathy.
13 Apex beat.
14 Asymmetry.
15 Expansion.
16 Percussion (don't forget clavicles, axillae).
17 Tactile vocal fremitus.
18 Breath sounds.
19 Vocal resonance.
20 Repeat 14–19 on back of chest (feel for lymph nodes in the neck).

7 / 'Spot' Diagnosis

1 *Visual survey*
2 Retrace the same ground more thoroughly
  (i) head (*Paget's, dystrophia myotonica*)
  (ii) face (*acromegaly, Parkinson's, hemiplegia,* dystrophia myotonica, tardive dyskinesia, hypopituitarism, Cushing's, hypothyroidism, systemic sclerosis)
  (iii) eyes (*jaundice, exophthalmos,* ptosis, Horner's, xanthelasma)
  (iv) neck (*goitre,* Turner's, spondylitis, torticollis)
  (v) trunk (pigmentation, ascites, purpuric spots, spider naevi, wasting, pemphigus)
  (vi) arms (choreoathetosis, psoriasis, Addison's, spider naevi, syringomyelia)
  (vii) hands (acromegaly, *tremor,* clubbing, sclerodactyly, arachnodactyly, claw hand, etc.)
  (viii) legs (bowing, purpura, pretibial myxoedema, necrobiosis)
  (ix) feet (pes cavus).
3 Abnormal colouring (*pigmentation, icterus,* pallor).
4 Break down and scrutinize (especially face).
5 Additional features.

8 / Eyes

Observe

1 Face (e.g. myasthenic, tabetic, hemiparesis).
2 Eyes (exophthalmos, strabismus, ptosis, xanthelasma, arcus senilis).
3 Pupils (Argyll Robertson, Horner's, Holmes-Adie, IIIrd nerve).

Test

4 Visual acuity.
5 Visual fields.
6 Eye movements (ocular palsy, diplopia, nystagmus, lid lag).
7 Light reflex (direct, consensual).
8 Accommodation reflex.
9 Fundi.

9 / Face

1 *Visual survey* of patient.
2 Scan the head and face.
3 Break down and scrutinize the parts of the face
  (a) eyelids (ptosis, rash)
     eyelashes (scanty)
     cornea (arcus, interstitial keratitis)
     sclerea (icteric, congested)
     pupils (small, large, irregular, dislocated lens, cataracts)
     iris (iritis)
  (b) face (erythema, infiltrates)
     mouth (tight, shiny, adherent skin; pigmented patches, telangiectasia, cyanosis).
4 Additional features.

10 / Arms

Observe

1 Face (hemiplegia, nystagmus, wasting, Parkinson's, Horner's).
2 Neck (pseudoxanthoma elasticum, lymph nodes).
3 Elbows (psoriasis, rheumatoid nodules, scars, deformity).
4 Tremor.
5 Hands (joints, nails, skin).
6 Muscle bulk.
7 Fasciculation.

Test

8 Tone.
9 Arms out in front (winging, sensory wandering).
10 Power
  (i) Arms out to the side (C5)
  (ii) Bend your elbows (C5, 6)
  (iii) Push out straight (C7)
  (iv) Squeeze fingers (C8, T1)
  (v) Hold the fingers out straight (radial nerve, C7)
  (vi) Spread fingers apart (ulnar nerve)
  (vii) Piece of paper between fingers (ulnar nerve)
  (viii) Thumb at ceiling (median nerve)
  (ix) Opposition (median nerve).
11 Coordination (rapid alternate motion, finger-nose).
12 Reflexes.
13 Sensation (light touch, pinprick, vibration, joint position).

11 / Neck

1 *Survey* the patient (eyes, face, legs).
2 Look at the neck (swallow).
3 Palpate the thyroid (swallow; size, consistency, etc., pyramidal lobes).
4 Lymph nodes (supraclavicular, submandibular, postauricular, suboccipital, axillae, groins, spleen).
5 Auscultate the thyroid (distinguish from venous hum and conducted murmurs).
6 Assess thyroid status.

12 / Ask Questions

1 *Visual survey* (from top to toe, ?obvious diagnosis).
2 Specific questions (Raynaud's, systemic sclerosis/CRST, hypo- or hyperthyroidism, Crohn's, nephrotic syndrome).
3 General questions (name, address).
4 Questions with long answers (last meal).
5 Articulation ('British Constitution', 'West Register Street', 'Biblical criticism').
6 Repetition.
7 Additional signs.
8 Comprehension ('put out your tongue', 'shut your eyes', 'touch your nose', 'smile').
9 Nominal dysphasia (keys).
10 Higher mental function.

13 / Pulse

Observe

1 Face (malar flush, thyroid facies).
2 Neck (Corrigan's pulse, raised JVP, thyroidectomy scar, goitre) and chest (thoracotomy scar).

Palpate and assess

3 Pulse.
4 Rate.
5 Rhythm (?slow atrial fibrillation).
6 Character (normal, collapsing, slow rising, jerky).
7 Carotid.
8 Opposite radial.
9 Radio-femoral delay.
10 All the other pulses.
11 Additional diagnostic features.

14 / Visual Fields

Observe

1 *Visual survey* (acromegaly, hemiparesis, cerebellar signs).

Test

2 Peripheral visual fields by confrontation.
3 Central scotoma with a red-headed hat pin.
4 Additional features.

15 / Skin

1 *Visual survey* (regional associations; scalp, face, mouth, neck, trunk, axillae, elbows, hands, nails, legs, feet).
2 Distribution (psoriasis on extensor areas, lichen planus on flexural areas, etc.).
3 Lesions: look for characteristic features (scaling, Wickham's striae, etc.).
4 Associated lesions (arthropathy, etc.).

16 / Gait

1 *Visual survey* (cerebellar signs, Parkinson's, Charcot–Marie–Tooth, ankylosing spondylitis).
2 Check patient can walk.
3 Observe ordinary walk (ataxia, spastic, steppage, Parkinsonian).
4 Arm swing (Parkinson's).
5 Turning (ataxia, Parkinson's).
6 Heel-to-toe (ataxia).
7 On toes (S1).
8 On heels (L5).
9 Romberg's test (sensory ataxia).
10 Gait with eyes closed.
11 Additional features.

17 / Rash

1 *Visual survey* (scalp to sole).
2 Distribution.
3 Surrounding skin (?scratch marks).
4 Examine the lesion (colour, size, shape, surface, character).
5 Additional features.

18 / Legs and Arms

As appropriate from *checklists* 5 and 10.

19 / Cranial Nerves

1 Look.
2 Smell and taste (I, VII, IX).
3 Visual acuity (II).
4 Visual fields (II).
5 Eye movements (III, IV, VI).
6 Nystagmus (VIII, cerebellum and its connections).
7 Ptosis (III, sympathetic).
8 Pupils (light, accommodation—III).
9 Discs (II).
10 Facial movements (VII, V).
11 Palatal movement (IX, X).
12 Gag reflex (IX, X).
13 Tongue (XII).
14 Accessory nerve (XI).
15 Hearing (Weber, Rinné—VIII).
16 Facial sensation (including corneal reflex—V).

20 / Thyroid Status

1 *Visual survey* (exophthalmos, myxoedematous facies, goitre, thyroid acropachy, pretibial myoedema).
2 Composure (fidgety, normal, immobile).
3 Pulse.
4 Ankle jerks.
5 Palms.
6 Tremor.
7 Eyes (lid retraction, lid lag).
8 Thyroid (look, palpate, auscultate).
9 Questions.

Short case	Frequency		Page
	Main focus (%)	Additional feature (%)	no.
1 Diabetic retinopathy	34	—	62
2 Hepatosplenomegaly	24	8	65
3 Mitral stenosis	20	—	66
4 Rheumatoid hands	17	7	68
5 Mixed mitral valve disease	16	—	72
6 Dullness at lung base	14	4	73
7 Splenomegaly	14	2	74
8 Optic atrophy	14	4	76
9 Chronic liver disease	13	3	78
10 Polycystic kidneys	12	2	80
11 Paget's disease	12	1	82
12 Psoriatic arthropathy psoriasis	11	1	84
13 Combinations of aortic and mitral valve disease	11	—	88
14 Mixed aortic valve disease	11	—	89
15 Systemic sclerosis/CRST syndrome	11	1	90
16 Exophthalmos	11	8	92
17 Hepatomegaly (without spleno megaly)	10	9	95
18 Spastic paraparesis	10	2	96
19 Fibrosing alveolitis	10	1	97
20 Aortic incompetence (lone)	9	1	98
21 Hemiplegia	9	3	100
22 Old tuberculosis	8	—	102
23 Acromegaly	8	1	104
24 Aortic stenosis (lone)	8	—	106
25 Graves' disease	8	8	108
26 Ocular palsy	8	3	110
27 Mitral incompetence (lone)	7	—	114
28 Motor neurone disease	7	1	116
29 Goitre	7	6	118
30 Ulnar nerve palsy	7	—	122
31 Visual field defect	6	3	124
32 Peripheral neuropathy	6	5	126
33 Hypertensive retinopathy	6	1	128
34 Cerebellar syndrome	6	6	130
35 Retinitis pigmentosa	6	—	131
36 Carcinoma of the bronchus	5	4	132
37 Parkinson's disease	5	—	134
38 Chronic bronchitis and emphysema	5	1	136
39 Hypothyroidism	5	1	138
40 Osler–Weber–Rendu syndrome	5	—	141
41 Abdominal mass	4	3	142
42 Dystrophia myotonica	4	—	144
43 Bronchiectasis	4	1	146
44 Wasting of the small muscles of the hand	4	11	148
45 Generalized lymphadenopathy	4	6	151

Short case	Frequency Main focus (%)	Additional feature (%)	Page no.
46 Papilloedema	3	2	152
47 Diabetic foot	3	2	154
48 Nystagmus	3	2	156
49 Old choroiditis	3	—	158
50 Neurofibromatosis	3	1	160
51 Erythema nodosum	3	—	162
52 Horner's syndrome	3	1	164
53 Old polio	3	1	166
54 Ankylosing spondylitis	3	—	168
55 Abnormal gait	3	3	170
56 Irregular pulse	3	22	174
57 Single palpable kidney	3	3	175
58 Ascites	3	5	176
59 Sturge–Weber syndrome	3	—	178
60 Necrobiosis lipoidica diabeticorum	3	—	180
61 Ventricular septal defect	3	1	182
62 Lower motor neurone VIIth nerve palsy	3	—	184
63 Clubbing	2	13	188
64 Retinal vein thrombosis	2	—	190
65 Eisenmenger's syndrome	2	1	192
66 Crohn's disease	2	—	194
67 Mitral valve prolapse	2	—	196
68 Cervical myelopathy	2	2	198
69 Patent ductus arteriosus	2	—	200
70 Tricuspid incompetence	2	2	201
71 Purpura	2	3	202
72 Xanthomata	2	2	204
73 Drug-induced extrapyramidal syndrome	2	—	206
74 Bilateral parotid enlargement/Mikulicz's syndrome	2	—	207
75 Primary biliary cirrhosis	2	—	208
76 Lupus pernio	2	—	210
77 Muscular dystrophy	2	—	212
78 Prosthetic valves	2	1	214
79 Addison's disease	2	—	216
80 Cushing's syndrome	2	3	218
81 Friedreich's ataxia	2	—	220
82 Peutz–Jeghers syndrome	2	—	221
83 Systemic lupus erythematosus	2	—	222
84 Superior vena cava obstruction	2	—	224
85 Vasculitis	2	2	226
86 Cor pulmonale	1	—	228
87 Myelinated nerve fibres	1	—	229
88 Charcot–Marie–Tooth disease	1	—	230
89 Cataracts	1	4	232
90 Idiopathic haemochromatosis	1	—	233
91 Chest infection/consolidation/pneumonia	1	?	234
92 Coarctation of the aorta	1	1	235

	Frequency		
Short case	Main focus (%)	Additional feature (%)	Page no.
93 Bulbar palsy	1	—	236
94 Choreoathetosis	1	2	237
95 Dysarthria	1	1	238
96 Dysphasia	1	1	239
97 Ehlers–Danlos syndrome	1	—	240
98 Erythema ab igne	1	—	242
99 Marfan's syndrome	1	—	244
100 Myasthenia gravis	1	1	246
101 Osteoarthrosis	1	—	248
102 Raised jugular venous pressure	1	?	249
103 Pretibial myxoedema	1	3	250
104 Retinal artery occlusion	1	—	252
105 Vitiligo	1	—	254
106 Tophaceous gout	1	—	256
107 Fallot's tetralogy with a Blalock shunt	1	—	258
108 Slow pulse	1	1	259
109 Dermatomyositis	0.9	—	260
110 Hypopituitarism	0.9	0.6	262
111 Swollen knee	0.9	1.5	264
112 Pseudobulbar palsy	0.9	—	265
113 Pemphigus/pemphigoid	0.9	—	266
114 Syringomyelia	0.9	—	268
115 Pseudoxanthoma elasticum	0.8	—	270
116 Radiation burn on the chest	0.8	4	272
117 Subacute combined degeneration of the cord	0.8	0.4	273
118 Holmes–Adie–Moore syndrome	0.8	—	274
119 Nephrotic syndrome	0.7	—	275
120 Jugular foramen syndrome	0.7	—	276
121 Herpes zoster	0.7	2	278
122 Polymyositis	0.6	—	280
123 Argyll Robertson pupils	0.5	0.4	281
124 Congenital syphilis	0.5	—	282
125 Carpal tunnel syndrome	0.5	0.8	284
126 Cerebello-pontine angle lesion	0.5	—	285
127 Dextrocardia	0.5	—	286
128 Down's syndrome	0.5	0.6	287
129 Gynaecomastia	1.5	1.6	288
130 Absent ankle jerks and extensor plantars	0.5	1	290
131 Lichen planus	0.5	—	292
132 Lateral popliteal nerve palsy	0.5	—	294
133 Ptosis	0.5	5	296
134 Osteogenesis imperfecta	0.5	—	298
135 Pulmonary stenosis	0.5	—	299
136 Raynaud's phenomenon	0.5	2	300
137 Turner's syndrome	0.5	—	302
138 Mycosis fungoides	0.5	—	304
139 Dermatitis herpetiformis	0.3	—	306
140 Urticaria pigmentosa (mastocytosis)	0.3	—	308
141 Pneumothorax	0.3	—	309

| Short case | Frequency | | Page |
	Main focus (%)	Additional feature (%)	no.
142 Tabes	0.3	0.8	310
143 Atrial septal defect	0.1	—	312
144 Pyoderma gangrenosum	0.1	—	314
145 Multiple sclerosis	—	16	316
146 Felty's syndrome	—	1	317
147 Hypertrophic obstructive cardiomy-opathy	—	—	318
148 Radial nerve palsy	—	—	319
149 Lateral medullary syndrome	—	—	320
150 Normal	see p. 322	see p. 322	322

Some short cases which occurred as 'main focus' only once in the survey

Hemiballismus

Diabetic with pallor

Nail-patella syndrome (anecdote 1, p. 340)

Repaired thoracic aortic aneurysm (experience 57, p. 338)

Hyperlipidaemia (xanthelasma, arcus, IHD)

Cyanosis

Primary pulmonary hypertension

Rash on hands and lower arm ?cause

Unilateral lower motor neurone XIIth nerve lesion

Absent knee jerk

Takayasu's disease

Multiple abcesses on the thigh

Juvenile chronic arthritis (Still's disease) (anecdote 14, p. 342)

Elbow flexion contraction due to haemophilia

Brisk reflexes and normal plantar responses

Pigeon chest, scoliosis and torticollis in a patient with ?pulmonary stenosis

Guillain–Barré syndrome

ECG with 2 : 1 block (anecdote 10, p. 341)

?Steele–Richardson syndrome (total parenteral nutrition was the subject of short case rather than the condition) (anecdote 11, p. 342)

Aortic sclerosis

Epidermolysis bullosa congenita

Deep venous thrombosis (experience 4, p. 329)

Acne rosacea

Glaucoma

Transplanted kidney in the right iliac fossa in a patient with polycystic kidneys and chronic renal failure (anecdote 7, p. 341)

Patient with proliferative diabetic retinopathy who also had a partial iridectomy

Thalidomide victim with psoriasis

Chest infection due to decreased immunity in a patient with hepatosplenomegaly (this may have occurred more than once)

Multiple surgical scars and hepatomegaly

A diabetic with cervical myelopathy and peripheral neuropathy (experience 56, p. 338)

Axillary vein thrombosis

Brachial artery aneurysm (anecdote 23, p. 343)

Left ventricular aneurysm

Sickle-cell stigmata

'Heart failure'

Aphakia

Senile dementia (anecdote 21, p. 343)

Torticollis

Left VIth, VIIth, XIIth cranial nerve lesions and nystagmus (experience 1, p. 327)

Absent radial pulse due to heart failure (experience 54, p. 337)

Old rickets

3 / Examination frequency of examiners' instructions

Instruction	Frequency (%)	Page no.	Instruction	Frequency (%)	Page no.
'Examine this patient's heart'	97	12	'Examine this patient's neck'	12	42
'Examine this patient's abdomen'	79	16	'Ask this patient some questions'	8	43
'Examine this patient's fundi'	67	19	'Examine this patient's pulse'	7	46
'Examine this patient's hands'	58	21	'Examine this patient's visual fields'	6	48
'Examine this patient's legs'	54	25	'Examine this patient's skin'	5	49
'Examine this patient's chest'	49	28	'Examine this patient's gait'	4	51
'What is the diagnosis?'	41	32	'Examine this patient's rash'	4	52
'Examine this patient's eyes'	32	35	'Examine this patient's arms and legs'	3	54
'Examine this patient's face'	20	37	'Examine this patient's cranial nerves'	3	54
'Examine this patient's arms'	15	39	'Assess this patient's thyroid status'	2	57

Some other instructions which occurred more than once in the survey

Instruction	Possible diagnoses (in order of frequency)
'Examine this patient's tongue' (2%)	1 Bilateral lower motor neurone XIIth nerve lesion 2 Motor neurone disease 3 Unilateral lower motor neurone XIIth nerve lesion 4 Pseudobulbar palsy
'Examine this patient's JVP' (2%)	1 Tricuspid incompetence 2 Raised JVP—cause not asked 3 Cor pulmonale
'Examine this patient's hands and chest' (2%)	1 Cryptogenic fibrosing alveolitis 2 Carcinoma of the bronchus 3 Pulmonary fibrosis and Raynaud's
'Examine this patient's mouth' (2%)	1 Osler–Weber–Rendu 2 Peutz–Jeghers syndrome
'Examine this patient's hands and face' (2%)	1 Systemic sclerosis/CRST 2 Cyanosis 3 Dermatomyositis 4 Systemic lupus erythematosus

Instruction	Possible diagnoses (in order of frequency)
'Examine this patient's abdomen and chest' (1%)	1 Myeloproliferative disease leading to immune deficiency and chest infection
'Examine this patient's arms and abdomen' (1%)	1 Polycystic kidneys with dialysis scars or fistulae 2 Chronic liver disease with spider naevi
'Examine this patient's hands, legs and eyes' (1%)	1 Thyroid acropachy, pretibial myxoedema, exophthalmos 2 Peripheral neuropathy, Charcot's joints, necrobiosis lipoidica diabeticorum, diabetic retinopathy, cataracts
'Look at the patient, now examine the abdomen' (1%)	1 Jaundice, hepatomegaly and related signs
'Look at the hands; now ask the patient some questions' (1%)	1 Raynaud's 2 Systemic sclerosis/CRST
'Examine this patient's pupils' (1%)	1 Optic atrophy (consensual reflex but not direct)
'Examine this patient's visual fields and fundi' (1%)	1 Retinal artery occlusion 2 Retinitis pigmentosa
'Examine this patient's knee/knees' (1%)	1 Swollen knee
'Examine this patient's feet' (1%)	1 Diabetic foot
'Examine this patient's gait and legs' (1%)	1 Spastic paraparesis 2 Charcot–Marie–Tooth disease
'Look at the patient; now examine the heart' (1%)	1 Fallot's tetralogy with a Blalock shunt
'Examine this patient's cerebellar system' (1%)	1 Cerebellar syndrome

4 / Clinical courses for the MRCP

Ashford, Middlesex—Ashford Hospital
2 day courses
Apply: The Medical Centre Secretary, Ashford Hospital, Ashford, Middlesex TW15 3AA. Tel: Ashford (Middx.) 51188 Ext. 4370

Birmingham—Dudley Road Hospital
2 week courses
Apply: Mrs J. Collins, Postgraduate Centre, Dudley Road Hospital, Birmingham B18 7QH. Tel: 021 554 3801 Ext. 4489

Birmingham—East Birmingham Hospital
1 week courses
Apply: Miss M. Wood, Postgraduate Medical Centre, East Birmingham Hospital, Bordesley Green East, Birmingham B9 5ST. Tel: 021 772 4311 Ext. 4259

Cardiff—University Hospital of Wales
1 week courses
Apply: Mrs Maureen Thomson, Area Postgraduate Administrator, University Hospital of Wales, Heath Park, Cardiff. Tel: 0222 755944 Ext. 2474

London—Central Middlesex Hospital
1 week courses
Apply (in writing only): Ms Seenar Deen, Postgraduate Administrator, The Avery Jones Postgraduate Medical Centre, Central Middlesex Hospital, Acton Lane, London NW10 7NS

London—Charing Cross Hospital
2 week courses
Apply: The Administrator, Postgraduate Medical Centre, Charing Cross Hospital, Fulham Palace Road, London W6 8RF. Tel: 01 748 2040 Ext. 3077/3037

London—Med Ed (UCH or Kensington) Dr John Davies
3 week evening courses
Weekend courses
One-day mock examinations
Apply: 'MED ED', c/o Mrs P. Robinson, 34 Ivere Drive, Barnet, London EN5 1AS

London—North Middlesex Hospital
1 week courses
Apply: Academic Secretary, North Middlesex Hospital, Silver Street, Edmonton, London N18 1QX. Tel: 01 807 3071 Ext. 481

London—Royal Northern Hospital
1 week courses
Apply: Postgraduate Secretary, Royal Northern Hospital, Holloway Road, London N7 6LD. Tel: 01 272 7777

London—Royal Northern Hospital
Weekend courses
Apply: Dr J. A. Cohen, 60 Theydon Grove, Epping, Essex CMQ16 4QA. Tel: Epping 74936 (after 7 p.m.)

London—West Middlesex, Hillingdon and Mount Vernon Hospitals
2 week courses
Apply: Postgraduate Administrator, Postgraduate Medical Centre, West Middlesex University Hospital, Twickenham Road, Isleworth, Middlesex TW 6AF. Tel: 01 560 2121 Ext. 294

Manchester—Consult-Ed.
Weekend courses
1 day courses
Apply: Consult-Ed, 24 Moorfield Road, West Didsbury, Manchester 20. Tel: 061 445 5401

Manchester—Withington Hospital, Manchester Royal Infirmary and Hope Hospital, Salford
1 week courses
Apply: Administrative Assistant, Department of Postgraduate Medical Studies, Gateway House, Piccadilly South, Manchester M60 7LP. Tel: 061 236 9456 Ext. 556

Newport, Gwent—Royal Gwent Hospital
Weekend courses
Apply: Mrs O. Palmer, Postgraduate Secretary, Royal Gwent Hospital, Newport, Gwent. Tel: 0633 52244 Ext. 4290

Pas Test—London, Manchester and Glasgow
Weekend courses
One day courses
Apply: Mrs Beverley Gower, Course Organiser, PO Box 81, Hemel Hempstead HP1 1UR. Tel: 0442 52113

Rochdale—Birch Hill Hospital
1 week courses
Apply: Administrative Assistant, Department of Postgraduate Medical Studies, Gateway House, Piccadilly South, Manchester M60 7LP. Tel: 061 236 9456 Ext. 556

Romford, Essex—Oldchurch Hospital (Regional Centre for Neurology/Neurosurgery)
Weekend course in clinical neurology
Apply: Dr L. J. Findley, Romford Medical Acadmic Centre, Oldchurch Hospital, Romford, Essex RM7 0BE. Tel: 0708 46090 Ext. 3100

Smethwick, West Midlands—Midland Centre for Neurosurgery and Neurology
1 week courses in Clinical Neurology

Apply: Dr J. A. Spillane, Postgraduate Clinical Tutor, Midland Centre for Neurosurgery and Neurology, Holly Lane, Smethwick, Warley, West Midlands B67 7JX. Tel: 021 558 3232 Ext. 351

Southampton—Southampton General Hospital
1 week courses
Apply: Regional Director of Postgraduate Studies, Wessex Regional Health Authority, Romsey Road, Winchester, Hants. S022 5DH. Tel: 0962 64149

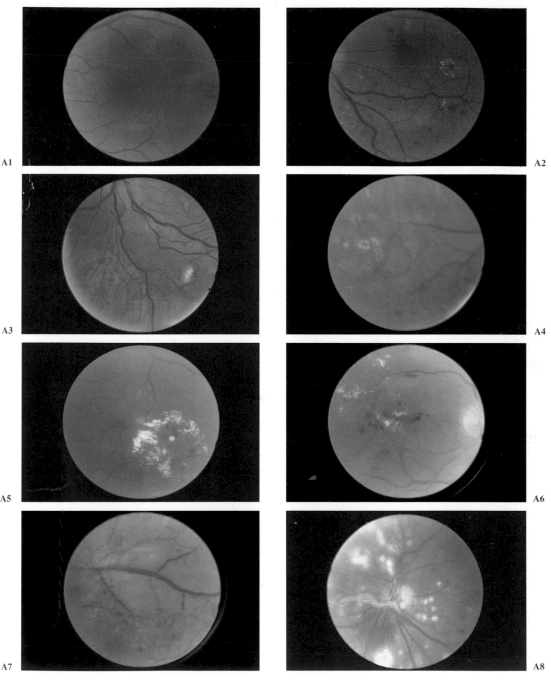

A1 Diabetic retinopathy—early background changes of microaneurysms and blot haemorrhages.

A2 Diabetic retinopathy—extensive background changes (note small circinate temporal to the macula).

A3 Diabetic retinopathy—the soft exudate in the lower right of the picture indicates ischaemia which is the stimulus to new vessel formation.

A4 Diabetic retinopathy (note photocoagulation scars).

A5 Diabetic retinopathy—the large circinate temporal to the macula indicates oedema in that area.

A6 Diabetic retinopathy—haemorrhages and exudates at the macula (maculopathy).

A7 Diabetic retinopathy—venous irregularity and beading (preproliferative signs).

A8 Diabetic retinopathy. The leash of new vessels protruding into the vitreous is in focus, whereas the retina with its photocoagulation scars is further away and therefore slightly out of focus. Note the leash of fibrous tissue accompanying the new vessels (previous haemorrhage).

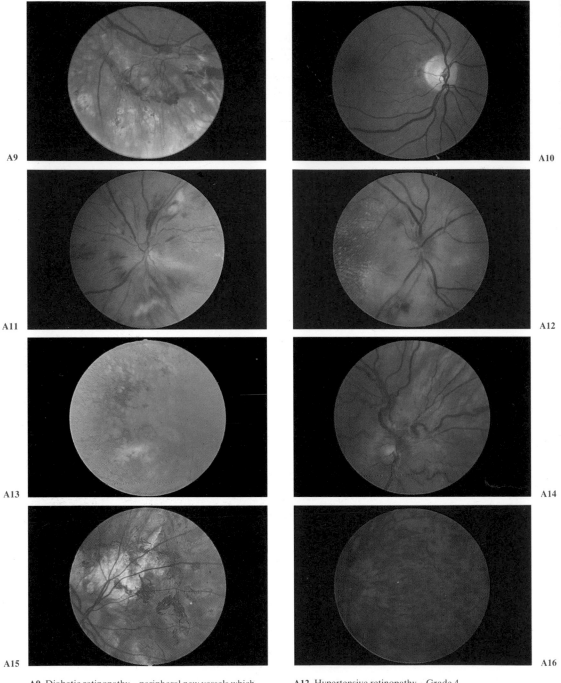

A9 Diabetic retinopathy—peripheral new vessels which are haemorrhaging (note photocoagulation scars—same patient as A8).

A10 Optic atrophy.

A11 Hypertensive retinopathy—Grade 4 (note papilloedema, flame-shaped haemorrhages and cotton wool spots).

A12 Hypertensive retinopathy—Grade 4.

A13 Retinitis pigmentosa.

A14 Papilloedema (benign intracranial hypertension).

A15 Choroidoretinitis.

A16 Central retinal vein thrombosis—haemorrhages scattered riotously like bundles of straw.

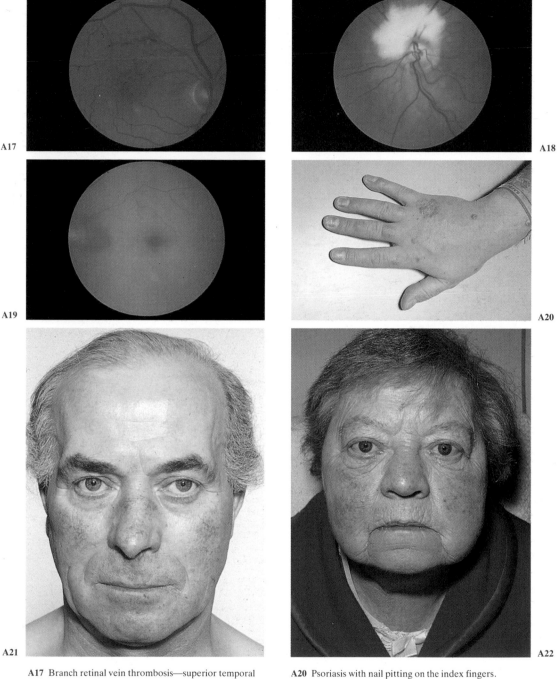

A17   Branch retinal vein thrombosis—superior temporal region.

A18   Myelinated nerve fibres.

A19   Central retinal artery occlusion. The fundus milky white due to retinal oedema and there was a cherry red spot at the macula. The triangular area temporal to the disc remains pink as it continues to be perfused by the ciliary circulation.

A20   Psoriasis with nail pitting on the index fingers.

A21   Malar flush (mitral stenosis).

A22   Malar flush (myxoedema).

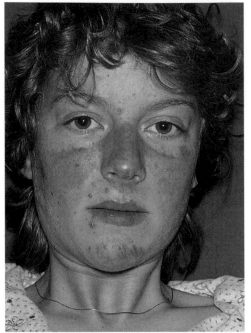

A23

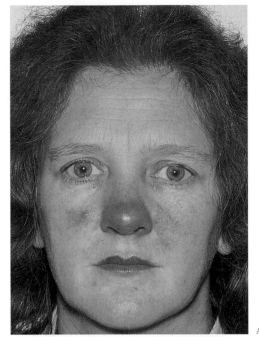

A24

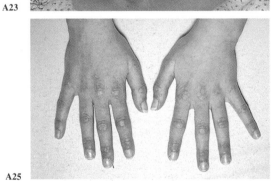

A25

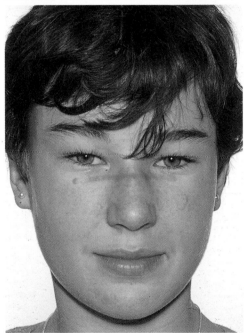

A26

A23 Systemic lupus erythematosus.

A24 Lupus pernio.

A25 Dermatomyositis—heliotrope rash on the knuckles.

A26 Dermatomyositis—note oedema and heliotrope discolouration around the eyes (same patient as A25).

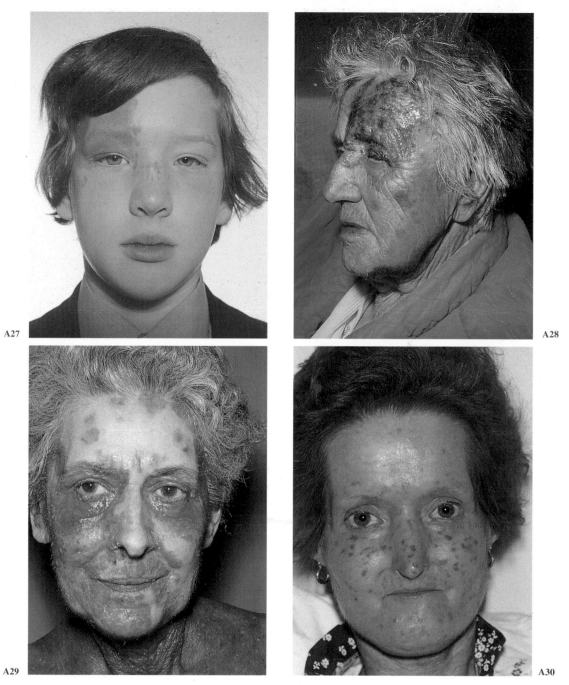

A27   Sturge-Weber syndrome.

A28   Herpes zoster ophthalmicus.

A29   Pemphigus.

A30   Systemic sclerosis (note the tight, shiny skin, pinched nose and telangiectasia).

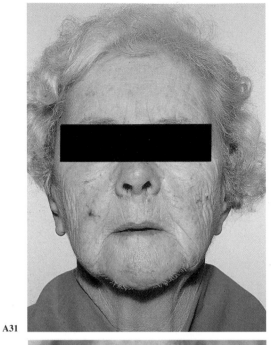

A31

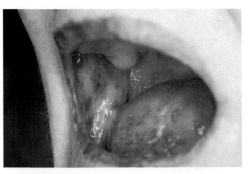

A32

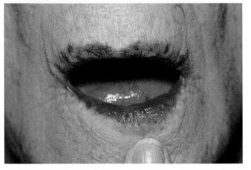

A33

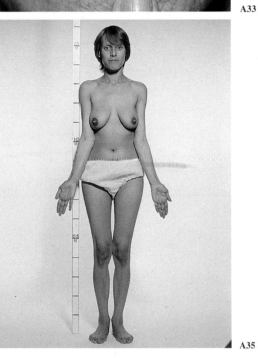

A35

A34

A31 Osler–Weber–Rendu syndrome—the diagnosis is confirmed on looking inside the mouth.

A32 Osler–Weber–Rendu syndrome—the soft palate of the same patient as A31.

A33 Peutz–Jeghers syndrome.

A34 Peutz–Jeghers syndrome—pigmentation of buccal mucosa.

A35 Addison's disease (note pigmentation of nipples).

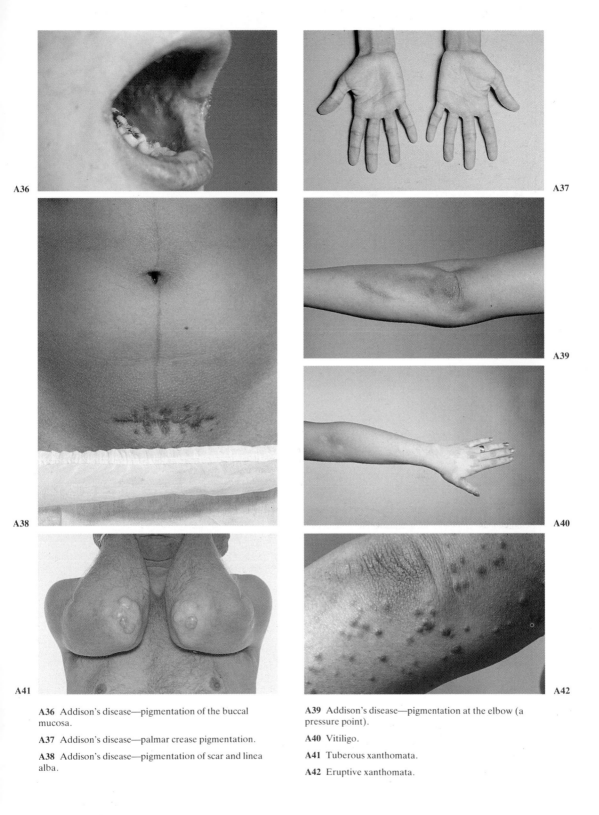

A36 Addison's disease—pigmentation of the buccal mucosa.

A37 Addison's disease—palmar crease pigmentation.

A38 Addison's disease—pigmentation of scar and linea alba.

A39 Addison's disease—pigmentation at the elbow (a pressure point).

A40 Vitiligo.

A41 Tuberous xanthomata.

A42 Eruptive xanthomata.

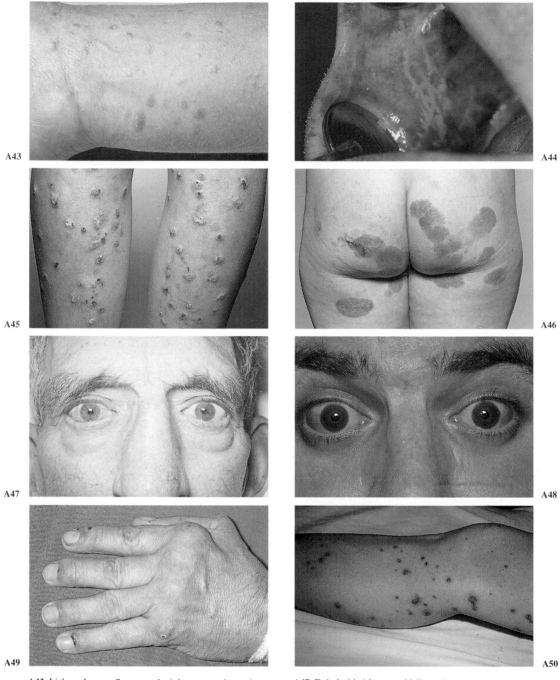

A43 Lichen planus—flat-topped, violaceous, polygonal papules on the wrist. Note Wickham's striae.

A44 Lichen planus—white, lacy pattern on buccal mucosa.

A45 Dermatitis herpetiformis.

A46 Mycosis fungoides.

A47 Episcleritis (rheumatoid disease).

A48 Blue sclerae of osteogenesis imperfecta.

A49 Vasculitis (rheumatoid arthritis).

A50 Vasculitis.

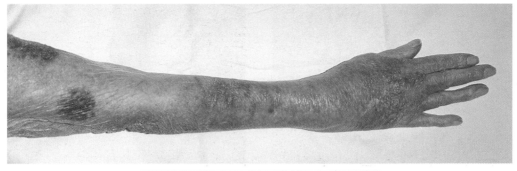

A51

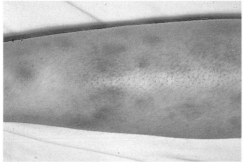

A52

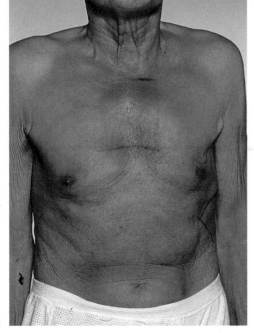

A53

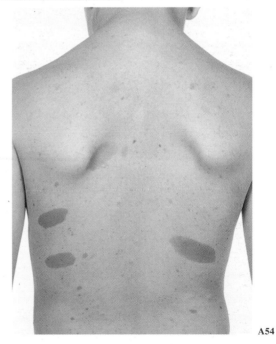

A54

A51 Purpura (steroid therapy for rheumatoid arthritis).

A52 Erythema nodosum.

A53 Radiotherapy field markings with radiation burns between the marks on the sternum (carcinoma of the bronchus).

A54 Neurofibromatosis—*café-au-lait* spots.

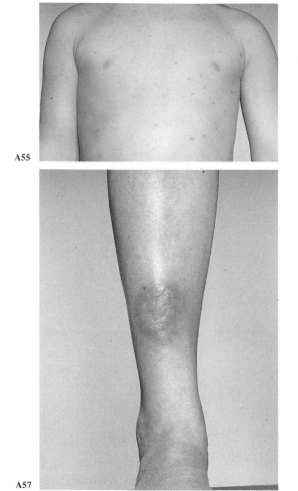

A55

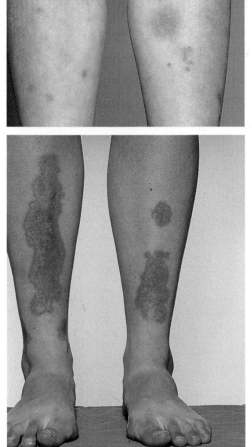

A56

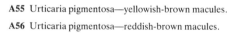

A57

A58

A55 Urticaria pigmentosa—yellowish-brown macules.

A56 Urticaria pigmentosa—reddish-brown macules.

A57 Pretibial myxoedema.

A58 Necrobiosis lipoidica diabeticorum.

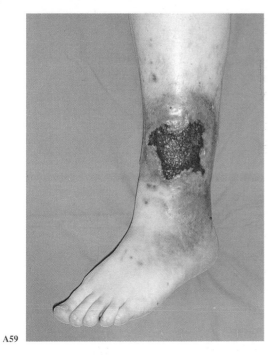

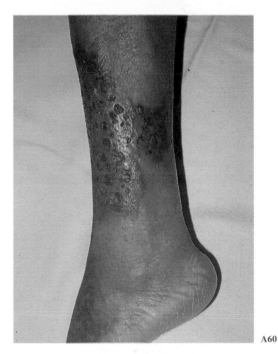

A59 Pyoderma gangrenosum (note ragged, bluish-red edge to the ulcer).

A60 Pyoderma gangrenosum.

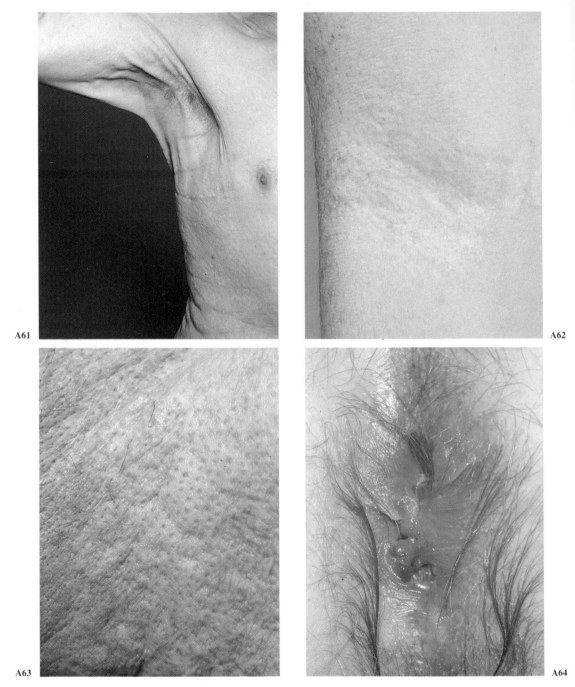

A61

A62

A63

A64

A61 Pseudoxanthoma elasticum—note loose skin.

A62 Pseudoxanthoma elasticum—antecubital fossa.

A63 Pseudoxanthoma elasticum—plucked chicken-skin appearance.

A64 Anal Crohn's disease—note purplish discolouration of the perianal skin, oedematous skin tags, fissuring, ulceration and fistula formation.

Index

Figures in bold refer to examination routines and short cases.

383

MRCP—'it teaches more than it tests'